Bioengineering and Biomaterials in Ventricular Assist Devices

Emerging Materials and Technologies

Series Editor:
Boris I. Kharissov

Recycled Ceramics in Sustainable Concrete: Properties and Performance
Kwok Wei Shah and Ghasan Fahim Huseien

Photo-Electrochemical Ammonia Synthesis: Nanocatalyst Discovery,
Reactor Design, and Advanced Spectroscopy
Mohammadreza Nazemi and Mostafa A. El-Sayed

Fire-Resistant Paper: Materials, Technologies, and Applications
Ying-Jie Zhu

Sensors for Stretchable Electronics in Nanotechnology
Kaushik Pal

Polymer-Based Composites: Design, Manufacturing, and Applications
V. Arumugaprabu, R. Deepak Joel Johnson, M. Uthayakumar, and P. Sivaranjana

Nanomaterials in Bionanotechnology: Fundamentals and Applications
Ravindra Pratap Singh and Kshitij RB Singh

Biomaterials and Materials for Medicine: Innovations in Research,
Devices, and Applications
Jingan Li

Advanced Materials and Technologies for Wastewater Treatment
Sreedevi Upadhyayula and Amita Chaudhary

Green Tribology: Emerging Technologies and Applications
*T V V L N Rao, Salmiah Binti Kasolang, Xie Guoxin,
Jitendra Kumar Katiyar, and Ahmad Majdi Abdul Rani*

Biotribology: Emerging Technologies and Applications
*T V V L N Rao, Salmiah Binti Kasolang, Xie Guoxin,
Jitendra Kumar Katiyar, and Ahmad Majdi Abdul Rani*

Bioengineering and Biomaterials in Ventricular Assist Devices
Eduardo Guy Perpétuo Bock

Semiconducting Black Phosphorus: From 2D Nanomaterial to
Emerging 3D Architecture
Han Zhang, Nasir Mahmood Abbasi, and Bing Wang

Bioengineering and Biomaterials in Ventricular Assist Devices

Edited by
Eduardo Guy Perpétuo Bock

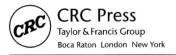

CRC Press
Taylor & Francis Group
Boca Raton London New York

CRC Press is an imprint of the
Taylor & Francis Group, an **informa** business

First edition published 2022
by CRC Press
6000 Broken Sound Parkway NW, Suite 300, Boca Raton, FL 33487-2742

and by CRC Press
2 Park Square, Milton Park, Abingdon, Oxon, OX14 4RN

© 2022 Taylor & Francis Group, LLC

CRC Press is an imprint of Taylor & Francis Group, LLC

Library of Congress Cataloging-in-Publication Data
Names: Bock, Eduardo Guy Perpétuo, editor.
Title: Bioengineering and biomaterials in ventricular assist devices / edited by Eduardo Guy Perpétuo Bock.
Description: First edition. | Boca Raton: CRC Press, 2022. | Includes bibliographical references and index. |
Summary: "Often associated with artificial hearts, Ventricular Assist Devices (VAD) are blood pumps that can provide circulatory assistance to the left ventricle, the right ventricle, or both biventricular. Bioengineering and Biomaterials in Ventricular Assist Devices details constructive details of VADs and the biomaterials used in their development and support. This advanced text is aimed at advanced students, researchers, and practicing engineers conducting work on VADs and will be of interest to a broad interdisciplinary group, including on bioengineers, materials engineers, chemical engineers, mechanical engineers, electrical engineers, and others"— Provided by publisher.
Identifiers: LCCN 2021029823 (print) | LCCN 2021029824 (ebook) |
ISBN 9780367686321 (hardback) | ISBN 9780367686338 (paperback) | ISBN 9781003138358 (ebook)
Subjects: LCSH: Cardiovascular instruments, Implanted. | Blood—Circulation, Artificial. |
Heart, Mechanical. | Biomedical engineering. | Biomedical materials.
Classification: LCC RD598.35.A77 B56 2022 (print) | LCC RD598.35.A77 (ebook) |
DDC 617.4/120645—dc23
LC record available at https://lccn.loc.gov/2021029823
LC ebook record available at https://lccn.loc.gov/2021029824

ISBN: 978-0-367-68632-1 (hbk)
ISBN: 978-0-367-68633-8 (pbk)
ISBN: 978-1-003-13835-8 (ebk)

DOI: 10.1201/9781003138358

Typeset in Times
by codeMantra

This book is dedicated to my parents, my wife, and my sons; Alice, who took me out of the rabbit hole keeping a piece of my heart with her; Eng. Sidney, who carved my technique in stone; Karen, who shares the daily trenches with me; and Ian and Eric, who filled this book with smiles and hugs waiting countless hours for their absent father.

Contents

PART I   Bioengineering in Ventricular Assist Devices

PART II   Biomaterials in Ventricular Assist Devices

Foreword

What Is "Social" about Artificial Hearts?

Marisol Marini[1]
UNICAMP

> The technique has a bad reputation; it may seem devoid of soul
>
> **Sennett (2019, p. 169)**

The question that gives title to this reflection is provocative. It is a rhetorical question, which nevertheless mirrors an understanding of (scientific) common sense that there are social aspects in scientific and technological production. Such an understanding would justify, for example, attempts to collaborate in multi- or interdisciplinary teams, assuming a division of labor. In the scientific and technological production line, each specialty should be responsible for a part of a whole, as if each one had an isolated "slice," which at the end is mechanically added to other parts to form a whole. It is to problematize the conception that there is a "slice" called "social" that I write the present text.

What is social about scientific and technological production besides the fact that every scientific and technological enterprise is inherently social?

Thinking of "social aspects" solely as the way patients/users deal with new technologies is not enough. Likewise, "social problems" cannot be reduced to listening to patients' demands to improve the devices. Scientific and technological production is a social activity before anything. Thinking of "social aspects" as isolated or reduced issues of scientific and technological production disregards the very fact that it is, by definition, a "social" activity. Society and research practices are all losing out when we treat the social merely as the improvement of the reception of previously made artifacts, closed and stabilized, which later would be submitted to patients/passive users.

From anthropological and science and technology studies (STS) point of view, approaches that inform the present reflection, the scientific and technological enterprise reveals specific forms of intertwining nature and culture. The definitions and boundaries around this division are central, a fundamental focus of anthropology. As Sarah Franklin suggests, "Anthropology is a science and has the tools to understand science as a form of culture" (Franklin, 1995, 165).

---

[1] Postdoctoral researcher in the Science and Technology Policy Department (DPCT – IG – UNICAMP). PhD and Master in Anthropology from the Postgraduate Program in Social Anthropology (PPGAS – FFLCH – USP). She idealized the audiovisual project "Unstable bodies" (https://www.youtube.com/watch?v=gIFCxclQ5H8).

Technoscientific production is a particular way of giving meaning and making up the world. If the relationship between nature and culture is a universal axis of understanding and performing the world, it is precisely the mapping and understanding of the particular modes of these relationships that are of interest to anthropological analysis. The task is to highlight these different cultural forms, the ways by which each group or culture finds to live and relate to the world.

Technology is a classic topic in anthropological studies, since humans have always produced and used artifacts and techniques to apprehend and transform the world.[2] However, the topic gained new outlines and meanings, becoming, alongside science, one of the main institutions of so-called modern societies.

In addition to problematizing science and society dualism, addressing an implantable technology in the body implies exploring the fusion between organism and machine. The theoretical strategy proposed by Donna Haraway (2000) is the concept of the cyborg. This calls into question some dualisms, such as animal and human, organism and machine, public and private, nature and culture, men and women, and primitive and civilized, dualisms that, since World War II, have been cannibalized, dichotomies that are dichotomies called into question (p.63)

The machine's understanding of the body through biomedicine is what enables the institution of a heart-device cyborg. Just as the emergence of new paradigms, regarding the definitions of death, allows the manipulation of "living" organs and tissues from one organism to another. Medical and biotechnological access and interventions coproduce material and cognitive transformations. New ways of circulating blood, new blood flows giving by mechanical devices, new energy possibility for the heart-device arrangement, characterizing a composition of heterogeneous entities—new material bodies coproduced by new understandings about the body, new materiality crossed by new definition of human, about the limits of life and the occurrence of death as an irreversible process.

Fear and anguish before the finitude of life are manifested in attempts to control chance, which in modernity is related to technoscientific production. This means that technoscience occupies a privileged and structuring place in the so-called modern cosmologies, which implies that they end up transforming worlds and their own power and political place.

These are efforts to transform the body and make up (new) physiological arrangements, seeking to prolong life, as a way of dealing with the high rate of deaths understood as early, characterized as a public health problem. In this sense, mechanical devices are a strategy for dealing with social and natural problems at the same time. It is about shaping matter and dilemmas, material body, and existential/social embodied conflicts. Such circulatory assist devices, therefore, are efforts to delay death, to deal with tired, worn, exhausted hearts that refuse to perform their pumping function, distributing blood properly, rendering flawed bodies. So more than "adjusting" these bodies, such devices potentially allow us to question our own understandings of what this "misfit" is and how it was produced within a society that treats them

---

[2] I am not suggesting technology should be understood as the mere production of artifacts. It is a complex and broad field, which would require a careful debate that does not fit the purposes of this text.

not only as mechanisms, but also as energy to feed a system (and therefore it needs to be profitable, productive).

The purpose of looking at these productions is to investigate whether artificial hearts produce ontological instabilities in terms of what are human and non-human, life and death, nature and culture. It is about addressing the constitution of technologies as a result of practices, that is, highlighting the centrality of material engagement, the heterogeneous arrangements through which circulatory assistance devices emerge. All modern technoscience can be taken as a hybrid, described through a vocabulary of "composition," "coproduction," and "construction," but artificial hearts pose specific questions and implications.

Technoscientific developments continually threaten breaking ethical boundaries. Anticipatory governance is a tool to deal with and control these risks. Faced with still unstable technologies, an ethical-constructive approach (Kiran et al., 2015) allows reflecting on the moral dimensions of technologies while they are still being designed. In this regard, it is about to take into account reflections on how to design desirable technologies, according to society's expectations. There is a mediation role essential to find answers and strategies that enable to design technologies capable of meeting society's demands, in order to make people's lives better, healthier, more just, and egalitarian. For this, it is necessary to know what society wants, after all.

Responsible innovation is simple and complicated. It is simple because, in general, it means taking responsibility for what is being done (not only individuals or institutions, but also governments and companies). Even so, it is complicated because what it means to be responsible implies a broader debate open to society, in general. A large part of capitalist societies lack infrastructure and conditions for this debate to take place.

Engaging the population, recognizing their needs, and meeting these demands are something structurally lacking in Brazil. What about the difficulties surrounding more democratic and dialogical practices of technoscience, in a country that has not even managed to debate the greatest social disease, which is the scandalous wound of social inequality, resulting from not facing the mitigation of the slave regime? How to promote debates in a society that produces systematic extermination of marginal populations, a society whose scientific production is still done and reserved for an elite? Health, welfare state, and life cannot be achieved without proper working conditions, guarantees of rights, income distribution, and access to guarantees established by the constitution.

An aggravating factor is that, in our market-based democracies, the dialogic and participatory dimension is not central to the regulation of technoscience, scientific knowledge, and product development (Pestre, 2008). Furthermore, on a path different from the ideal, we witness a dismantling of the regulations implemented in the previous century (e.g., the welfare state) in favor of an extension of property rights, together with an attack on "common goods," for instance, the privatization of scientific knowledge through patent policy.

There is a widely shared assumption in the field of engineering and science that knowledge production is something that responds to specific and simplified demands and problems. This cannot be an excuse, however, to be blind to real and systemic empirical problems. In this sense, responsible innovation begins with an honest and open questioning about the need and adequacy of the technology that is intended to be developed.

Engineering and science operate by simplifying and isolating problems so that they can be addressed. Complexity can make any partial or possible treatment unfeasible. However, it is imperative that, in the face of democratic responsibility, we understand the processes in which partial and specific problems are inserted. It is groundless to claim that the effects and potential developments of what is being produced are unknown. Science and technology are not done outside society, but emerge from specific political and epistemological projects.

Although being aware of the complex and ambivalent scenario in which we live may not seem to be related to the "purely technical" solutions sought in biomedical research, at this point, we should be aware that there is nothing purely technical, there is nothing neutral, there is no science and technology produced in a vacuum, apart from relations and policies. There is no generic body. There is no neutral technology.

We can find collective paths that allow us to walk more comfortably in the paradox that is to develop technologies to prolong certain lives in a scenario of refusal of the recognition of the legitimacy of the end of some other lives. We live in a society that announces technological miracles capable of "saving" lives and miraculous techniques to prevent death and prolong life as long as possible and that refuses to accept the possibility that a terminal patient can choose to die, or decide how and when his death will be. Since Foucault's understanding of biopolitics, it became clear that what is at stake is the state's control of death.

We build artifacts, which carry morals and concepts that are fundamental to being who we are. The intertwining between humans and technology is undeniable. This means that technologies express and build our morals and our worldviews.

I do not mean to suggest that scientists should be individually blamed and disregard the unequal responsibility of companies and governments. Ravetz's aphorism tells us: Scientists take credit for penicillin, but does society take the blame for the atomic bomb?

How can we distribute these responsibilities more equally?

REFERENCES

Franklin, Sarah. Science as Culture, Cultures of Science. *Annual Review of Anthropology.* 1995; 24: 163–184. JSTOR, www.jstor.org/stable/2155934

Haraway, Donna. "Manifesto Ciborgue: ciência, tecnologia e feminismo-socialista no final do século XX". In: Silva, T. T. (org.). *Antropologia do Ciborgue: as vertigens do pós-humano.* Belo Horizonte: Autêntica, 2000.

Kiran, Asle; Nelly E. Oudshoorn; Peter P. Verbeek. Beyond checklists: toward an ethical-constructive technology assessment. *Journal of Responsible Innovation.* 2015; 2(1): 5–19. doi: 10.1080/23299460.2014.992769

Pestre, Dominique. Challenges for the democratic management of technoscience: Governance, participation and the political today. *Science as Culture,* 17(2): 101–119. doi: 10.1080/09505430802062869, 2008.

Sennett, Richard. 2019. *O Artífice.* Rio de Janeiro: Record.

Editor

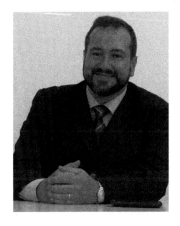

Eduardo Guy Perpétuo Bock, Eng. PhD., graduated in Mechanical Engineering from Universidade São Judas Tadeu (2003), master's and PhD in Mechanical Engineering from Universidade Estadual de Campinas—UNICAMP (2007 and 2011). He is an associate professor (class D-IV) at the Laboratory of Bioengineering and Biomaterials (BIOENG; www.labbioeng.com) and teaches at the Department of Mechanics in Institute Federal of São Paulo (IFSP). Eduardo is a board member of the Latin American Society for Artificial Organs (LASAO). He studied with Dr Yukihiko Nosé at Baylor College of Medicine and has experience in the field of biomedical engineering with emphasis on bioengineering, working mainly on the following topics: biomaterials, tribology, numerical simulation, artificial organs, artificial heart, circulatory assistance, left ventricular assistance, and extracorporeal circulation. He has published 4 books, 15 book chapters, and 45 papers with 469 citations received and had advised 16 students. He is founder of The Academic Society (TAS; www.theacademicsociety.net/tasj) and is part of the TAS Journal editorial board.

Email: eduardobock@gmail.com

Contributors

Aron J. P. Andrade
Department of Bioengineering
Instituto Dante Pazzanese de
    Cardiologia
Sao Paulo, Brazil

Gustavo C. Andrade
Department of Bioengineering
Instituto Dante Pazzanese de
    Cardiologia
São Paulo, Brazil

César A. Antônio
Faculdade de Tecnologia
FATEC – SO
São Paulo, Brazil

Rosana F. Antônio
Department of Chemical Engineering
Centro Universitário FACENS
São Paulo, Brazil

Sergio Y. Araki
Department of Mechanics
Member of the Mechanics Department
Instituto Federal de São Paulo
São Paulo, Brazil

Marcelo Barboza
Department of Mechatronics
Polytechnic School of the University of
    São Paulo
São Paulo, Brazil

Luben Cabezas-Gómez
Mechanical Engineering Department
University of Sao Paulo
Sao Paulo, Brazil

André César Martins Cavalheiro
Fundação Santo André University
    Center
Santo André, Brazil

Nilson C. Cruz
Laboratory of Technological Plasmas
São Paulo State University
São Paulo, Brazil

Jeison Willian Gomes da Fonseca
Institute "Dante Pazzanese" of
    Cardiology
University of Sao Paulo
Sao Paulo, Brazil
and
Technological Institute of Aeronautics
Sao Judas Tadeu University
Sao Paulo, Brazil

Gustavo C. de Andrade
Institute "Dante Pazzanese" of
    Cardiology
Sao Judas Tadeu University
Sao Paulo, Brazil

Adriana Del Monaco De Maria
Engenharia Biomédica
Centro Universitário das Américas
São Paulo, Brazil

Rosa Corrêa Leoncio de Sá
Laboratório Associado de Sensores e
    Materiais
INPE National Institute for Space
    Research
Sao Paulo, Brazil

José Ricardo de Sousa Sobrinho
Department of Mechatronics
Polytechnic School of the University of
    São Paulo
São Paulo, Brazil

Rogerio L. de Souza
Department of Mechanics
Institute Federal of São Paulo
Sao Paulo, Brazil

Jonatas Dias
Department of Mechatronics
Polytechnic School of the University of
    São Paulo
São Paulo, Brazil

Bruno Jesus dos Santos
Department of Electrical Engineering
Instituto Federal de São Paulo
São Paulo, Brazil

Diolino José dos Santos Filho
Department of Mechatronics
Polytechnic School of the University of
    São Paulo
São Paulo, Brazil

Fernando dos Santos Ortega
Faculdade Israelita de Ciências da
    Saúde Albert Einstein
Hospital Israelita Albert Einstein
São Paulo, Brazil

Juliana dos Santos Solheid
Institute for Applied Materials –
    Applied Materials Physics
Karlsruhe Institute of Technology
Karlsruhe, Germany

Evandro Drigo
Engenharia Biomédica
Centro Universitário das Américas
São Paulo, Brazil

Wesley L. Fotoran
Genetic Department
Butantan Institute
São Paulo, Brazil

Isac K. Fujita
Department of Mechanics
Member of the Mechanics Department
Instituto Federal de São Paulo
São Paulo, Brazil

Guilherme B. Lopes Junior
Mechanical Engineering Department
Federal University of Pernambuco
Recife, Brazil

Tarcísio F. Leão
Department of Electrical Engineering
Instituto Federal de São Paulo
São Paulo, Brazil

Juliana Leme
Product Development
Dental Morelli
Sorocaba, Brazil

Raquel J. Lobosco
Mechanical Engineering Department
Universidade Federal do Rio de Janeiro
Rio de Janeiro, Brazil

Marisol Marini
Science and Technology Policy
    Department
UNICAMP
Sao Paulo, Brazil

Breno Y. T. Nishida
Department of Bioengineering
Institute Dante Pazzanese of Cardiology
Sao Paulo, Brazil

Breno T. Y. Nishida
Institute "Dante Pazzanese" of
  Cardiology
University of Sao Paulo
Sao Paulo, Brazil

Henrique Stelzer Nogueira
Department of Electrical
Instituto Federal de São Paulo
São Paulo, Brazil

Wilhelm Pfleging
Institute for Applied Materials –
  Applied Materials Physics
Karlsruhe Institute of Technology
Karlsruhe, Germany

Elidiane C. Rangel
Laboratory of Technological Plasmas
São Paulo State University
São Paulo, Brazil

Bruno U. Silva
Anima Education
Universidade São Judas Tadeu
São Paulo, Brazil

Rodrigo Lima Stoeterau
Mechatronic Engineering Department
Polytechnic School of the University of
  São Paulo
São Paulo, Brazil

Introduction

Eduardo Guy Perpétuo Bock
Instituto Federal de São Paulo

The aim of this book is to establish an area of intersection between engineering and medicine, more precisely between cardiology and engineering. In a more specific form of engineering, still in two complementary topics, this book takes two approaches, one in the field of *bioengineering* and another in the field of *biomaterials*.

The idea is to be a fundamental book for translational science, both in cardiology courses that need to go into the constructive details of the *ventricular assist devices* and the applied biomaterials and in Biomedical Engineering graduation during Biomaterials and Bioengineering courses, showing the whole process development from mechanical design to automation and control.

What to expect from this book? The book aims to have a didactic aspect for both scientists and professionals looking for a specific chapter to solve problems; or undergraduate students that need to acquire a basic knowledge to later go deeper into the subject.

However, this does not imply treating topics just as introductory or superficial way, but serving as absolute reference for each theme, giving a comprehensive approach, and always leaving a solid and updated bibliography.

The authors are a group of friends who have collaborated on average for 10 years and have interacted and sought solutions to problems that require knowledge in several multidisciplinary areas. Those contributors are mainly Brazilians, researchers who also teach, young PhD students, and recent doctors. Only about a third of this group is a compound of professors with more than 10 years of PhD. If it were possible to trace the genealogy of this research group, it would certainly lead to Yukihiko Nosé from Baylor College of Medicine (Nosé, Schauman, and Kantrowitz 1963) (see Figure 0.1). The authors constitute two groups: (i) VAD researchers who are students, or students of Nosé's students; and (ii) researchers with a solid background in their fields who approached the group because of their interest in collaborating with VAD research.

Dr. Yukihiko Nosé passed away on October 13, 2011, at the age of 79. This year, in memory of the 10 years since his death, we would like to dedicate this book to his career and his example book *Yukihiko Nosé: Life Long Dream*.

The idea of writing this book is an old dream, but I confess that it started to become a reality when I assumed the chair of Biomaterials at the Instituto Federal de São Paulo in 2013. Naturally, like many others who teach this course, I adopted as basic bibliography the book "Biomaterials Science: An Introduction to Materials in Medicine" (Ratner et al. 2013).

Our book does not claim to address the theme of Biomaterials as extensively as this colleague, obviously. But I took the courage to think more seriously when I personally met Prof. Ratner at a conference playing the guitar and telling him about teaching experiences in a developing country. I spent years telling my students, from

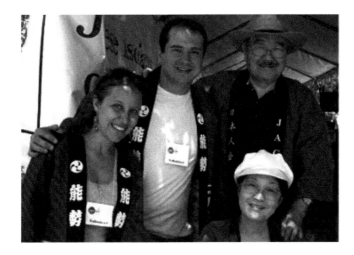

FIGURE 0.1   The beloved "Mr Artificial Organs," the pioneer Prof. Dr. Yukihiko Nosé with Eduardo Bock with respective wives, Ako Nosé and Karen Bock, in 2006.

different classes, that aura of simple nobility and elegant thoughts permeated this contact. Until one day, at a conference in Maresias, I met Prof. Ratner. More than this, I met Prof. Hoffman and, together with my students, confirmed the guitar story, laughing and celebrating the reunion.

Our book begins with a thought-provoking prologue. Marisol Marini proposes an anthropological reflection on the role of our research, where we intend to reach, what is the impact on our lives, and how we can make science better for everyone.

Aron Andrade starts Chapter 1 with his group from Instituto Dante Pazzanese de Cardiologia talking about VAD design. He is not just the most experienced of our group; he was my advisor. Nobody better than him to deal with the theme of design and, thus, be able to share decades of experience in the subject (Andrade et al. 1989).

Breno Nishida and Rogerio Souza are solidly trained engineers who know how to calculate and design machines and became great researchers. In Chapter 2, they conduct a didactic explanation that begins with the constructive details of VAD electromechanical actuators and goes on to the mathematical modeling necessary for the computational numerical analysis of the affected electromagnetic phenomena, their construction, and validation (Nishida et al. 2017; de Souza et al. 2020; Osa et al. 2015; Pohlmann and Hameyer 2013; Fenercioğlu 2016).

In the last two decades, Jeison Fonseca has become a great specialist in cardiovascular simulators, not just gaining recognition with international awards from ASAIO, but becoming a reference in the art of creating conditions similar to physiological to assess the requirements for circulatory assistance (Fresiello et al. 2015; Shi, Korakianitis, and Bowles 2007; Fonseca et al. 2011).

Tarcisio Leão and Bruno Santos are control engineers, but I like to call them "VAD-robotic scientists." In many projects, I am proud to be their colleague, but I find it difficult to keep up with their minds. They brilliantly conduct the narrative of Chapter 5 on control systems by explaining what types are possible and how we can make control smarter (Santos et al. 2020; Leao et al. 2020).

Diolino Santos Filho's group from the University of São Paulo is avant-garde proposing the solution of problems that are not debated by the majority, but are being reported in INTERMACS year after year. In Chapter 5 on supervisory systems, they make a broad and didactic approach to the problem and propose modern architecture linked to future problems such as IoT protocols (Sobrinho, 2016; Barboza et al. 2020; Neto et al. 2020).

André César Martins Cavalheiro has been working with VAD security for over 10 years and has made bold proposals to address the issue from the point of view of safety control. In Chapter 6, he manages to be didactic and concise, opening up possibilities for new research (Cavalheiro et al. 2011).

We open Part II of this book with Chapter 7 on hemocompatibility, hemolysis, and cell viability that underlies all the concepts in the following chapters. Wesley Fotoran brilliantly explains several concepts of biology in a didactic way giving aspects of biomaterials and their future trends (Fotoran et al. 2019).

Luben Gomez, Raquel Lobosco, and Guilherme Lopes entered this book project through Chapter 8 with a very special mission, to build material that serves as a reference on the subject of CFD in VADs. In my opinion, this topic is the most difficult to start in research, precisely because there are no didactic chapters on the specific topic (Telyshev et al. 2020; Shida, Masuzawa, and Osa 2020; Chen et al. 2019; Wang, Tan, and Yu 2019; Lopes Jr et al. 2016; Lopes, Bock, and Gómez 2017).

Rosa Sá deals with biofunctional materials in Chapter 9 showing how we can still improve the VADs' biomaterials that are currently being used and how we could have new generations of devices that would escape the titanium hegemony (de Sá et al. 2017).

Fernando Ortega wrote a remarkable chapter on ceramic materials (Chapter 10). I believe it will serve as a guide for everyone who intends to start, improve, or master the processing of ceramic materials for VADs (Ortega et al. 1999).

Rodrigo Stoeterau deals with the subject of tribology in Chapter 11. His partnership has brought new approaches to the subject that has been very well received in academic circles. His future projects are promising and are expected to show results soon. He tells us a little about how to achieve it in his chapter (Hernandes et al. 2017).

In Chapter 12, Nilson Cruz and his group from UNESP give a complete explanation of film and material deposition and illustrate a still little explored possibility of obtaining high-performance biomaterials in VADs (Momesso et al. 2021).

Adriana Del Monaco and Evandro Drigo, authors of Chapter 13, are highly trained researchers of excellence who explain the technologies and demonstrate ways of using the three-dimensional technologies of additive manufacturing in VADs (Del Monaco et al. 2018).

Wilhelm Pfleging is an internationally renowned researcher, his research center is a reference in Germany and outside. His participation in our book is an honor. Chapter 14 deals with laser additive manufacturing for the realization of new material concepts (Pfleging et al. 2015).

Bruno Santos and Henrique Nogueira take a very interesting approach on the use of biosensors in Chapter 15. The material presented serves as a basis for researchers who want to start developing biosensors; in addition, it can serve for new perspectives for those who already research the topic (Nogueira et al. 2020).

Chapter 16 closes this book with a *grand finale*. My companions and veterans, Isac Fujita and Sergio Araki describe their research in optics and VADs. In a very creative way, they propose solutions for testing and controlling VADs with optical methods (Loiola et al. 2019).

Finally, I would like to say that this book is not just a book of Brazilians waving to the world saying we are here and we want to be seen. Science in Brazil is inventive because it is done without resources. We believe that this book has a special way of looking at this area of multidisciplinary research. As all the authors here do a little bit of everything, everyone needs to know a lot about all topics. The VAD market may not be favorable to entrepreneurs, but our science is here, more alive than ever, waiting to be financed.

REFERENCES

Andrade, Aron, José Biscegli, Denys Nicolosi, Henrique Gómez, and José Sousa. 1989. "Estudo comparativo das características fluidodinâmicas de próteses valvulares biológicas de pericárdio bovino de perfil alto e baixo." *Revista Brasileira de Cirurgia Cardiovascular* 4 (3): 231–36.

Barboza, Marcelo, Fabricio Junqueira, Eduardo Bock, Tarcisio Leão, Jeferson Dias, Jonatas Dias, Marcosiris Pessoa, José Ricardo Souza, and Diolino dos Santos. 2020. "Ventricular assist device in Health 4.0 context." In IFIP Advances in Information and Communication Technology, 577: 347–54, Springer.

Cavalheiro, André, Diolino J. Santos Fo, Aron Andrade, José Roberto Cardoso, Osvaldo Horikawa, Eduardo Bock, and Jeison Fonseca. 2011. "Specification of supervisory control systems for ventricular assist devices." *Artificial Organs* 35 (5): 465–70.

Chen, Zengsheng, Sofen K. Jena, Guruprasad A. Giridharan, Michael A. Sobieski, Steven C. Koenig, Mark S. Slaughter, Bartley P. Griffith, and Zhongjun J. Wu. 2019. "Shear stress and blood trauma under constant and pulse-modulated speed CF-VAD operations: CFD analysis of the HVAD." *Medical & Biological Engineering & Computing* 57 (4): 807–18.

de Souza, Rogerio Lima, Ivan Eduardo Chabu, Evandro Drigo da Silva, Aron Jose Pazin de Andrade, Tarcisio Fernandes Leao, and Eduardo Guy Perpetuo Bock. 2020. "A strategy for designing of customized electromechanical actuators of blood pumps." *Artificial Organs* 44 (8): 797–802.

Fenercioğlu, A. 2016. "Design and analysis of a magnetically levitated axial flux BLDC motor for a Ventricular Assist Device (VAD)." *Turkish Journal of Electrical Engineering & Computer Sciences* 24 (4): 2881–92.

Fonseca, Jeison, Aron Andrade, D. E. C. Denys, E. C. Nicolosi, José F. Biscegli, Juliana Leme, Daniel Legendre, Eduardo Bock, and Julio Cesar Lucchi. 2011. "Cardiovascular simulator improvement: Pressure versus volume loop assessment." *Artificial Organs* 35 (5): 454–58.

Fotoran, Wesley L., Thomas Müntefering, Nicole Kleiber, Beatriz N.M. Miranda, Eva Liebau, Darrell J. Irvine, and Gerhard Wunderlich. 2019. "A multilamellar nanoliposome stabilized by interlayer hydrogen bonds increases antimalarial drug efficacy." *Nanomedicine: Nanotechnology, Biology, and Medicine* 22 (November): 102099.

Fresiello, Libera, Gianfranco Ferrari, Arianna Di Molfetta, K. Zieliński, A. Tzallas, Steven Jacobs, Marek Darowski, Maciej Kozarski, Bart Meyns, and Nikolaos S. Katertsidis. 2015. "A cardiovascular simulator tailored for training and clinical uses." *Journal of Biomedical Informatics* 57: 100–112.

Hernandes, Mariana Maria Aparecida Pinto, Joaquim Antonio Ferreira Da Rocha, Michele Aparecida Saito, Sérgio Yoshinobu Araki, Pamela Silva, Rodrigo Lima Stoeterau, and Eduardo Guy Perpetuo Bock. 2017. "Dimensional control in pre-sintered zirconia machining for double pivot micro bearings of blood pumps." *In Proceedings of the 17th International Conference of the European Society for Precision Engineering and Nanotechnology*, Hannover, *EUSPEN* 2017, 483–84.

Leao, Tarcisio, Bruno Utiyama, Jeison Fonseca, Eduardo Bock, and Aron Andrade. 2020. "In vitro evaluation of multi-objective physiological control of the centrifugal blood pump." *Artificial Organs* 44 (8): 785–96.

Loiola, Monyze T. C., Sergio Y. Araki, Eduardo G. P. Bock, and Isac K. Fujita. 2019. "Aplicação Da Técnica Óptica de Moiré de Projeção Para Análise de Deformação Nos Mancais Cerâmicos Do Dispositivo de Assistência Ventricular (DAV)." *The Academic Society Journal* 3 (3): 246–55.

Lopes Jr, Guilherme B., Luben C. Gómez, and Eduardo Bock. 2016. "Mesh independency analyses and grid density estimation for ventricular assist devices in multiple reference frames simulations." *Technische Mechanik* 36 (3): 190–98.

Lopes, Guilherme., Eduardo. Bock, and Luben Gómez. 2017. "Numerical analyses for low reynolds flow in a ventricular assist device." *Artificial Organs* 41 (6): E30–E40.

Momesso, Gustavo Antonio Correa, Tarik Ocon Braga Polo, William Phillip Pereira da Silva, Stéfany Barbosa, Gileade P. Freitas, Helena Bacha Lopes, Adalberto Luiz Rosa, et al. 2021. "Miniplates coated by plasma electrolytic oxidation improve bone healing of simulated femoral fractures on low bone mineral density rats." *Materials Science and Engineering C* 120 (January): 111775.

Del Monaco, Adriana, Evandro Drigo, J. C. M. Lautert, S. S. Margarido, and T. Y. Miyashiro. 2018. "Case report: Auxiliary device for recreational use in a child with upper limb malformation, made by additive manufacture (3D printing)." *The Academic Society Journal* 2 (4): 242–47.

Neto, Silva, J. R. C. Sousa Sobrinho, C. da Costa, T. F. Leão, S. A. M. M. Senra, E. G. P. Bock, G. A. Santos, et al. 2020. "Investigation of MEMS as accelerometer sensor in an implantable centrifugal blood pump prototype." *Journal of the Brazilian Society of Mechanical Sciences and Engineering* 42 (9): 1–10.

Nishida, B. Y. T., G. A. Pereira, E. Drigo, M. Fonseca, R. B. B. Santos, M. A. G. Silveira, and E. G. P. Bock. 2017. "Prototype for optical applications that microscopically affect the cancer cell diagnosis in biological sciences." *In Proceedings of the* 17th *International Conference of the European Society for Precision Engineering and Nanotechnology,* Hannover, *EUSPEN 2017.*

Nogueira, Henrique Stelzer, D. M. S. D. Duque, Vagner de Mendonça, Wladecir Lima, and Eduardo Bock. 2020. "Monitoring the level of infection by COVID-19: An previous experiment to possibility of future application to the C-reactive protein detection by bioelectric signals." *The Academic Society Journal* 4 (June): 104–22.

Nosé, Yukihiko, Martin Schamaun, ÁdrianKantrowitz. 1963. Experimental use of an electronically controlled prosthesis as an auxiliary left ventricle. *Transactions – American Society for Artificial Internal Organs* 9(1): 269–274.

Ortega, Fernando S., R. G. Pileggi, P. Sepulveda, and V. C. Pandolfelli. 1999. "Optimizing particle packing in powder consolidation." *American Ceramic Society Bulletin* 78 (8): 106–11.

Osa, Masahiro, Toru Masuzawa, Naoki Omori, and Eisuke Tatsumi. 2015. "Radial position active control of double stator axial gap self-bearing motor for pediatric VAD." *Mechanical Engineering Journal* 2 (4): 15–105.

Pfleging, Wilhelm, Renu Kumari, Heino Besser, Tim Scharnweber, and Jyotsna Dutta Majumdar. 2015. "Laser surface textured titanium alloy (Ti-6Al-4V): Part 1-surface characterization." *Applied Surface Science* 355: 104–11.

Pohlmann, André, and Kay Hameyer. 2013. "Design of an BLDC drive with iron core to improve the efficiency of ventricular assist devices." In 2013 *International Conference on Electrical Machines and Systems (ICEMS)*, Busan, South Korea, 888–91. IEEE.

Ratner, Buddy D., Allan S. Hoffman, Frederick J. Schoen, and Jack E. Lemons. 2013. *Biomaterials Science: An Introduction to Materials: Third Edition.* Academic Press: San Diego, CA.

de Sá, Rosa Corrêa Leoncio de, Nilson Cristino da Cruz, João Roberto Moro, Tarcísio Leão, Aron José Pazzin de Andrade, and Eduardo Guy Perpétuo Bock. 2017. "Modification surface in medicine: Techniques with plasma in a centrifugal blood pump implantable." *Sinergia* 18 (2): 91–94.

Santos, Bruno J., Rachel P. Tabacow, Marcelo Barboza, Tarcisio F. Leão, and Eduardo G. P. Bock. 2020. "Standard protocols for IoT and supervisory control systems." *Cyber Security in Health*, 0: 313–29. doi: 10.4018/978-1-7998-2910-2.ch015.

Shi, Yubing, Theodosios Korakianitis, and Christopher Bowles. 2007. "Numerical simulation of cardiovascular dynamics with different types of VAD assistance." *Journal of Biomechanics* 40 (13): 2919–33.

Shida, Shuya, Toru Masuzawa, and Masahiro Osa. 2020. "Dynamic motion analysis of impeller for the development of real-time flow rate estimations of a ventricular assist device." *International Journal of Artificial Organs*, 1–8. doi: 10.1177/0391398820984485.

Sobrinho, José Ricardo Corrêa de Sousa. 2016. "Detecção de trombos em uma bomba de sangue centrífuga implantável por análise de vibração com MEMS."

Telyshev, Dmitry, Maxim Denisov, Aleksandr Markov, Libera Fresiello, Tom Verbelen, and Sergey Selishchev. 2020. "Energetics of blood flow in Fontan circulation under VAD support." *Artificial Organs* 44 (1): 50–57.

Wang, Shuai, Jianping Tan, and Zheqin Yu. 2019. "Comparison and experimental validation of turbulence models for an axial flow blood pump." *Journal of Mechanics in Medicine and Biology* 19 (8): 1–14.

MATLAB® is a registered trademark of The MathWorks, Inc. For product information, please contact:

The MathWorks, Inc.
3 Apple Hill Drive
Natick, MA 01760-2098 USA
Tel: 508-647-7000
Fax: 508-647-7001
E-mail: info@mathworks.com
Web: www.mathworks.com

Part I

Bioengineering in Ventricular Assist Devices

1 VAD Design

Aron J. P. Andrade and Gustavo C. Andrade
Instituto Dante Pazzanese de Cardiologia

Juliana Leme
Dental Morelli

Bruno U. Silva
Universidade São Judas Tadeu

CONTENTS

In this chapter, the theoretical framework for better understanding the process of ventricular assist device (VAD) design will be presented.

1.1 AUTHORS' EXPERIENCES—HOW IT BEGAN[1]

Dr. Aron Andrade is a co-editor for Central and South America for Artificial Organs. Dr. Aron Jose Pazin Andrade is one of the pioneers in mechanical circulatory support in Latin America. Before finishing mechanical engineering school in 1983, he began his student-training program at the Institute Dante Pazzanese of Cardiology (IDPC), an important research and healthcare center maintained by the Government of the State of São Paulo. There he developed a cardiovascular simulator for prosthetic heart valve evaluation. After getting his diploma in 1985, he was admitted as an engineer at IDPC—Department of Bioengineering—and also began his master's degree program at the University of Campinas, performing comparative assessment studies with different cardiac prosthetic valves. He became the head of the Biomechanical Laboratory in 1990, where the development of many types of prostheses, medical devices, and surgical instruments occurred—great contributions to

---

[1] Presented by Paul S. Malchesky, DEng Editor-in-Chief of *Artificial Organs.*

DOI: 10.1201/9781003138358-2

Brazilian cardiology. In 1995, Dr. Andrade's PhD thesis sent him to the Department of Surgery at Baylor College of Medicine in Houston, TX. There, under the tutelage of Prof. Yukihiko Nosé, Dr. Andrade began the evaluation of a new model of centrifugal blood pump for cardiopulmonary bypass (CPB), which became known and patented as the Spiral Pump. At Baylor, he had the opportunity to join Prof. Nosé's research group. He helped to improve and to evaluate an electromechanical total artificial heart (TAH) and to test an implantable centrifugal pump under development at that time. Just before returning to Brazil, Dr. Andrade proposed a new project of an artificial heart to Dr. Nosé, but not an orthotopically implanted device such as Baylor's model: Dr. Andrade proposed a heterotopic artificial heart, the so-called auxiliary TAH (ATAH). Back at IDPC, he began to work on this new ATAH based on the same electromechanical principle as Nosé's TAH, but with new design features, technologies, and different applied materials. The main purposes of the ATAH were to have easier and faster implantation without removing the patient's natural heart; to have a more effective device controller as it would need only to follow the natural heart rate using a full empty control mode; to provide safer application as the natural heart still can maintain a patient's blood circulation in case of a catastrophic device failure; and to maintain the possibility of native heart reverse remodeling. The ATAH project grew and became his main PhD thesis subject, which was concluded in 1998. A few years later, the first ATAH prototypes were prepared for initial preclinical trials and the external components as the batteries system and controlling system were completely functional. During ATAH development, Dr. Andrade also started his work on the dissemination of artificial organs information in Latin America. In 1998, he founded a scientific society called LASAO—Latin American Society for Artificial Organs and Biomaterials, with important help from his colleagues. In the same year, the first LASAO congress was held in Belo Horizonte, Brazil, with 409 attendants and 107 presentations. From 2001 to 2004, Dr. Andrade was the head of LASAO and after that became a member of its Board of Trustees. LASAO has published three peer-reviewed special issues for Artificial Organs, presenting selected articles from its congresses. During this period, Dr. Andrade, his students, and colleagues started several other projects in mechanical circulatory support, biomedical engineering, and cardiology. These projects, including the ATAH, caused Dr. Andrade to become renowned as a successful professional, professor, and researcher in Brazil and in Latin America. In 2009, Dr. Andrade created and became the head director of the "Engineering Center of Circulatory Assistance" (ECCA), the first center in Latin America exclusively dedicated to the development of blood pumps and devices for mechanical circulatory assistance. At ECCA, his research associates and students began new projects such as implantable centrifugal pumps and mixed flow blood pumps for left ventricle assistance, CPB and temporary ventricular assist devices, device controllers and controlling system software, and a hybrid cardiovascular simulator for blood pump evaluations. The implantable centrifugal blood pump is in preclinical trials, and a new remodeled version of the Spiral Pump is approved for CPB. Currently, Dr. Andrade is a professor teaching materials science and biomedical technology at FATEC—College of Technology (since 1992)—and USP—University of São Paulo (since 2007), where he is a PhD program adviser in Cardiovascular Technology. He has published over 240 articles, 5 book chapters, 15 technological products, and 8 patents and has received 20 awards and titles. Dr. Andrade continues to organize the COLAOB Special Issue in collaboration with Artificial Organs.

1.2 VENTRICULAR ASSIST DEVICE (VAD)

The development of blood pumps goes through design steps, prototype construction, *in vitro* evaluation, in vivo evaluation, clinical evaluation, and release for use. These items are included in the international standard ISO 14708—Implants for Surgery—Active implantable medical devices—Part 5: Circulatory support devices, 2010 (ISO 14708-5, 2010). This standard deals with a regulatory item of definitions, specifications, tests, and documentation for the development of all procedures and is already applied in Brazil as ABNT NBR ISO 14708-5: 2017.

Regarding the development (geometry and dimensions), the standard is not specific. It shows a methodology of step-by-step development, based on the progression of experiments and improvement of the project through preliminary results, the same proposed by Dr. Nosé in 1998 (ISO 14708-5, 2010; Nosé, 1998). In other words, the development is at the discretion of the ideology of the researcher, and from the results of the tests proposed by ISO 14708-5, changes are made in the project, which may result in a product different from the original and even for other applications.

For the development of blood pumps, it is necessary to understand how they are classified, which may be in terms of the type of pumping, the mode of activation, its location in the patient, and its applicability.

As for the type of pumping, the pumps can be pulsatile and nonpulsatile.

- Pulsatile: The blood flow occurs due to the movement of a diaphragm associated with the use of mechanical or biological artificial valves, which allow the unidirectional passage of blood (Nosé & Motomura, 2003);
- Nonpulsatile: The continuous flow can be generated by radial or axial drive:
  - Nonpulsatile radial drive pumps (centrifuges) promote a blood flow perpendicular to the pump rotation axis. Intake is performed by the center of the pump where the inlet connector is placed. The blood acquires a rotation movement and is forced by the centrifugal effect to its lateral portion, where the outlet connector is placed;
  - Nonpulsatile axial flow pumps promote the flow of blood parallel to the rotation axis of the pump. Intake is performed by one end of the tubular body. The blood is pumped by a screw-threaded impeller, being pushed to the other end of the tubular body.

An axial VAD can also be classified according to implantation surgical procedure: transcatheter (TC), open-heart surgery (OHS), and minimally invasive surgery (MIS). In TC, the axial flow pump is inserted through the femoral artery and positioned, for example, inside the aorta to increase arterial blood flow. In OHS, the surgeon makes a large incision at the sternum, pulls the ribs apart, and implants the VAD. The VAD can be either directly implanted to the ventricle or connected to the ventricle by a cannula. MIS is an alternative to OHS, where surgeons can perform the procedure using laparoscopy or through very small incisions.

Table 1.1 shows some well-known models of axial VADs currently in use or under development, along with some parameters.

TABLE 1.1

Models of Axial Pumps and Summary of Some Parameters

Model	Company	Pressure (mmHg)	Flow (L/min)	Rotation (rpm)	Types	Diameter (mm)
Valvo-pump	-	100	5	7,000	OHS	38
Streamliner	UPMC	100	6	7,000	OHS	-
INCOR I®	Berlin Heart	100	5	8,000	OHS	30
HeartMate II™	Thoratec Corporation	100	4	9,000	OHS	40
Jarvik 2000®	Jarvik Heart Inc.	100	7	12,000	OHS	25
DeBakey VAD®	Micromed	100	6	12,500	OHS	25
IVAP	SUN Med. Tec. Corp.	-	8	13,000	OHS	13.5
LongHorn	HeartWare Inc.	60	6	21,000	MIS	20
Hemopump	Medtronic Inc.	-	5	26,000	TC	8.1
Impella®	Abiomed	100	7	30,000	TC	6.4

Source: Adapted from Song et al. (2003) and Connellan et al. (2013).

As for the drive mode, the pumps can be (i) pneumatic, where the device uses one or two flexible diaphragms positioned between two chambers isolated from each other, the pumping chamber containing blood and an antechamber containing air. An air compressor is used to pump the air to the antechamber, promoting the movement of the diaphragms resulting in the ejection of blood (Oshiro et al., 1995); (ii) electrohydraulic, this type of device uses two blood-pumping chambers that are separated by diaphragms from two other antechambers containing a fluid. A high rotation pump is used for pumping fluid from one antechamber to the other, moving the diaphragms and ejecting the blood from one pumping chamber to the other (Leme, 2015); (iii) electromechanical, this type of drive has as the operating principle the transformation of the rotation movement of an electric motor into linear movement of one or two diaphragms. A mechanical system pushes one or two propeller plates, displacing one or two diaphragms. This type of device promotes alternate ejection of the right and left chambers (Leme, 2015); and (iv) electromagnetic, this type of device is composed of an electromagnet positioned between two metal plates that, with its attraction, compress a polyurethane bag, acting as a blood-pumping chamber.

Regarding the pump location in the patient, they can be paracorporeal, where all the components of the pump are implanted externally to the patient's body using transcutaneous cannulas for blood transportation; or intracorporeal, where the pump is implanted inside the patient's body, and can be in the thoracic or abdominal cavity. The positioning of each of the components of a blood-pumping system is related to the duration of its use (Nosé and Okubo, 2004).

As for their applicability, the pumps can be classified according to the patient's needs:

- Extracorporeal circulation (ECC): The pump is used during the surgical act, when there is a need for momentary replacement of the functions of the heart and lungs, being the function of pumping the heart performed by a mechanical pump and the functions of the lungs replaced by a device capable of performing gas exchange with the blood.

- Recovery bridge: The pump is used to assist the cardiac function, facilitating the patient's recovery, that is, giving circulatory support until the pump can be removed or until some surgical procedure can be performed.
- Bridge for decision: A disposable pump is used to easily and quickly implant a candidate patient for a blood pump for prolonged assistance or other interventions to be defined. In this case, a temporary circulatory support is used, with or without a blood oxygenator, and the patient does not need heart surgery to implant the pump, but a procedure to introduce catheters percutaneously via an artery and/or femoral vein.
- Bridge for transplantation: The pump is used when the patient needs an immediate heart transplant and the pump helps to keep the patient alive until the organ is obtained.
- Destination therapy: A blood pump is used on patients who are not indicated for a heart transplant. The patient needs a pump to help the weakened heart and thus improve its clinical conditions and quality of life. In this case, the patient needs continuous monitoring and, if necessary, pump replacement.

There is also the classification of the device as orthotopic or total artificial heart, heterotopic or auxiliary artificial heart, artificial ventricle or ventricular assistance device, and temporary circulatory support device.

- Orthotopic or total artificial heart: It is a pulsatile flow blood pump with two pumping chambers that totally replace the patient's natural heart (removing the native heart), called TAH. TAHs are long-lasting, implantable pumps. Currently, some institutions are studying a continuous flow TAH using centrifugal pumps.
- Artificial ventricle or ventricular assistance device (VAD): It is a univentricular blood pump with pulsatile or continuous flow, centrifugal or axial, used to assist the sick ventricle. The VAD is mostly used for the left ventricle, but two devices can be used simultaneously for biventricular assistance. For this type of application, a pump and a controller are used for each ventricle. The VADs are devices of medium to long duration, and their function is to support the life of the patient, assisting the natural heart in pumping blood during all assistance time (Bock et al., 2008).
- Temporary circulatory support device: In this case, the following are used disposable centrifugal pumps with continuous flow being subdivided in ECMO and Temporary Circulatory Support (TCS).
- Extracorporeal circulation with membrane oxygenator (ECMO): This application uses disposable centrifugal pumps and a membrane oxygenator, currently made of polymethyl pentene, with a low gradient of pressure, for cardiopulmonary support (Formica et al., 2008).
- Temporary Circulatory Support (TCS): For this application, disposable centrifugal pumps are used, and their use is limited to 30 days (temporary). However, they must have hydrodynamic characteristics and durability superior to CPB pumps. The implant of this type of pump must be fast and easy and can be used as a decision bridge or recovery bridge.

1.3 ROTOR GEOMETRY

The optimization of flow machines ranges from the selection of materials to the definition of the best shapes for the blades and their positioning on the rotor. Many papers in the literature evaluate the optimization of these machines from different points of view, obtaining results that show significant efficiency gains. For example, in Wen-Guang, 2011, an inverse problem-based methodology is used to design pump rotor blades, performing simulations in computational fluid dynamics (CFD) to measure hydrodynamic performance and obtaining results that demonstrate efficiency improvements of around 5%.

There is a large amount of data in the literature demonstrating the efficiency of the CFD study in minimizing hemolysis and thrombosis. The ABNT NBR ISO 14708-5: 2010 standard proposes computer simulation as a tool for the validation of circulatory support devices. It determines test guidelines seeking results in hydrodynamic performance, hemolysis, or thrombus formation.

Regarding the rotor design, the first relevant aspect is related to the pitch, i.e., the distance between two consecutive blades. A low blade pitch results in high pumping pressure and low flow (Sudhamshu et al., 2016).

According to Mizuguchi et al. (2008), rotors with continuous blades, that is, without any division in the blade, result in the elimination of zones of high negative pressure, reducing hemolysis in the pump. However, according to Wampler (1987), the best combination of blades consists of a noncontinuous rotor with three blades spaced 120 degrees apart and divided into two columns. The three-bladed arrangement provides the best compromise between flow orientation and drag loss. To confirm which model is the best, tests were performed on both continuous and column-divided rotors.

The number of blades in the rotor appears to be a relevant factor in the study of the efficiency of flow machines, as the intuition leads to the belief that a larger number of propellers allow a higher interaction between rotor and fluid and thus allow a better transfer of energy. However, experiments presented in Gölcü and Pancar (2005) show that efficiency tends to decrease as the number of blades is increased, since there is a bottleneck in the flow between the blades and an increase in friction between the fluid and the structure in the paths between the blades, with the highest losses occurring due to the congestion generated at the rotor inlet. The usual number of blades is between 2 and 8 (Kanpur, 2018).

In terms of the gap between the rotor and the pump housing, in an axial turbine, such gap is generally around 1%–2% of the blade height. An increase in the gap implies an increase in fluid leakage and consequent degradation of the pump performance (Schabowski and Hodson, 2007; Oliveira, 2014). However, a change in the gap will promote important changes in the shear stress in the fluid, so it is necessary to find the best combination between performance and shear stress.

1.4 HEMOLYSIS AND THROMBOSIS

Artificial pumping of blood requires certain precautions due to the problems generated by this type of procedure. Inconveniences related to blood pumping that concern the formation of clots or thrombosis, trauma to the blood cells, and the formation

TABLE 1.2
Values of NIH and Its Clinical Results

NIH (g/100L)	Clinical Results
>0.06	Increased level of PFH
>0.04	No increase in PFH, but requires blood transfusion
<0.04	Physiologically satisfactory
<0.02	Clinically satisfactory
<0.01	Ideal level for extended mechanical assistance

Source: Nosé (1998) and Chan et al. (2014).

of bubbles inside the devices are reported by Nosé (1971). Those problems must be minimized and conducted to physiologically acceptable levels (Nosé, 1971).

Blood clotting has long been known to involve three factors, the Virchow triad: the nature of the surface, the condition of the blood, and local flow conditions. Slow, stagnant, or recirculating flow and low shear stress promote thrombosis (Hochareon et al., 2004).

A problem commonly associated with blood pumping is the occurrence of hemolysis, i.e., a rupture of the red blood cell membrane, releasing hemoglobin into the plasma, constituting plasma-free hemoglobin (PFH). Hemoglobinuria is the phenomenon generated by the increase of PFH, as a consequence of hemolysis (Silva et al., 2013). A high concentration of PFH can cause kidney dysfunction (Olsen, 2000).

The hemolysis rates depend on the levels of stress to which the cells are submitted and the time of exposure of these cells to the agents that cause trauma (Legendre et al., 2003).

Hemolysis occurs when the product of shear stress acting on the cell and the exposure time to this shear stress exceeds a critical threshold (Leverett et al., 1972).

When developing a blood pump, it is desirable to maintain the normalized index of hemolysis (NIH) at values that do not cause clinical problems for the patient. It is important to evaluate these values during the blood pump development process so that design changes can be made if necessary (Chan et al. 2014). The NIH values and their corresponding clinical results are shown in Table 1.2 (Nosé, 1998; Chan et al., 2014).

Some parameters were considered by Morales (2017), considering the time of exposure of red blood cells to shear stresses. For that, the trajectories of the particles where the shear stress occurs were considered. Table 1.3 presents reference values of shear stress and exposure time that cause red blood cells to rupture, according to the type of flow.

An exposure time vs shear curve was generated with these values, Figure 1.1, and the area in blue represents the values where there is no mechanical-induced hemolysis.

TABLE 1.3

Shear Stress and Exposure Time for Rupture of the Red Cell

Flow Type	Exposure Time (s)	Shear (Pa)	Flow Type	Exposure Time (s)	Shear (Pa)
Laminar	$>10^2$	150	Capillary	10^{-2}	450~700
Turbulent	10^2	150	Turbulent	$\leq 10^{-2}$	≥ 600
Laminar	10^{-1}	150–400	Laminar	10^{-1}~10^0	600
Turbulent	10^2	150–250	Turbulent	10^{-3}	800
Laminar	10^0	400	Turbulent	10^{-6}	1,000
Turbulent	$\leq 10^{-2}$	400	Turbulent	10^{-4}	1,000
Turbulent	10^{-3}	450	Turbulent	10^{-5}	4,000
Capillary	10^{-2}	500	Turbulent	10^{-5}	4,000

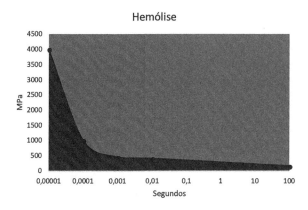

FIGURE 1.1 Exposure time vs shear curve.

1.5 COMPUTATIONAL FLUID DYNAMICS (CFD)

Computational simulation for fluid flow problems is commonly referred to as computational fluid dynamics (CFD). The simulation of a diversity of types of flow pumps is made from CFD tools to assist in their projects, promoting an increase in their performance (Gulich, 1999; Burgreen et al., 2001; Voorde et al., 2004).

The element-based finite volume method was originally developed to solve flows described by the Navier–Stokes equations. The methods' general idea was initially proposed in Baliga et al. (1983), in the early eighties, for the solution of advection–diffusion equations. Later, the methodology was extended by these same authors to solve more general problems of fluid mechanics and heat transfer (Baliga et al., 1983). In these works, unstructured meshes of triangular elements were considered as a geometric base to build control volumes by joining the centroids of each triangle with the midpoints of its sides. The differential conservation equations were integrated into each of these control volumes to obtain approximate equations that respected the conservation of physical quantities at the discrete level. These authors also proposed the name control volume finite element method (CVFEM) for this method. However, as argued in Maliska (2004), this denomination is imprecise, since it suggests that it is a method that follows the philosophy of the finite element method and that also employs control volumes. However, as mentioned above, the reality is that it is a method that is built on the conceptual basis of the finite volume method and that only uses the element concept for the geometric representation of the solution domain. For this reason, the name element-based finite volume method (EbFVM) is more appropriate, which is used in this paper.

The equation that rules this simulation system is equation I, this is the integral form of the transport equation, and it involves continuity, the amount of movement, and the energy:

$$\frac{\partial}{\partial t}\underbrace{\int_V \rho\varnothing \cdot dV}_{\text{Transient}} + \underbrace{\oint_A \rho\varnothing \, dV \cdot dA}_{\text{Convective}} = \underbrace{\oint_A \Gamma_\varnothing \nabla\varnothing \cdot dA}_{\text{Diffusive}} + \underbrace{\int_V S_\varnothing \cdot dV}_{\text{Root}} \qquad (1.1)$$

where $\varnothing$ is the variable (described below as speed) transported through a site of density ρ and constant of diffusion Γ that moves in a volume V with a root term $S_\varnothing$. The equation is the same as Navier–Stokes equation, but applied to the amount of motion. Table 1.4 shows values of the speed components (in every three dimensions) that are then placed in the variable "$\varnothing$".

This formula is deduced by obtaining a control volume, and for this volume, a balance was made of continuity, amount of movement, and energy.

This equation has a transient term (which varies with time), convective term, diffusive term, and a root term (it involves everything that does not adapt well to this common structure, to generalize these equations, and it is placed inside the root term).

In the equations below, it can be seen that there were divergences and gradients in the equation. It is the same equation, but in a discrete or not continuous way, not working with integral, because the computer does not solve them, so the equation is simplified from divergences and gradients (Maliska, 2004).

$$\text{Continuity:} \quad \frac{\partial \rho}{\partial t} + \text{div}(\rho u) = 0 \qquad (1.2)$$

$$X \text{ momentum:} \quad \frac{\partial(\rho u)}{\partial t} + \text{div}(\rho\mu u) = -\frac{\partial p}{\partial x} + \text{div}(\mu \, \text{grad } u) + S_{Mx} \qquad (1.3)$$

TABLE 1.4
Velocity Components

Equation	$\varnothing$
Continuity	1
X momentum	u
Y momentum	v
Z momentum	w
Energy	i

$$Y \text{ momentum:} \quad \frac{\partial(\rho v)}{\partial t} + \text{div}(\rho v u) = -\frac{\partial p}{\partial y} + \text{div}(\mu \,\text{grad}\, v) + S_{My} \quad (1.4)$$

$$Z \text{ momentum:} \quad \frac{\partial(\rho \omega)}{\partial t} + \text{div}(\rho \omega u) = -\frac{\partial p}{\partial z} + \text{div}(\mu \,\text{grad}\, \omega) + S_{Mz} \quad (1.5)$$

$$\text{Energy:} \quad \frac{\partial(\rho i)}{\partial t} + \text{div}(\rho i u) = -p\,\text{div}\, u + \text{div}(k\,\text{grad}\, T) + \Phi + S_i \quad (1.6)$$

where t is time, ρ is density, and μ is viscosity, which is constant for a Newtonian fluid and for a non-Newtonian fluid varies according to Carreau's law:

$$\mu = \mu_\infty + (\mu_0 - \mu_\infty)\left[1 + (\lambda\gamma)^2\right]^{\frac{n-1}{2}} \quad (1.7)$$

The viscosity at a high shear rate (μ_∞) is equal to the value for the Newtonian model (i.e., 0.0035 Pa.s), while the initial shear value (μ_0) is 0.25 Pa.s and the shear rate (γ) varies over time. And the relaxation time (λ) is 25 s and the power index (n) is 0.25 according to Vosse (1987). This equation will be used to calculate the effective shear stress for each rotor as proposed in Hernandes (2017).

1.6 TRANSVENTRICULAR ASSIST DEVICE (TVAD)

The Dante Pazzanese Institute of Cardiology (IDPC, São Paulo, Brazil) has recently started a research and development project aiming an axial flow blood pump to be fully implanted within the heart. This pump, called transventricular assist device (TVAD), can be implanted surgically through a small left intercostal incision in a minimally invasive manner (Figure 1.2). The objective of this research is to develop and analyze the rotor of the TVAD, aiming at the best conditions to support the circulatory system and to achieve minimum areas of recirculating/stagnating flow and minimum shear stresses. The study is conducted through computational fluid dynamics (CFD) and *in vitro* tests. Based on the literature, a sort of rotors featuring different geometries and number of blades are defined and tested. The hydrodynamic characteristics of the rotors are compared with each other so as to determine the best one. Besides, studies are performed to determine the importance of volute vanes in the TVAD pumping characteristics. Finally, studies are carried out to verify the influence of the gap reduction between the periphery of the blade and the volute on the pumping characteristics as well on the hemolysis. The study showed that the rotor that presented the best performance was the rotor with two blades of constant pitch arranged each other at 180°. This presented, at a speed of 12,500 rpm, a manometric head of 80 mmHg and a flow rate of 3 L/min, which is considered acceptable for a TVAD. At this speed, the maximum manometric head was 126 mmHg and the maximum flow rate was 4.5 L/min. It is expected to have a low NIH (Andrade, 2019).

According to a study conducted by Andrade, G. (2019) and joining all the data obtained, it is assumed that the best rotor, among the rotors tested and studied, was the rotor with two blades arranged at 180°, continuous (only one column of blades), and

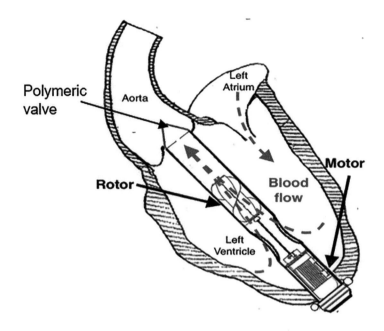

FIGURE 1.2 Schematic drawing of TVAD placement in the left ventricle.

with the blade pitch being constant. This one presented an elevated maximum head pressure and a high maximum flow. It suggests that (i) the higher the blade pitch, the higher the pressure load; and the lower flow rate, it increases the shear stress; (ii) a variable pitch decreases the pump efficiency, and (iii) a noncontinuous blade decreases significantly the pump's hydrodynamic performance and decreases the shear stress.

Also, according to CFD analysis conducted in the same study, this blade geometry presents an acceptable shear rate and exposure time. In a nutshell, it is expected that better conditions to pump blood are achieved using rotors with constant pitch, high pitch value, and low number of blades.

1.7 APICAL AORTIC BLOOD PUMP (AABP)

This study presents an assessment for long-term use of the apical aortic blood pump (AABP), focusing on wear reduction in the bearing system. AABP is a centrifugal left ventricular assist device (LVAD) initially developed for bridge-to-transplant application. To analyze AABP performance in long-term applications, a durability test was performed, and this test indicated that wear in the lower bearing pivot should be causing device failure. A wear test in the bearing system was conducted to demonstrate the correlation of the load in the bearing system with wear. The results from the wear test showed a direct correlation between load and wear at the lower bearing pivot. In order to reduce load, thus reducing wear, a new stator topology has been proposed; in this topology, a radial stator would replace the axial stator previously used. Another durability test with the new stator has accounted twice the time without failure comparing with the original model (Silva et al. 2013).

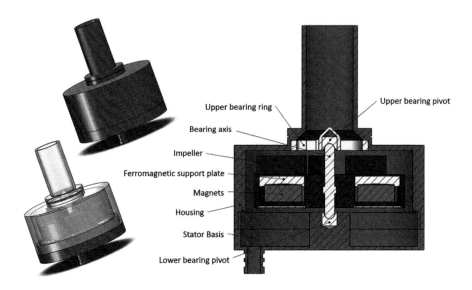

FIGURE 1.3 Apical aortic blood pump (AABP): external views and internal components.

AABP (Figure 1.3) is a centrifugal LVAD whose inlet cannula remains fixed at the left apex and outlet cannula connects to a PTFE graft anastomosed to the ascendant portion of the aorta artery. AABP concept is an idea of a renowned Brazilian surgeon, Dr. Adib Domingos Jatene (*1929–†2014), based on other similar devices. Since the initial concept AABP development included several studies, Silva et al. (2011) presented AABP concept validation through *in vitro* tests including impeller geometry and hydrodynamic performance optimization, hemolysis assessment, anatomical positioning, and analysis in a cardiovascular simulator; those studies indicated a satisfactory device performance for its use as a LVAD. In 2015, Leão presented a control algorithm for AABP and similar devices automated rotational speed control based on a natural heart rate estimator.

Original AABP concept was mainly for bridge to transplantation exclusively; however, in order to further study AABP performance in long term, a durability test was conducted. The results from the durability test indicated the main point for device improvement. This study presents results from this durability test, improvement development, and implementation (Silva et al., 2013).

There was no significant wear at the bearing axis. Previous tests indicated that load has a direct effect on the lower bearing pivot wear; thus, reducing the load could improve system durability. Our group adopted a new stator topology in order to reduce the load in the bearing system. This new topology consists of a radial stator (Figure 1.4), which should reduce the load in the bearing system, as presented in Figure 1.5, which presents a scheme from the distribution of forces comparing both models.

A prototype of the model with radial stator was constructed for a new durability test with this model, so far in an ongoing test this prototype has accounted ~7,200 hours of testing with the same conditions as the model with axial stator. However, the model with radial stator is under ongoing vane optimization studies for improvement of the hydrodynamic performance and hemolysis index.

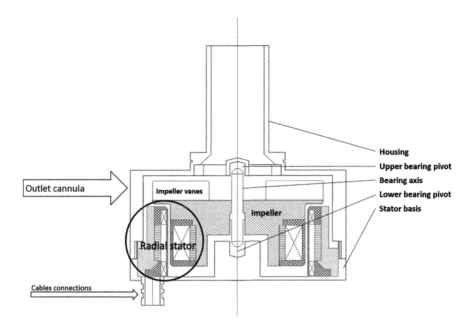

FIGURE 1.4 Drawing of AABP with radial stator topology.

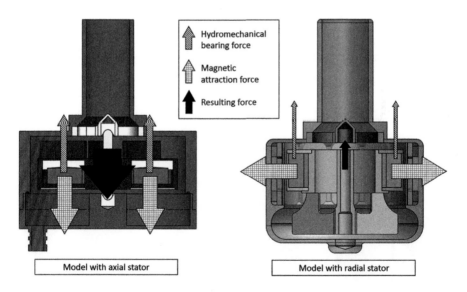

FIGURE 1.5 Scheme of force distribution on both models.

1.8 TEMPORARY VENTRICULAR ASSIST DEVICE (TVAD)

The Department of Bioengineering at Institute Dante Pazzanese of Cardiology has been developing and evaluating a new model of centrifugal blood pump for bridge to decision or recovery. This pump can be used extracorporeally as temporary circulatory support device (TCSD) with or without membrane oxygenator. During the development of the TCSD (Figure 1.6), different rotors were created using the golden ratio, specifically the value of "phi" (ϕ) to calculate the measures and the golden spiral curvature of blades. To choose the ideal model, tests were conducted: hydrodynamic performance and *in vitro* hemolysis.

Three different types of blades were modeled: straight blades—reference (Figure 1.7a), curved blades—model 1 (Figure 1.7b), and curved blades—model 2 (Figure 1.7c). Rapid prototyping technology has been used for the prototype production of rotors. Hydrodynamic performance tests were conducted with those three pumps, using a mock loop system composed of Tygon® tubes, flexible reservoir (500 mL), digital flow meter, pressure monitor, and adjustable clamp. Flow versus pressure curves were obtained at five different rotational speeds (1,000, 1,500, 2,000, 2,500, and 3,000 rpm). Hemolysis tests were conducted using a closed circuitry with bovine blood, and flow was 5 L/min against total pressure head of 100 mmHg.

The results showed (Figure 1.8) that rotors with straight blades and model 1 and model 2 curved blades provided similar hydrodynamic performance for lower rpm; however, rotors with straight impellers and model 2 curved blades showed better hydrodynamic performance for higher rpm.

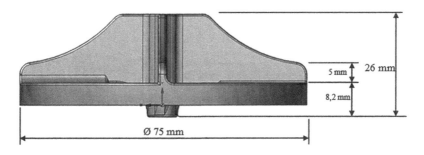

FIGURE 1.6 TCSD measures of development.

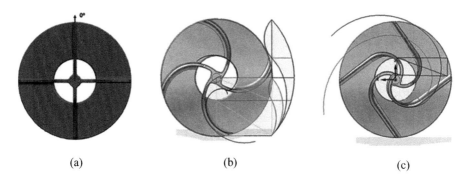

FIGURE 1.7 Three different types of blades were modeled: (a) straight blades—reference; (b) curved blades—model 1; and (c) curved blades—model 2.

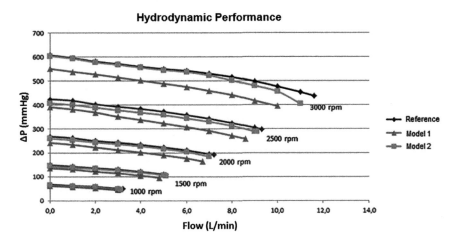

FIGURE 1.8 Hydrodynamic performance results.

TABLE 1.5
INH Test Results

Curved Blades	NIH (g/100L) Mean	p = 0.24 SD
Straight (reference)	0.03951	0.03031
Model 1	0.05115	0.03147
Model 2	0.00332	0.00136

The results from hemolysis tests (Table 1.5) showed better INH result for rotor with curved blades—model 2, INH = 0.003 ± 0.001 g/100L (mean $\pm$ SD). Those results are very important for the proper selection of the best blades' design to be used at the rotor of this centrifugal blood pump (Leme, 2015).

REFERENCES

Andrade AJP. "Cardiovascular simulator for prosthetic heart valve tests" *Braz Engin J* 1989;6:480–7.

Andrade A. 4th "Latin American congress for artificial organs and biomaterials". *Artif Organs* 2008;32:261.

Andrade, GC. "Rotor for a trans ventricular blood pump". Master dissertation, University of São Paulo, 2019.

Andrade A, Bock E. "Selected contributions from 6th Latin American congress for artificial organs and biomaterials". *Artif Organs* 2011;35:435–6.

Andrade AJP, Pinotti M. "First Latin American congress for artificial organs and biomaterials". *Artif Organs* 2000;24:167.

Andrade AJP, Pinotti M. "The 2nd Latin American congress for artificial organs and biomaterials". *Artif Organs* 2003;27:397.

Andrade AJP, Biscegli JF, Dinkhuysen JJ, et al. "Characteristics of a blood pump combining the centrifugal and axial pumping principles: The spiral pump". *Artif Organs* 1996;20:605–12.

Andrade AJP, Biscegli JF, Sousa JE, Ohashi Y, Nosé Y. "Flow visualization studies to improve the spiral pump design". *Artif Organs* 1997;21:680–5.

Andrade AJP, Nicolosi D, Lucchi J, Biscegli J, Arruda A, Nosé Y. "Auxiliary total artificial heart: A compact electromechanical artificial heart working simultaneously with the natural heart". *Artif Organs* 1999;23:876–80.

Andrade AJP, Fonseca J, Legendre D, et al. "Improvement on the auxiliary total artificial heart (ATAH) left chamber design". *Artif Organs* 2003;27:452–6.

Baliga BR, Patankar, SV. "A control-volume finite-element method for two-dimensional fluid flux and heat transfer". *Numer Heat Transfer* 1983;6(1):245–61.

Bock E, Ribeiro A, Silva M, Antunes P, Fonseca J, Legendre D, Leme J, Arruda C, Biscegli J, Nicolosi D, Andrade, A. "New centrifugal blood pump with dual impeller and double pivot bearing system: Wear evaluation in bearing system, performance tests and preliminary hemolysis tests". *Artif Organs* 2008;32(4):329–33.

Bock E, Antunes P, Uebelhart B, et al. "Design, manufacturing and tests of an implantable centrifugal blood pump". *IFIP AICT* 2011a;349:411–7.

Bock E, Utiyama B, Silva C, et al. "Implantable centrifugal blood pump with dual impeller and double pivot bearing system: Eletromechanical actuator, prototyping and anatomical studies". *Artif Organs* 2011b;35:437–42.

Burgreen GW, Antaki JF, Wu ZJ, Holmes, AJ. "Computational fluid dynamics as a development tool for rotary blood pumps". *Artif Organs* 2001;25(1):336–40.

Cavalheiro A, Santos D, Andrade AJP, et al. "Specification of supervisory control systems for ventricular assist devices". *Artif Organs* 2011;35:465–70.

Chan CH, Pieper IL, Hambly R, Radley G, Jones A, Friedmann Y, Hawkins KM, Westaby S, Foster G, Thornton CA. "The centrimag centrifugal blood pump as a benchmark for *in vitro* testing of hemocompatibility in implantable ventricular assist devices". *Artif Organs* 2014. doi: 10.1111/aor.12351.

Connellan M, Iyer A, Robson D, Granger E, Dhital K, Spratt P, Jansz, P. "The heartware transvalvular miniature ventricular assist device used for right ventricular support". *ISHLT 33rd Annual Meeting & Scientific Sessions*, 24 to 27 April, Montreal, 2013.

Felipini C, Andrade AJP, Lucchi J, Fonseca J, Nicolosi D. "An electro-fluid-dynamic simulator for the cardiovascular system". *Artif Organs* 2008;32:349–54.

Fonseca J, Andrade AJP, Nicolosi D, et al. "A new technique to control brushless motor for blood pump application". *Artif Organs* 2008;32:355–9.

Fonseca J, Andrade AJP, Nicolosi D, et al. "Cardiovascular simulator improvement: pressure versus volume loop assessment". *Artif Organs* 2011;35:454–8.

Formica F, Avalli L, Martino A, Maggioni E, Muratore M, Ferro O, Pesenti A, Paolini G. "Extracorporeal membrane oxygenation with a poly-methypentene oxygenator (Quadrox D). The experience of a single Italian center in adult patients with refractory cardiogenic shock". *ASAIO J* 2008;54(1):89–94.

Gölcü M, Pancar Y. "Investigation of performance characteristics in a pump impeller with low blade discharge angle". *World Pumps* 2005;2005(468):32–40.

Gulich JF. "Impact of three-dimensional phenomena on the design of rotodynamic pumps". *Proc Inst Mech Eng Part C J Mech Eng Sci* 1999;213(1):59–70.

Hemmings S, Gaylor J, Andrade AJP, Ohashi Y, Takatani S, Nosé Y. "Improvement of the control mechanism of the electromechanical total artificial heart". *Artif Organs* 1996;20:71.

Hernandes M, Lopes G, Bock E. "Escoamento Sanguíneo Em Dispositivos De Assistência Ventricular: Simulação Computacional E Validação". *In 5ª Edição Do Workshop De Biomateriais, Engenharia De Tecidos E Orgãos Artificiais - Obi*, 2017, Maresias, 2017.

Hochareon P, Manning KB, Fontaine AA, Tarbell JM, Deutsch S. "Correlation of in vivo clot deposition with the flux characteristics in the 50 cc penn state artificial heart: A preliminary study". *ASAIO J* 2004;50(3):537–542.

Horikawa O, Andrade AJP, Silva I, Bock EGP. "Magnetic suspension of the rotor of a ventricular assistance device of mixed flow type". *Artif Organs* 2008;32:334–41.

ISO 14708-5. International Standard. Implants for Surgery – Active implantable medical devices – Part 5: Circulatory support devices. 2010.

Kanpur I. extracted from http://nptel.ac.in/courses/112104117/37 in 03rd July 2018.

Legendre D, da Silva OL, Andrade A, Fonseca J, Nicolosi D, Biscegli J. "Endurance tets on a textured diaphragm for the Auxiliary Total Artificial Heart (ATAH)". *Artif Organs* 2003;27(5):457–60.

Legendre D, Antunes P, Bock E, Andrade AJP, Biscegli J, Ortiz JP. "Computational fluid dynamics investigation of a centrifugal blood pump". *Artif Organs* 2008a;32:342–8.

Legendre D, Fonseca J, Andrade AJP, et al. "Mock circulatory system for the evaluation of left ventricular assist device, endoluminal prothesis and vascular diseases". *Artif Organs* 2008b;32:461–7.

Leme J, Fonseca J, Silva C, et al. "A new model of centrifugal blood pump for cadiopulmonary bypass: design, improvement, performance and hemolysis tests". *Artif Organs* 2011;35:443–7.

Leme J. "Desenvolvimento e estudo *in vitro* de um dispositivo de suporte circulatório temporário". Doctoral thesis, University of São Paulo, 2015.

Leverett LB, Hellums JD, Alfrey CP, Lynch EC. "Red blood cell damage by shear stress". *Biophys J* 1972;12(3):257–72.

Maliska, C. *Transferência de calor e mecânica dos fluidos computacional* (Segunda Edição). Livros Técnicos e Científicos Editora S. A., Rio de Janeiro, 2004.

Mizuguchi K, Damm G, Benkowsky R, Aber G, Bacak J, Svjkovsky P, Glueck J, Takatani S, Nosé Y, Noon GP. "Development of an axial fluxo ventricular assist device: *In vitro* and *in vivo* evaluation". *Artif Organs* 2008;19(7):653–9.

Morales MM. "Modelagem Matemática da Fluidodinâmica Não-Newtoniana e Bifásica Simplificada da Hemólise Induzida Mecanicamente em Sistemas de Bombeamento Centrífugo de Sangue". Doctoral thesis, USP - Instituto Dante Pazzanese de Cardiologia, São Paulo, 2017.

Nosé Y. "Cardiac prosthesis utilizing biological material". *J Thorac Cardiovasc Surg* 1971;62(1):714–24.

Nosé Y. "Design and development strategy for the rotary blood pump". *Artif Organs* 1998;22(6):438–46.

Nosé Y, Motomura, T. *Cardiac Prosthesis: Artificial Heart and Assist Circulation*. ICMT Press, Houston, TX, 238 p., 2003.

Nosé Y, Okubo H. "Current status of the Gyro centrifugal blood pump: Development of the permanently implantable centrifugal blood pump as a biventricular assist device (NEDO project)" *Artif Organs* 2004;28(10):953–8.

Ohashi Y, Andrade AJP, Mueller J, Nosé Y. "Control system modification of an electromechanical pulsatile total artificial heart". *Artif Organs* 1997a;21:1308–11.

Ohashi Y, Andrade AJP, Mueller J, Nosé Y. "The effect of respiration on the performance of the total artificial heart" *Artif Organs* 1997b;21:1121–5.

Ohashi Y, Nakata K, Muller J, Andrade AJP, Nosé Y. "Selection of proper valves for the total artificial heart (TAH) from pulse power index (PPI)". *Artif Organs* 1997c;21:515.

Ohashi Y, Andrade AJP, Mueller J, Nosé Y. "Augmented destruction test with an electromechanical pulsatile total artificial heart". *Artif Organs* 1999;23:884–7.

Ohashi Y, Andrade AJP, Nosé Y. "Hemolysis in an electromechanical driven pulsatile total artificial heart". *Artif Organs* 2003;27:1089–93.

Oliveira ACA. Metodologia de Projeto Aerodinâmico de Rotores Axiais e Otimização da Pá com base nos Efeitos de Sweep e Dihedral. Master dissertation, Universidade Federal de Itajubá Programa de Pós-Graduação em Engenharia Mecânica, Itajubá, 2014.

Olsen DB. "The history of continuous-flow blood pumps". *Artif Organs* 2000;24(6):401–4.

Oshiro MS, Hayashida SA, Maizato MJ, et al. "Design, manufacturing, and testing of a paracorporeal pulsatile ventricular assist device: São Paulo heart institute VAD". *Artif Organs* 1995;19(3):274–9.

Schabowski Z, Hodson H. "The reduction of over tip leakage loss in un- shrouded axial turbines using winglets and squealer", ASME Turbo Expo 2007, Paper No. GT2007-27623, Montreal, Canada, pp. 663–675, 2007.

Silva I, Horikawa O, Cardoso J, Camargo F, Andrade AJP, Bock E. "Single axis controlled hybrid magnetic bearing for left ventricular assist device: Hybrid core and closed magnetic circuit". *Artif Organs* 2011;35:448–53.

Silva C, Silva BU, Leme J, Uebelhart B, Dinkhuysen J, Biscegli JF, Andrade A, Zavaglia C. "In vivo evaluation of centrifugal blood pump for cardiopulmonary bypass: Spiral Pump". *Artif Organs* 2013;37(11):954–7.

Song X, Throckmorton AL, Untaroiu A, Patel S, Allaire PE, Wood HG, Olsen DB. "Axial fluxo blood pumps". *ASAIO J.* 2003;49(1):355–64.

Sudhamshu AR, Pandey MC, Sunil N, Satish NS, Mugundhan V, Velamati, RK. "Numerical study of effect of pitch angle on performance characteristics of a HAWT". *Eng Sci Technol Int J* 2016;19(1):632–41.

Takami Y, Andrade AJP, Nakazawa T, et al. "Eccentric inlet port of the pivot bearing supported gyro centrifugal pump". *Artif Organs* 1997;21:312–7.

Tayama E, Nakazawa T, Takami Y, et al. "The hemolysis test of the gyro c1e3 pump in pulsatile mode". *Artif Organs* 1997;21:675–9.

Voorde JV, Vierendeels J, Dick E. "Fluxo simulations in rotary volumetric pumps and compressors with the fictitious domain method". *J Comput Appl Math* 2004;168(1):491–9.

Vosse, FNV. "Numerical analysis of carotid artery flow". (1987).

Wampler RK. "Single-stage axial flow blood pump", United States patent US4846152A, Medtronic Inc., 24 November 1987.

Wen-Guang L. "Inverse design of impeller blade of centrifugal pump with a singularity method". *Jordan J Mech Ind Eng* 2011;5:119–28.

2 Electromechanical Actuators

Breno Y. T. Nishida
Instituto Dante Pazzanese de Cardiologia

Rogerio L. de Souza
Instituto Federal de São Paulo

CONTENTS

2.1   BRUSHLESS DIRECT CURRENT (BLDC) MOTOR

Brushless direct current (BLDC) motors, Figure 2.1, have a simple design (less components) compared to common brushed motors. As they do not have brushes, they have a low noise level, high reliability, and high durability. That is the main reason why they are chosen as VADs actuators. Another important factor is the high power density that can be achieved with the application of materials with a high magnetic flux density. The increase in the magnetic flux density is possible with the application of rare earth

DOI: 10.1201/9781003138358-3

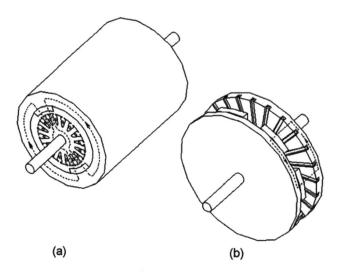

(a)   (b)

FIGURE 2.1 Comparison of topology: (a) radial motor and (b) axial motor. (Adapted from Gieras et al., 2008.)

elements such as neodymium (Nd), samarium (Sm), mixture of samarium and cobalt (SmCo), and mixture of neodymium, iron, and boron (NdFeB), used in the manufacture of permanent magnets and used in the construction of the rotor, contributing to reduce volume and increase efficiency (BLDC, 2003; Chabu, 1997; Osa et al., 2018).

2.2 AXIAL FLOW BRUSHLESS MOTORS

Axial flow brushless motors are permanent magnet synchronous machines. The rotation is synchronized with the supply current, and there is no slip. The fundamentals of electromagnetism are similar to those applied to radial flow motors, but they are more compact and applied in projects with restricted physical space, as shown in Figure 2.1 (Gieras et al. 2008).

Axial motors are divided into two groups: single- or double-sided motors. Single-sided motors have the following constructive configurations: stator with or without grooves and stator with protruding pole. The double-sided motors have the following constructive configurations: stator with or without grooves, stator with or without core, or stator and rotor without core. There are two ways to control the activation of BLDC motors: with sensor and without sensor. Most drivers use Hall effect sensors to determine the position of the rotor. These sensors are inserted in the stator (Leão et al., 2014).

The sensor sends the position to the control system, which energizes in sequence the phases to promote controlled rotational movement. In actuator designs, the tendency is to develop increasingly smaller devices and the insertion of yet another component (Hall sensor) implies more space or volume and a greater number of conductors. Other important factors are reliability and maintenance. In the event of failure, immediate replacement of the component in question is not possible, which can have serious consequences in the case of a VAD. The use of a redundancy system is necessary in case of failure or error in the sensor. Thus, the system will continue to receive rotor positioning information (Horikawa et al., 2008; Fonseca et al., 2008).

The sensorless driver control means the absence of sensors that indicate the position of the rotor. The techniques for detecting the position of the rotor are mainly as follows:

- Detection of the induced voltage (zero crossing point of the voltage in the coil that is de-energized).
- Detection of the third harmonic.
- Detection of the conduction interval of the return diodes of the three-phase inverter.

2.3   ELECTROMAGNETISM

The operating principle of BLDC is the conversion of electrical energy into a magnetic field and, finally, into mechanical energy. The magnetic field combined with geometric characteristics, such as the mean radius of the stator, is an essential variable for determining the motor torque. As the magnetic field plays a fundamental role in determining the torque, it is necessary to know its distribution and compute it (Gieras and Wing, 2013; da Silva et al., 2011).

Dealing with BLDC motors means measuring and analyzing their dispersion. Today, there are several ways to determine the distribution of the magnetic field. For complex geometries, advanced mathematical methods are used, but for simple geometries, analytical methods are applied.

The equations below represent the almost static form of Maxwell's equations, relating the magnetic fields to the currents that produce them.

Equation (2.1) states that the line integral of the tangential component of the magnetic field strength, along a closed contour C, is equal to the total current that passes through any surface S bounded by that contour. In Equation (2.1), we see that the origin of H is the current density J (de Souza et al., 2020).

$$\oint_C H\,dl = \int_S J \cdot da \tag{2.1}$$

Equation (2.2) states that the magnetic flux density B is conserved; that is, on a closed surface, there is no net inflow or outflow of the flux (which is to say that monopoly magnetic charges of magnetic fields do not exist).

$$\int_S B \cdot da = 0 \tag{2.2}$$

Two vectors that describe the magnetic field are $\vec{B}$ and $\vec{H}$. The vector $\vec{B}$ represents the density of the magnetic flux flowing through any area, and the vector $\vec{H}$ is the intensity of the magnetic field. The relationship between these vectors is a property of the material. In the construction of motors that use magnetic materials, for these materials, $\vec{B}$ and $\vec{H}$ are collinear, oriented in the same direction, within the material. The magnetic flux density is described by Equation (2.3):

$$\vec{B} = \mu \cdot \vec{H} \tag{2.3}$$

μ is the magnetic permeability of the material. Another important variable is the relative permeability described by Equation (2.4):

$$\mu_r = \frac{\mu}{\mu_0} \tag{2.4}$$

2.4 ANALYTICAL DESIGN

Several methods for the analytical calculation of the actuator are presented. These calculations are used to obtain the dimensions of the actuator, adopting some values for the parameters, such as torque and current. In order to obtain an optimized design, a numerical analysis is also carried out using the finite element method (FEM).

For a preliminary analysis, Figure 2.2 was used, which represents the characteristic curves of the Cardiac Assistance Recovery of Life (CARoL) pump, a CFVAD developed at Laboratory of Bioengineering and Biomaterials of Instituto Federal de São Paulo (IFSP). Average flow and pressure values were extracted from Figure 2.2. The operating range (*n*) analyzed is 2,100 rpm.

Figure 2.2 shows the characteristic curves obtained in the "mock loop" circuit workbench (Bock et al., 2008). Normally, the mean parameters (in red) are the flow rate (Q_s) around 5 liters per minute and (h) the difference in level indicated by the differential pressure gauge equal to 100 mm of mercury. The workbench was built with a (z_2) height of the fluid inlet in the reservoir in relation to the pump center line equal to 700 mm and (*d*) the pipe diameter equal to 9.5 mm. The reservoir was filled

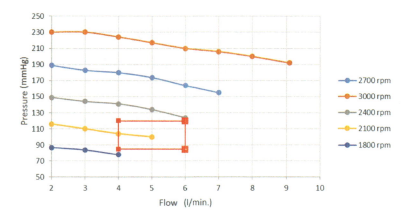

FIGURE 2.2   Characteristic curves of the CARoL CFVAD developed in IFSP.

with 10L of the water/glycerin mixture composed of 66% water and 34% glycerin for specific gravity similar to the blood (γ_s) 10395.049 N/m³ (Legendre et al., 2008).

In Equation (2.5), the pump power is obtained by the product of specific gravity of the blood, blood flow, and manometric height divided by the efficiency.

$$N_B = \frac{\gamma_s \cdot Q_S \cdot H_B}{\eta_B} \ [W] \tag{2.5}$$

The head H_B is the sum of the kinetic energy, pressure energy, and difference between dimensions. Kinetic energy is the ratio of speed differences. Pressure energy is the ratio of pressure differences divided by the blood specific gravity. The difference between dimensions is (z) height of the fluid. The adopted efficiency was obtained as a product of the hydraulic, volumetric, friction, and mechanical efficiency. The hydraulic efficiency value is obtained according to the manufacturing process. For small pumps without a sophisticated process, the efficiency value is 0.70, and for large pumps with a sophisticated manufacturing process, the yield value is 0.96. The volumetric efficiency is a function of the working pressure, low values for high-pressure pumps and high values for low-pressure pumps; these values range from 0.83 to 0.98. The friction efficiency occurs according to the specific rotation; for 60 is 0.93; for 180 is 0.98; and for 350 is 0.99. The mechanical efficiency is a function of power and varies from 0.96 to 0.99, with lower values for pumps with low power and higher values for pumps with high power (de Souza et al., 2020).

The specific rotation is given by Equation (2.6).

$$n_{qA} = 10^3 \cdot n \cdot \frac{Q_S^{1/2}}{Y^{3/4}} [-] \tag{2.6}$$

The specific energy is given by Equation (2.7).

$$Y = g \cdot H_B \ [J/kg] \tag{2.7}$$

The motor torque is estimated by the relationship between the pump power and the angular speed of the rotor, Equation (2.8) (Table 2.1):

$$T_m = \frac{N_B}{\omega} [N \cdot m] \tag{2.8}$$

2.5 ACTUATOR WINDING

The winding or number of turns per phase, the current supplied by the power source, air gap length, stator/rotor core, magnetic properties, and dimensions of the magnet are the parameters that determine the torque of the actuator. With these parameters, it is possible to determine the winding of the actuator.

TABLE 2.1
Estimated Pump Parameters for Analytical Calculation First Estimation

Variable	Description	Value	Units
Y	Specific energy	11.6	J/kg
$n_q A$	Specific rotation	319.3	-
η_B	Estimated pump efficiency	0.5	-
$P_2 - p_1$	Manometric equation	5,021	N/m²
H_B	Manometric height	1.2	m
N_B	Estimated pump power	2.2	W
ω	Angular speed	220	rad/s
T_m	Estimated torque	10×10^{-3}	Nm

The air gap (l_g) is defined in 2 mm, the magnet thickness (l_{pm}) is 5 mm, and the magnet N35 Ø 10 × 5 mm has remanence (B_r) of 1.21 T and coercive force (H_c) of 859.437 kA/m.

The magnetic flow in the air gap is related to the magnet's remnant flow, distance from the air gap, and thickness of the magnet. In order to avoid the dispersion of the flow between the magnets and the actuator, the air gap must be as short as possible, increasing its efficiency. Neglecting the reluctance and dispersion of the flux in the rotor core made of titanium, actuator without magnetic core, we can calculate the magnetic flux (B_{mg}) using Equation (2.9) (Gieras et al., 2008):

$$B_{mg} = \frac{B_r}{1 + \dfrac{\mu_{re} \cdot l_g}{l_{pm}}} \quad [\text{T}] \tag{2.9}$$

The relative permeability of the magnet (μ_{re}) is defined by the relationship between (μ) [H/m] permeability of the magnet and the constant (μ_o) relative permeability in vacuum whose value is $4\pi \times 10^{-7}$ H/m. The permeability of the magnet is defined by the relation between the magnet remnant and the coercive force. Applying the values of the magnetic properties of the N35 magnet mentioned above, we obtained the permeability of the magnet as $\mu = 1.408 \times 10^{-6}$ H/m. With the flow density value in the air gap, the magnetic load is calculated.

Following the calculations, it is necessary to determine the number of turns of each coil, but first, it is necessary to adopt some parameters for the actuator, as given in Table 2.2.

The external and internal radii and the number of poles were previously defined in the CARoL rotor design, and the operating range (n) was defined according to the characteristic curves and the nominal torque as already shown.

The calculation sequence described below was established by Batzel et al. (2014), in addition to variables defined previously. The shear stress in the air gap τ is the relationship between the force produced in the torque and the area of the active surface of the rotor. The active area of the rotor is delimited by the external and

TABLE 2.2

Parameters Adopted for the Actuator after First Calculations

Variable	Description	Value
T_n	Rated torque	12×10^{-3} Nm
r_e	External radius	20×10^{-3} m
r_i	Internal radius	10×10^{-3} m
U	Voltage	12 V
I_{rms}	Current per phase	0.5 A
M_{fase}	Number of phases	3
N_p	Number of poles	6
N_b	Number of coils	9
n	Rotations per minute	2,100 rpm

internal radii of the rotor. The shear stress can also be expressed by the product of magnetic loading and the linear current density. The linear current density is defined by the phase number, the number of turns per phase, current per phase, and average radius, Equation (2.10):

$$T_n = \frac{B_{mg} \cdot m_{fase} \cdot N_{ph} \cdot I_{rms} \cdot N_p \cdot d_i^2}{2 \cdot \pi} \; [\text{N/m}^2]$$ (2.10)

The number of turns per phase is given by Equation (2.11):

$$N_{ph} = \frac{2 \cdot \pi \cdot T_n}{B_{mg} \cdot m_{fase} \cdot I_{rms} \cdot N_p \cdot d_i^2} \; [-]$$ (2.11)

2.6 ELECTRICAL CONDUCTOR

The electrical conductor used is enameled copper, and it is used for winding motors and transformers. The standard used for selection is the AWG (American Wire Gauge Conductor Size Table). The design of the conductor will depend on the current density per area. According to Batzel et al. (2014) and Gieras et al. (2008), the variation range of this parameter for axial flow machine designs is from 3×10^6 to 9×10^6 A/m².

The construction details of the actuator (a), its coils (b), the conductor cross section (c), and the wiring diagram for the coils (d) are shown in Figure 2.3.

2.7 COMPUTATIONAL MODELING

In order to make the numerical analysis by the FEM, the prototype was modeled in the Inventor software (Professional v., 2018, Autodesk, San Rafael) and exported to the Maxwell software (v. 3D, Ansys, Canonsburg), and Figure 2.4 shows the 3D model.

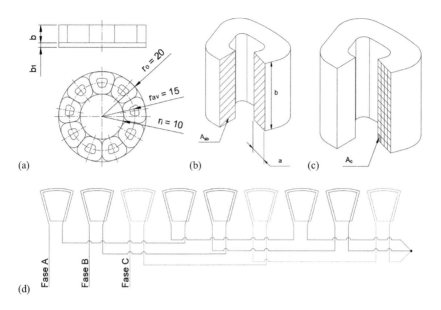

FIGURE 2.3 (a) Front view and top view of the actuator. (b) Isometric view of the coil cross section. (c) Isometric view of the cross section of the conductor. (d) Wiring diagram for the coils.

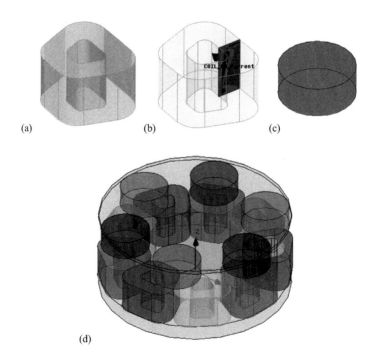

FIGURE 2.4 Tridimensional model of coils (a), cross section of conductor (b), permanent magnets (c), and the final actuator and rotor assembly (d).

The magnetic properties of the permanent magnet (from the previous tables) were added to the Maxwell FEM software library.

2.8 MAGNETIC FLOW DENSITY ANALYSIS

Using the governing equations in the permanent magnet synchronous motor (PMSM) module, computational numerical simulations were performed to calculate the magnetic flow density as can be seen in the flow distribution diagrams as shown in Figure 2.5.

After the numerical simulation, the prototype was built and validated on a dynamometer. The indicator instrument (A) has two displays; the torque generated by the actuator appears in the display (B) of the indicator instrument in (mN·m) and the axial

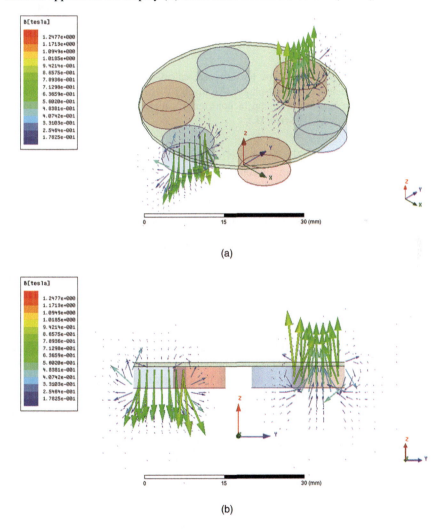

(a)

(b)

FIGURE 2.5 Magnetic flow density distribution and (a) isometric analysis for rotor and (b) ross section view of the magnetic flow.

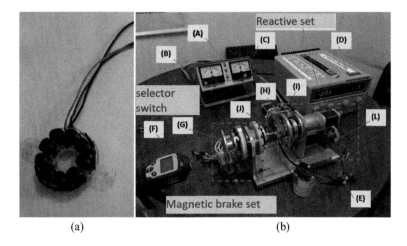

(a)   (b)

FIGURE 2.6 The BLDC prototype (a) designed, calculated, simulated, assembled, and validated in a dynamometer (b): Display 1 (A), display 2 (B), display 3 (C), power supply panel (D), controller board (E), digital tachometer (F), magnetic brake disc (G), actuator (H), adapter plate (I), rotor (J), screw (L).

force in the display (C) in (N). Below each reading display is a scale selection switch. The display (B) has two scaling options, 25 and 100 mN·m, and the display (C) also has two scaling options, 25 and 100 N. The voltage and current were obtained from the power supply panel (D), input from the controller board (E). The digital tachometer (F) was positioned to measure the rpm speed of the magnetic brake disc (G). The actuator (H) and the adapter plate (I) were mounted on the reactive subset of the dynamometer, which measures the reactive torque, and the rotor (J) on the magnetic brake subset, which applies restrictive load on the rotor, making it possible to vary the speed. The air gap is regulated by the screw (L), as specified in the project as shown in Figure 2.6.

2.9   VENTRICULAR ASSIST DEVICES (VADs)

Ventricular assist devices (VADs) are pumps used to assist patients with severe heart failure. The entrance of the VAD is implanted in the apex of the left ventricle, and the exit is implanted in the aorta. Their system has electrical component consisting of a brushless motor, a motor controller that is responsible for switching and detecting or estimating the position and speed of the motor, a supervisory control that measures the condition of the patient and the condition of the pump (motor), and a power supply system made by batteries, as shown in Figure 2.7.

Using Figure 2.7 as an example, the control output of the VAD system is the pump speed, which is responsible for the required flow and pressure of the implanted patient. However, as the flow and blood pressure of the human body do not have a linear behavior, it is necessary to use advanced control techniques for the pump to have a satisfactory response. For this reason, the feedback variables are connected to the supervisory system of the controller, which also receives current conditions from the motor controller, such as speed, torque, position, voltage, and current.

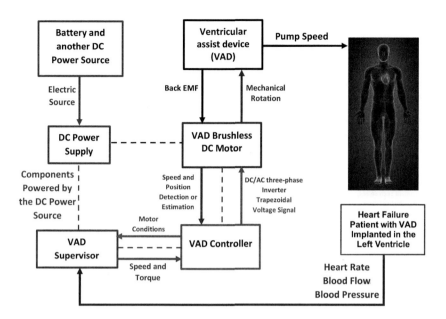

FIGURE 2.7   Schematic of general VAD components' energy path and control relations.

In the case of the brushless motor controller, it is responsible for switching the phases of the BLDC motor with trapezoidal voltage signals according to commands provided by the supervisory system. In addition, the controller uses estimators through voltage and current to measure the pump speed and the position of the rotor to develop the mechanical rotation to create the outflow requested in the feedback conditions (heart rate, blood pressure, and blood flow).

BLDC motors are highly efficient motors due to their high torque/weight ratio, compact design, high-speed operation capability, and higher power density. In BLDC applications, the electric motor may have sensors, or it may be sensorless; in the case of VAD, the motors are sensorless; the reason for this application is to reduce the pump size in the best possible way so as not to affect the other surrounding organs from the heart.

The evolution of VAD has a great influence on the technology of electric motors, although other factors also collaborate as the area of engineering of biomaterials (special surfaces) and the area of mechanical engineering that can develop more complex geometries of blood pumps (the VADs are also called blood pumps). Returning to the evolution of blood pumps with electric motors, the factors that most influenced motor technology are the development of permanent magnets with more flow concentration, more flexible copper wires, and less electrical resistance that makes it possible to manufacture coils with complex geometries and the development of simulation software technology and open access that allows greater access for users and, consequently, a greater number of projects.

Therefore, as shown in Figure 2.8, the passing of generations of VAD is according to the challenges from generation to generation. The first generation, which is the HeartMate I, which is a pulsatile flow pump and uses a brushless motor to perform the displacement of the fluid and the pump and the controller is outside the body,

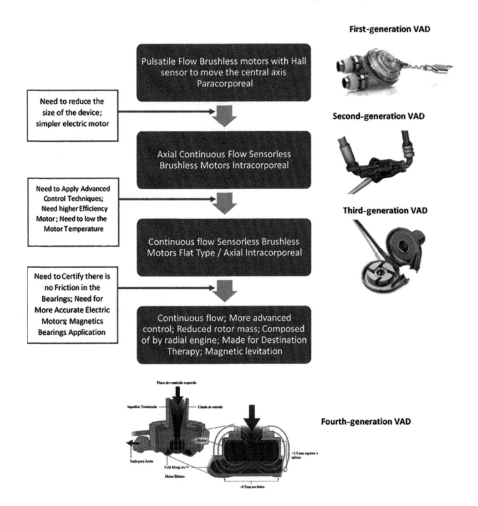

FIGURE 2.8   Generation of VAD, characteristics of each type, and requirements by stage.

needed to design a pump of smaller size and capable of being intracorporeal, which led to the second generation of VAD.

The second generation of VAD, showing the HeartMate II, has an axial flow BLDC motor. This engine can reach high rotation speeds (21,000 rpm), but there are cases of thrombosis, it has a temperature problem, it needs to apply more advanced control techniques.

This led to the development of the third generation of VAD using a BLDC motor with a flat configuration.

This generation of VAD can be called a third or a 2.5 generation, because the HeartWare pump was not developed by Thoratec (the company responsible for HeartMate II).

However, the pump that uses the BLDC motor with a flat configuration, which is widely used in HD motors, has the stator (part that has the phases with the coils) at the bottom and the rotor with the magnets at the top. To prevent the two parts from touching, there are two bearings that maintain the centering and the distance between stator and rotor.

As the wear of the bearings ends up being high in the long run, for example, the application of the device for target therapy (in which case the patient has the implanted pump), this led to the development of the next generation of VAD.

The current generation is the third generation of Thoratec blood pumps, but the fourth generation in general. It has magnetic bearings that prevent the contact of the bearing at the top and bottom of the device housing.

It uses a complex BLDC motor geometry that manages to maintain the flow of the pump and at the same time the magnetic levitation that is influenced by the flow of the pump inlet.

To develop an application at this level, it is necessary to apply more advanced control techniques.

Considering what has already been seen, the design of a VAD is complex and time-consuming and involves an engineering and medical team that works in a synchronous manner. A VAD project can be considered a cycle as shown in Figure 2.8.

Figure 2.8 shows in general terms the stages of a VAD project.

The first step, which is the study of the state of the art, implies which are the most up-to-date technologies in the world and also access to that same technology. The second stage consists of the simulation and construction of prototypes of engines and pump housings to carry out the bench tests. The third stage is the part where the bench tests start, and the projects of the engineering teams come together to form the prototype of the blood pump. The fourth step is to study the dynamic behavior of the prototype. The fifth stage is the beginning of the multidisciplinary project and involves the medical and engineering team. In this stage, the prototype is discussed, and the professionals are trained to apply the device in tests involving animals or in vivo. The sixth stage is the implantation of the device in animals; this experiment is carried out in a quantity of samples defined by the governmental organizations responsible for the inspection of materials that involves the health area. The last step is the moment when the results of the tests are discussed and if more development and research is needed (a new cycle) or the results are sufficient to advance to the clinical evaluation where the designed device is implanted in patients.

Considering the second and third phases of Figure 2.9, it is possible to establish a fact that there are at least two engineering teams working on the design of the blood pump. The first team can be considered responsible for the mechanical construction of the VAD; in this part of the project, the special surfaces that will be fixed on the blood pump are studied, the geometry of the pump so that there is a balance between the best performance and the impact of the device on the blood tissue. The second team, however, is responsible for the development of the BLDC engine and that it is in accordance with the geometry of the first team mentioned. In this design group, engineers must design the BLDC motor assembly and the controller.

Therefore, by studying the dynamics of the team responsible for the electric motor and controller, it is possible to divide the research and construction process of the prototype into stages, as shown in Figure 2.10.

The construction project for a BLDC engine can be divided into four stages. The first stage is the study of the state of the art of the engine and the application. In this

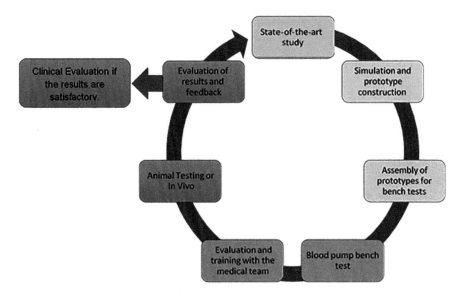

FIGURE 2.9 Ventricular assist devices' project cycle.

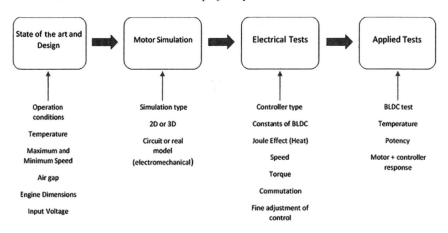

FIGURE 2.10 Linear process of BLDC project.

stage, information about the application is researched and collected. At these times, operating conditions such as ambient temperature, application location, engine working area, the speed range the engine should have, air gap, and the system supply voltage are studied.

The second stage is the simulation of the BLDC motor. The choice of the simulation software must be made. At that moment, the level of detail must be raised; this means which type of mesh should be simulated, in this case, first order (triangular mesh) or second order (quadratic mesh). It is necessary to check whether the available equipment has the capacity to compile the program. After these substeps, the type of simulation is chosen, whether it is electrical or electromechanical modeling.

The third stage consists of building the prototype and performing the bench tests to synchronize the controller and the engine built. In this stage, tests are performed to calculate the engine's findings, the speed range, the Joule effect, the phase switching, and fine adjustments of acceleration and rotor position.

The last stage of the project is after joining the projects of the engineering team responsible for the mechanical part of the blood pump. In this stage, application tests are performed; in the case of VAD, performance and dynamic lessons are used to study the performance of the device.

Thus, the objective of this chapter is to show the reader the knowledge necessary to develop a BLDC engine for the application of VAD. The types of electric motors, the analytical design of BLDC motors, and the method used to simulate BLDC motors will be explained.

2.10 PERMANENT MAGNET DIRECT CURRENT (PMDC) MOTOR

Before explaining BLDC motors, it is necessary to understand the working principle of direct current electric motors with permanent magnets.

These types of motors that have permanent magnets in the structure have many advantages over inductive motors, some of which are simplified construction, mechanical efficiency, dynamic performance, high torque, and have no excitation losses (Singh, 2009).

The use of permanent magnets in electric motors started in the 19th century, but it was neither developed nor adopted because of the poor quality of magnetic materials. In the 1930s, with the development of the Alnico material (aluminum, nickel, and cobalt alloy), the research on permanent magnet motors was opened again.

Currently, the use of electric squirrel-cage induction motors is still the most popular, but the development and advances in power electronics and digital processing technology have made the area of permanent magnet motors more and more prominent in the industry.

The reason for this highlight is that inductive motors have a disadvantage in relation to the power factor and efficiency in relation to synchronous motors; on the other hand, synchronous motors have limitations in nominal speed and noise. These problems led to invest in the technology of brushless motors of permanent magnets (Singh, 2009).

Thus, the permanent magnet brushless (PMBL) motors can be considered as a type of three-phase motor, considering the rotor with magnets instead of the brushes. Switching takes place via the transistors that supply the current required in the motor phases to synchronize and rotate the axis.

2.11 CLASSIFICATION OF PMBL MOTORS

PMBL motors are powered by a three-phase inverter voltage or current source that is controlled by the position of the rotor. The position of the rotor can be measured in two ways: The first way can be done using position sensors (Hall sensors, encoders, or optics), and the second way is done by measuring the voltage and current of the force against the electrator of the stator in relation to the engine positioning (Singh, 2009).

Thus, PMBL engines can be divided into two subgroups. The first subgroup uses sinusoidal electromotive force, making the torque ripple low; this type of motor is called the PMSM.

The second subgroup provides square current waves that, consequently, the signal that the voltage shows is a trapezoidal wave and are called BLDC motors.

BLDC motors have losses in the stator region due to construction; in addition, the heat generated by eddy currents due to resistance in the phases is concentrated in copper and in the back iron. As the counter-electromotive force is directly proportional to the motor speed and the torque is related to the current of the phases, it is necessary to study the application of the BLDC motor to see whether there is not a large variation in torque or the motor is over-dimensioned (Shafiei, 2015).

2.12   BRUSHLESS DC MOTORS

BLDC motors have a simple design (less components) compared to brushed motors. They operate in a wide range of speeds, which can be >10,000 rpm. in a vacuum or with constant resistant load (conjugate). They have an internal rotor with low moment of inertia, which allows to accelerate, decelerate, and invert the direction of rotation quickly.

As they do not have brushes, they have a low noise level, high reliability, and high durability. Another important factor is the high power density that can be achieved with the application of materials with a high magnetic flux density. The increase in the magnetic flux density is possible with the application of rare known chemical elements. Examples of these elements are rare earth elements, neodymium (Nd), samarium (Sm), mixture of samarium and cobalt (SmCo), and mixture of neodymium, iron, and boron (NdFeB), used in the manufacture of permanent magnets and used in the construction of the rotor, contributing to reduce volume and increase efficiency.

Most manufacturers of VADs use BLDC actuators because, in addition to the features mentioned above, they are reliable, perform well, are compact, and allow the use of different types of control logic. There are major manufacturers of BLDC engines that have products for various applications, in which VADs are also included.

In the development of a VAD, the search for an optimized product is inevitable. With regard to design, weight and volume are essential constraints. For this reason, designers seek to devise a device in which the pump and the actuator are integrated into a single body, as shown in Figure 2.11 (Chabu, 1997).

In the area of engine development, it is necessary to make some design decisions. The reason for these decisions is that there are different types of electric motors and different types of magnetic materials. The switching method is also an important decision to be resolved, as it affects the engine design. The choice of a motor with an external rotor, internal rotor, or axial rotor must also be chosen beforehand. The number of phases, poles, type of winding, number of coils in the stator, and arrangement of magnets in the rotor must also be discussed (Hendershot & Miller, 1994).

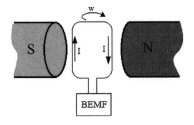

FIGURE 2.11 Schematic of Faraday's law, the turn that varies in area according to the angle.

2.13 ANALYTIC STUDY OF BLDC

To design a BLDC motor, it is necessary to understand the operation of the electric machine and demonstrate it in quantitative methods. Initially, the general mathematical model of the engine is made and then the more specific models are made (Shafiei, 2015).

2.13.1 MATHEMATICAL MODEL OF BLDC MOTOR

The mathematical model of a BLDC motor is similar to a conventional DC motor. The differential equations that characterize the BLDC engine can be derived by the equation:

$$V = i * R + L * \frac{di}{dt} + \text{BEMF} \tag{2.12}$$

$$\text{BEMF} = K_e * \omega \tag{2.13}$$

where
   V—direct current voltage in Volts (V),
   i—current in Amperes (A),
   L—phase inductance in Henry (H),
   R—phase resistance in Ohms (Ω),
   BEMF—back-electro motor force in Volts (V),
   K_e—motor constant in V s/rad,
   ω—motor speed in rad/s.
   Equation (2.1) can be rewritten as follows:

$$\frac{di}{dt} = (V - \text{BEMF} - i * R) * \frac{1}{2} \tag{2.14}$$

The relationship between speed, torque of electrical origin, and load torque can be expressed as follows:

$$T = J * \frac{d\omega}{dt} + B * \omega + T_c \tag{2.15}$$

where
   T—torque of electromagnetic origin in Newtons per meter (Nm)
   J—moment of inertia in Kg m^2
   T_c—load torque
   B—friction coefficient in Kg/ms

Isolating the coefficient that represents the change in angular velocity over time in Equation (2.4):

$$\frac{d\omega}{dt} = (T - T_c - B*\omega)*\frac{1}{J} \tag{2.16}$$

Considering the reinforcement stresses as Equation (2.1) and applying in their respective phases:

$$V_a = R*i_a + L*\frac{di_a}{dt} + e_a \tag{2.17}$$

$$V_b = R*i_b + L*\frac{di_b}{dt} + e_b \tag{2.18}$$

$$V_c = R*i_c + L*\frac{di_c}{dt} + e_c \tag{2.19}$$

where
   V_a, V_b, V_c—voltage of phase a, phase b, and phase c,
   i_a, i_b, i_c—current of phase a, phase b, and phase c,
   e_a, e_b, e_c—voltage of the counter-electromotive force of phase a, phase b, and
      phase c.

The counter-electromotive forces of phases A, B, and C have a phase difference of 120°, and the back-electromotive force (BEMF) of each phase can be represented by the equations:

$$e_a = K_e * f(\theta_e, \omega) \tag{2.20}$$

$$e_b = K_e * f\left(\theta_e + \frac{2\pi}{3}, \omega\right) \tag{2.21}$$

$$e_b = K_e * f\left(\theta_e + \frac{4\pi}{3}, \omega\right) \tag{2.22}$$

where
   K_e—voltage constant by speed,
   $f(\theta, \omega)$—angular frequency of the motor as a function of speed and initial position in electrical degrees in Hertz (Hz).

The total torque can be defined as follows:

$$T_e = \frac{P}{\omega} = \frac{\left(e_a * i_a + e_b * i_b + e_c * i_c\right)}{\omega} \qquad (2.23)$$

2.13.2   MATHEMATICAL CONSTANTS OF **BLDC** MOTORS

In the BLDC motor industry, commercial motor works with constants that represent the rated speed and torque. There are four constants that through them you can equate and calculate the speed and torque of the motor. The first constant relates the voltage of the motor's counter-electromotive force to the speed. The second constant relates the torque to the motor current. The third relates the motor size index to the power produced by the resistance of the motor phases (Hendershot, 2010).

2.13.3   VOLTAGE INDEX (K_t) AND VELOCITY INDEX (K_v)

The voltage constant for velocity (K_e) can be calculated using the mathematical deduction of BEMF. Through Faraday's law that mathematically determines that through a magnetic field that varies over time and that is in the center of a coil, a current induced by the field occurs that consequently generates an induced voltage (Hendershot, 2010).

Figure 2.11 demonstrates the same phenomenon, only that the variation of the magnetic field does not happen with the movement of the permanent magnets, but with the variation of the loop area in relation to the angle of the magnetic flux of the magnets and the inside of the loop.

To better understand the physical phenomenon that performs the induced tension, first, it is necessary to understand the case of Figure 2.11, which shows the variation of the magnetic field in relation to the angle of the face of the loop in relation to the magnetic flux that passes between the poles of the magnets (Hendershot, 2010).

This variation of the internal area of the coil with the magnetic field is the magnetic flux.

Then, Φ flow in Webers will be as follows:

$$\Phi = B * A * \cos(\theta) \qquad (2.24)$$

where
 Φ—magnetic flux,
 B—total magnetic field,
 A—total area.

Consider a speed with a certain angular frequency f in Hertz, like Figure 2.12, and the variation of the magnetic field as shown in Equation (2.25).

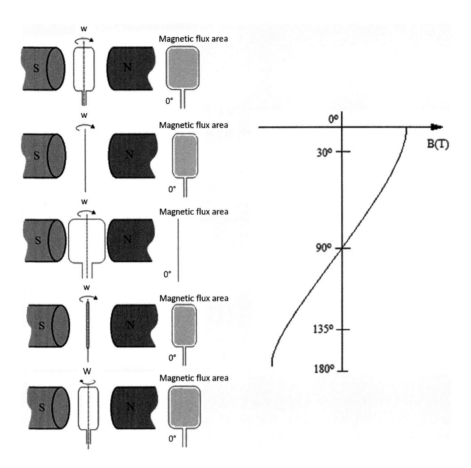

FIGURE 2.12   Variation of magnetic field with angle.

Faraday's law states that the induced voltage is calculated by varying the magnetic flux over time:

$$\epsilon = -\frac{\Delta\Phi_m}{\Delta t} \tag{2.25}$$

However, to obtain the induced voltage, it is necessary to vary the position (degrees) by the time (s). Then, the derivative of the flow over time is made as follows:

$$\epsilon = \frac{d(B*A*\cos(\theta))}{dt} \tag{2.26}$$

Since the magnetic field is constant and the total area too, so they are not variable to derive:

$$\epsilon = B*A*\frac{d(\cos(\theta))}{dt} \tag{2.27}$$

$$\epsilon = B * A * (-\omega * sen(\omega t)) \tag{2.28}$$

$$\epsilon = -B * A * \omega * sen(\omega t) \tag{2.29}$$

Since the multiplication of $(-B \times A)$ is constant:

$$\frac{\epsilon}{\omega} = -B * A = K_e \tag{2.30}$$

where
  ϵ—induced voltage (V),
  ω—angular velocity (rad/s),
  A—coil total area (m²),
  K_e—voltage/frequency constant (V s/rad).

$$\omega = 2\pi * f \tag{2.31}$$

Then,

$$\frac{\epsilon}{2\pi * f} = -B * A = K_e \tag{2.32}$$

The velocity constant is the inverse of K_e:

$$K_v = \frac{2\pi * f}{\epsilon} \tag{2.33}$$

where
  K_v—velocity constant (rad/V s)

And the maximum engine speed can be calculated as follows:

$$\omega_n = K_v * V_{cc}$$

where
  V_{cc}—voltage of DC source supply.

2.13.4 TORQUE INDEX (K_t)

To calculate the torque (τ), it is necessary to understand the principle of the magnetic force of the coils and the acting region of the forces (Hendershot, 2010). Figure 2.13 shows the forces acting on the loop; considering the y-axis as central, it can be

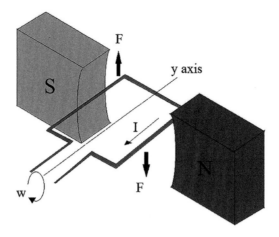

FIGURE 2.13   Drawing of loop with torque.

concluded that there are two forces in the clockwise direction of the loop. So you can calculate the forces like:

$$F = I * L * B \qquad (2.34)$$

F—magnetic force of the loop,
I—current in the loop,
L—height of the loop,
B—magnetic field of the magnet.
Considering the general torque equation:

$$\tau = F * d \qquad (2.35)$$

where
τ—torque (Nm),
F—actuating force (N),
d—distance of action (m).

The torque distance is the half of width of the loop in relation to the angle:

$$\tau = 2 * I * L * B * d \qquad (2.36)$$

Replacing the variables:

$$\tau = 2 * I * L * B * \frac{C}{2} * \mathrm{sen}(\omega t) \qquad (2.37)$$

where
C—loop length.

How $C * L = A$, then:

$$\tau = I * B * A * sen(\omega t) \tag{2.38}$$

$$\tau = I * \frac{60}{2\pi * f} * \epsilon \tag{2.39}$$

where
  f—angular frequency.
  And the $60/2\pi$ is the conversion to SI.

In a BLDC engine, the torque will be maximum when the engine starts. In addition, the torque is dependent on the number of turns and the current supplied:

$$\tau = I * N * B * A * \cos(\theta) \tag{2.40}$$

where
  N—number of loops in the coil.

Considering Equation (2.28), it can be said that the constant K_t is equal to:

$$K_t = \frac{60}{2\pi f} * \epsilon = 60 * K_e \tag{2.41}$$

2.13.5 Motor Size Index (K_M)

The motor size index is used to study the relationship between the power dissipated by the resistance of the phases in relation to the maximum torque of the motor. And it can be calculated as follows:

$$K_m = \frac{\text{Torque}}{\text{Raiz (potenciadissipada)}} \tag{2.42}$$

As the dissipated power can be calculated by multiplying the phase resistance by the squared current (Ohm's law):

$$\text{Potd} = I^2 * R \tag{2.43}$$

Replacing values:

$$K_m = \frac{60}{2\pi * K_v * \sqrt{R}} \tag{2.44}$$

where
  R—phase resistance.

2.14   FINITE ELEMENT METHOD

In the area of science and engineering research, the objective is to calculate the physical effects of a particular structure, which may be airplanes, buildings, a set of molecules, or even an organism.

When these structures are stimulated by some external variable, there is a system response.

Therefore, any physical process can be described mathematically if the process allows it to be dependent on space and time.

The cornerstone of the mathematical descriptions of any physical phenomenon is the state variables that describe the state of the system and allow mathematical modeling to cause variation in that of the system.

The mathematical modeling is represented by a set of equations and that through the state variables results from the analytical investigation of the physical process. In most analyses, mathematical equations are represented by differential equations. This means that the mathematical formulation is demonstrated by derivations of the functions and according to the variables (Koutromanos, 2017).

The reason for working with differential equations is to use the conservation principle. This principle determines that there are quantitative elements that must be preserved in the physical process. In the case of simulation of electric motors, the elements that are conserved in nature are as follows:

- Magnetic field of permanent magnets,
- Number of coil turns,
- Mass,
- Energy,
- Spiral Area, and
- Electrical resistance.

2.14.1   FINITE ELEMENT METHOD

With the need to use computer simulators to perform analysis of the physical systems described in differential equations, it was necessary to establish a method to solve these problems in an approximate way.

The most used method is the FEM, and this method uses differentiation that involves the values of the functions in specific spaces.

These spaces are called gridpoints, and the set of these gridpoints makes the finite differential mesh of the domain (Koutromanos, 2017).

An example to discuss gridpoints is to consider Figure 2.14. Consider a space of only one dimension with total size D and consider that the space variable is S.

When the space is divided into elements through the gridpoints as shown in Figure 2.14, through each gridpoint, an interaction can occur that in this case can be represented by the equation below:

$$\left.\frac{dF}{ds}\right|_{s=S_0} \approx \frac{S_{s_2} - F_{s_1}}{S_{s_2} - S_{s_1}} = \frac{S_{s_2} - F_{s_1}}{2 * \Delta S}$$

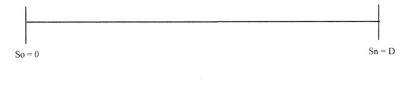

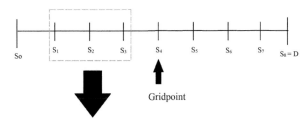

Gridpoint

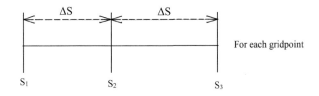

For each gridpoint

FIGURE 2.14   FEM gridpoint example, 1D method.

In the area of BLDC electric motors, the precision of the analysis and design process of electric machines is increasingly necessary and together with the popularization of numerical models specialized in electromagnetism.

These numerical methods are based on the calculation of the electric or magnetic field in structures, based on Maxwell's equations.

An analytical study is difficult to perform, due to the complex geometry of the electric machines and the nonlinear characteristics of the materials; however, in the case of the numerical study, it is possible.

The analysis of the distribution of electromagnetic fields has many advantages. It is possible to analyze meticulously certain regions of the motor, amplitude of the magnetic field, and saturation. You can have a good estimate of the performance of electromagnetic equipment. In addition, it substantially reduces the number of prototypes built.

However, there are disadvantages as well. Because the simulation is of a numerical nature, then the solution will be approximate. If the technique is not used correctly, it can generate inaccurate results. And as the process is quantified in the space domain, the simulation time is long (Bianchi, 2017).

The precise result of the simulation is dependent on the finite element mesh sizing and the uniformity of the element division; however, the increase of the mesh elements increases the simulation time. Hence, it is necessary to study the level of precision of the simulation of the electric motor and that it is according to the

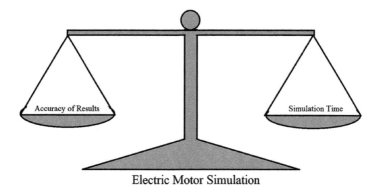

Electric Motor Simulation

FIGURE 2.15 Scale of the simulation time and simulation precision, demonstrating the need to find the balance of the two measures to obtain a favorable process.

computational process that determines in time, this situation it can be compared as a scale where one side is the simulation time and on the other the precision and the foot of the scale is the simulation itself, as shown in Figure 2.15.

Despite the advancement of computational processing technology, it facilitates and substantially decreases the simulation time, and it is still necessary to carry out this time vs. simulation.

REFERENCES

Batzel, Todd D, Andrew M Skraba, and Ray D Massi. 2014. "Design and test of an ironless axial flux permanent magnet machine using a halbach array." *International Journal of Modern Engineering*, 15 (1): 52–60.

Bianchi, Nicola 2017. *Electrical Machine Analysis Using Finite Elements*. CRC Press: Boca Raton, FL.

Bock, Eduardo, Adriana Ribeiro, Maxwell Silva, Pedro Antunes, Jeison Fonseca, Daniel Legendre, Juliana Leme, et al. 2008. "New centrifugal blood pump with dual impeller and double pivot bearing system: Wear evaluation in bearing system, performance tests, and preliminary hemolysis tests." *Artificial Organs* 32 (4): 329–33.

Brushless DC (BLDC). 2003. *Motor Fundamentals Application Note,* AN885. Microchip: Chandler, AZ.

Chabu, Ivan Eduardo. 1997. "Contribuicao Ao Estudo e Projeto Dos Motores Sincronos de Relutancia."

da Silva, Isaías, Oswaldo Horikawa, Jose RJR Cardoso, Fernando A Camargo, Aron JP de Andrade, Eduardo Bock, Isaias Silva, et al. 2011. "Single axis controlled hybrid magnetic bearing for left ventricular assist device : Hybrid core and closed magnetic circuit." *Artificial Organs* 35 (5): 448–53.

de Souza, Rogerio Lima, Ivan Eduardo Chabu, Evandro Drigo da Silva, Aron Jose Pazin de Andrade, Tarcisio Fernandes Leao, and Eduardo Guy Perpetuo Bock. 2020. "A strategy for designing of customized electromechanical actuators of blood pumps." *Artificial Organs* 44 (8): 797–802.

Fonseca, Jeison, Aron Andrade, Denys Emilio Campion Nicolosi, José Francisco Biscegli, Daniel Legendre, Eduardo Bock, and Julio Cesar Lucchi. 2008. "A new technique to control brushless motor for blood pump application." *Artificial Organs* 32 (4): 355–9.

Gieras, Jacek and Mitchell Wing. 2013. *Permanent Magnet Motor Technology: Design and Applications*. CRC Press: Boca Raton, FL.

Gieras, Jacek F, Rong-Jie Wang, and Maarten J Kamper. 2008. *Axial Flux Permanent Magnet Brushless Machines*. Springer Science & Business Media: Berlin, Germany.

Hendershot Jr, James, and Miller, Tim. 1994. *Design of brushless permanent-magnet motors*. Magna Physics Pub: Madison, WI.

Hendershot Jr., James. 2010. *Design of Brushless Permanent-Magnet Machines*. Motor Design Books: Venice, FL.

Horikawa, Oswaldo, Aron José Pazin De Andrade, Isaías Da Silva, and Eduardo Guy Perpetuo Bock. 2008. "Magnetic suspension of the rotor of a ventricular assist device of mixed flow type." *Artificial Organs* 32 (4): 334–41.

Koutromanos, Ioannis. 2017. *Fundamentals of Finite Element Analysis: Linear Finite Element Analysis*. John Wiley & Sons: Hoboken, NJ.

Leão, Tarcísio, Jeison Fonseca, Eduardo Bock, Rosa Sá, Bruno Utiyama, Evandro Drigo, Juliana Leme, and Aron Andrade. 2014. "Speed control of the implantable centrifugal blood pump to avoid aortic valve stenosis: Simulation and implementation." *In 5th IEEE RAS/EMBS International Conference on Biomedical Robotics and Biomechatronics*, Sao Paulo, Brazil, pp. 82–86, IEEE.

Legendre, Daniel, Pedro Antunes, Eduardo Bock, Aron Andrade, José F Biscegli, and Jayme Pinto Ortiz. 2008. "Computational fluid dynamics investigation of a centrifugal blood pump." *Artificial Organs* 32 (4): 342–8.

Osa, Masahiro, Toru Masuzawa, Takuya Saito, and Eisuke Tatsumi. 2018. "5-DOF control miniaturized self-bearing motor for paediatric ventricular assist device." *Journal of the Japan Society of Applied Electromagnetics and Mechanics* 26 (1): 95–101.

Shafiei, Mehdi, Mozaffari Niapour, Shokri Garjan, Reza Feyzi, Saeed Danyali, and Mojtaba Bahrami Kouhshahi. 2015. Review of permanent-magnet brushless DC motor basic drives based on analysis and simulation study. *International Review of Electrical Engineering* 9 (5): 930–957.

Singh, Bhim and Sanjeev Singh. 2009. "State-of-art on permanent magnet brushless DC motor drives." *Journal of Power Electronics* 9: 1–17.

3 Cardiovascular System Simulators

Jeison Willian Gomes da Fonseca
University of Sao Paulo
Sao Judas Tadeu University

Breno T. Y. Nishida
University of Sao Paulo

Gustavo C. de Andrade
Sao Judas Tadeu University

CONTENTS

3.1 INTRODUCTION

This chapter presents a literature review of cardiovascular system simulators applied for "in vitro" tests with assistance pumps and artificial heart. Although there are many simulators worldwide—far beyond those that will be presented, the concern of this chapter is to discuss some "better known" exploring the peculiar characteristics of each one of these tools in terms of operation and mode of activation. Additionally, at the end of this chapter, a hybrid simulator of the cardiovascular system that was developed at our research institution is presented in greater detail including its experimental evaluation. Such a simulator has been used for the development of research with circulatory assistance devices in our institution.

DOI: 10.1201/9781003138358-4

49

3.2   HISTORY OF CARDIOVASCULAR SIMULATORS

The first simulators were developed to evaluate artificial heart valves. These equipment were simple pulse duplicators, driven by linear motors and actuators, to create the pressure pulse morphology, in general of the aorta [1].

The first simulator of the cardiovascular system developed to evaluate blood pump performance, Figure 3.1, was reported by Ref. [2]. According to the author, the equipment was built with the primary objective of minimizing the number of animal experiments and contemplated both the systemic and pulmonary circulation. The two ventricles were powered by compressed air, and the pressures in the aorta and pulmonary artery were obtained by water columns −82 cm H_2O (60 mmHg) for the aorta and 26 cm H_2O (20 mmHg) for the pulmonary artery.

The afterloads of the left and right ventricles were obtained through water columns [2]: AE—left atrium; AD—right atrium; Ao—aorta; AP—pulmonary artery; VE—left ventricle; and VD—right ventricle.

In 1971, Rosenberg presented a prototype of a physical simulator of the cardiovascular system developed at the University of Pennsylvania, Figure 3.2. This equipment simulated both systemic and pulmonary circulation and was composed of a

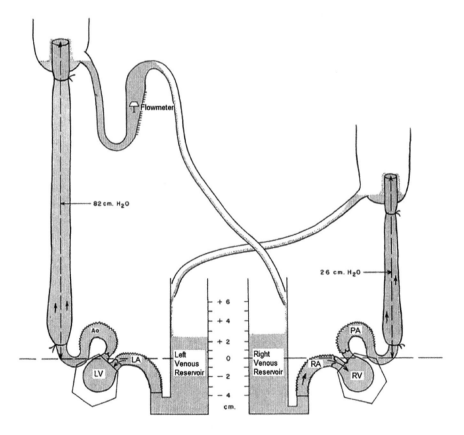

FIGURE 3.1   Kolff's simulation circuit.

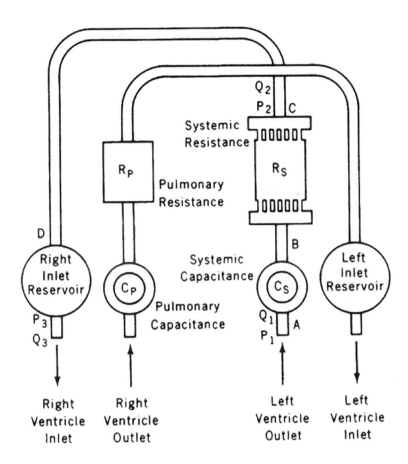

FIGURE 3.2   Penn State University simulator diagram [Ref. 3].

piston–cylinder–spring arrangement to simulate arterial compliance and by a set of tubes between flat plates to simulate flow resistance, conformed in a similar way to a serpentine. An open reservoir at atmospheric pressure was located near the entrance of the ventricle to simulate the veins and the atrium.

The physical arrangement of the components on the systemic side of the simulator is shown in Figure 3.3. In this arrangement, the elements that make up the vascular impedance are modeled in a concentrated way where the systemic compliance is reproduced between points A and B, the systemic vascular resistance between points B and C, and the inertance is represented between points C and D. The reservoir downstream of point D was considered large so that the pressure at the pump inlet was constant [3].

Pioneer works in Brazil, more specifically in the Technological Institute of Aeronautics, with the support of the Institute "Dante Pazzanese" of Cardiology, date back to the 1970s, as in Ref. [4], where a system of artificial heart control is presented in which the ventricle is modeled as a variable elastance in time. The functioning of the system is simulated in an analogical computer and its regime solution

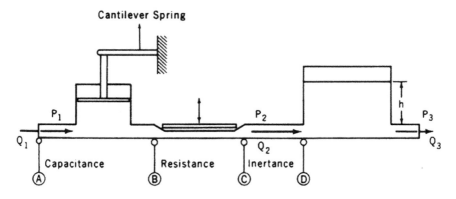

FIGURE 3.3   Details of the design of the Penn State University simulator components [Ref. 3].

is calculated analytically. A method for the control of artificial hearts is proposed: to make the pressure/volume relations of the artificial ventricular cavities vary in a similar way to the elastances of the natural ventricles. For this, the volume of each cavity is measured and its value multiplied by the desired elastance. The result of this product, which is the pressure in the ventricular chamber, serves as a reference to a servomechanism formed by speakers and responsible for ventricle pumping.

Rosenberg et al. [3] described some characteristics that a simulation of the cardiovascular system must have, to evaluate the functioning of circulatory assistance pumps: The simulator must be a system capable of reproducing analogously the cardiovascular apparatus from the adjusted hydraulic impedance operation point; it must have adjustable and measurable elements of resistance and compliance so that several physiological conditions can be simulated from a configured operation point; it must have the capacity to simulate the "in vivo" connection and the environment of the device to be tested; the simulator must be built from an analytical model that can be developed to assure the confidentiality of the results obtained; and the simulator must be easy to operate.

Arabia and Akutsu [5] report the construction of a physical simulator to study the human circulatory system and the effects obtained from variations in the systemic and pulmonary impedances and can be used for evaluation of artificial hearts, making it possible to simulate several physiological or pathological situations. Following the characteristics presented by Ref. [3], the simulator is constructed from an electrical analog model and a mathematical analysis is made to show its properties and how it can be controlled. The operator initially fixes the desired situation by adjusting the systemic and pulmonary resistances as well as the pump characteristics and then registers the system behavior. It allows to observe the mutual influence between the characteristics of the circulatory system (simulator) and the artificial heart and in particular the distribution of blood volume, pressure, and flow.

The concentrated parameter simulator presented in the work of Williams et al. [6], Figure 3.4, uses three-leaf valves, and, similar to the work of [4], the pumping action of the left ventricle is performed by a piston actuated by a speaker that has the function of mimicking the left ventricle pressure–volume ratio based on the variable

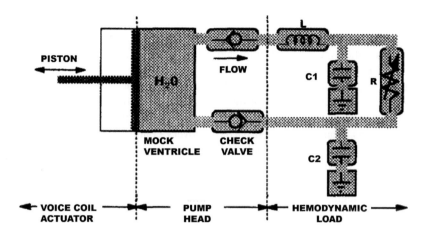

FIGURE 3.4 Simulator diagram presented by Ref. [6].

elastance model in Sagawa's time [6]. This simulator was used as a tool to assist in the development of a left ventricular assist device (LVAD) control algorithm, and through load variation, it was possible to evaluate the interaction between existing ventricular assist devices (VADs) and the left ventricle.

Probably, the first hybrid simulator was presented by Ref. [7]. This hybrid simulator, Figure 3.5, is obtained from an adaptation of the physical models presented by Ref. [7] to study the interaction of the cardiovascular system with circulatory assistance devices—the study presented results and discussions about the insertion of an intra-aortic balloon and a VAD connected between the left atrium and aorta (parallel). In this hybrid simulator, the numerical section's purpose is to perform

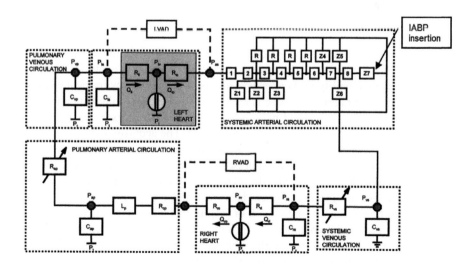

FIGURE 3.5 Diagram of the hybrid simulator presented by Ref. [7]. LVAD, left ventricular assist device; RVAD, right ventricular assist device; IAB, intra-aortic balloon.

calculations, based on the variable elastance model proposed by Suga and Sagawa, to "adjust" the outflow produced by a gear pump through a digital–analog interface. In this way, the systemic and pulmonary circulation and also the right heart are hydraulically modeled.

In Ref. [8], a simulator composed of the atrium, ventricle, systemic, pulmonary, and coronary circulation was built for VAD testing. The objective of the study was to evaluate the volume and pressure relation $(P \times V)$ of the ventricle built in normal conditions, heart failure, and partial recovery conditions. The artificial atrium was made of a flexible polymer ball with a diameter of 50 mm and connected to the ventricle inlet through a valve. An air compressor insufflated the pressure chamber during systole to simulate a normal or insufficient ventricle. A 25-mm-diameter polyurethane segment connected to the ventricle outlet by a valve was connected to the systemic and coronary vascular simulation module. This module had four integrated chambers to represent the grouped proximal resistance, systemic compliance, peripheral resistance, and venous compliance. The inertial effects were observed due to the cross-sectional area, length of the pipe, and internal fluid. Pressure points were installed in the atrium, ventricle, aorta, and in the pressurization chamber, as well as flow measurement points in the aorta, coronary artery, and in the VAD. Variations in ventricular preload and afterload were imposed, and the resulting $P \times V$ curves were analyzed. The results showed that the $P \times V$ relation obtained with a simulator reproduced the behavior of the natural heart in the same conditions in which the tests were performed.

In Ref. [9], the construction of a simulation circuit is described and the results obtained from preliminary "in vitro" experiments for the evaluation of a centrifugal pump are explained. In this simulator, the peripheral resistance is adjusted by 1.5-inch "gate valves." The venous and arterial complacencies are considered in the circuit and modeled using chambers of 1.5 inches diameter and 16 inches high, containing water and air.

In Ref. [10], a simulation method of the cardiovascular system that is a computer-controlled hydraulic model is presented, as shown in Figure 3.6. The drive of the propellant, which simulates the systolic and diastolic effects of the left ventricle, is done by an air compressor coupled to an electrovalve system to control the airflow. For fluid direction, ball-type check valves are used. An acrylic cylindrical chamber with a rubber diaphragm at the base is the model used for arterial compliance. The peripheral resistance is modeled by a "gate valve" with the cursor attached to the shaft of a step motor, which is computer-controlled. The acquisition of pressure and flow data is done by the data acquisition board, and on the computer, an application developed in LabVIEW® environment presents both the data obtained, the activation of the ventricular electrovalves, and the adjustment of the circuit resistance.

A comparative study of the characteristics of circulatory assistance to continuous and pulsatile flow is shown in the work of [11]. In this work, a pneumatic simulator composed of ventricular chamber, left atrium, and systemic and coronary vascular components was evaluated, where the continuous flow assistance pump used was Bio-Medicus (Medtronic, Eden Prairie, MN) and the pulsatile flow pump used was UTAH-100 (University of Utah, Salt Lake City.)

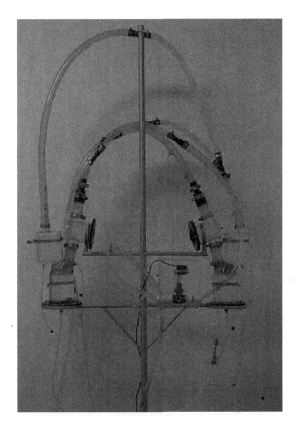

FIGURE 3.6   Physical model of the DynaSim cardiovascular system [Ref. 10].

The work presented by Ref. [12] reports a hydrodynamic study of the interaction between a VAD and the left ventricle from a mathematical and "in vitro" model. The results obtained were compared to those with animals' experiments. The VAD used in the work was the Medos rotating pump (Deltastream, Stolberg, Germany), in which some pump failure conditions were simulated, as well as characteristics of rotation variation and drive for pulsatile flow production. Additionally, the VAD PUCA II was evaluated, which is formed by a valved catheter and a positive displacement pump, to verify the effect of reducing the left ventricle load.

In Ref. [13], the construction of a cardiovascular system simulator to evaluate VADs is reported. This simulator consists of two pulsatile chambers, water/air tanks to simulate venous and arterial compliance, tubes to model the flow resistance, and a tourniquet to model the systemic resistance variation for several flows and pressure conditions. Measurements of the system without ventricular assistance were made to verify the model in situations of healthy people sleeping, resting, physical activity, and on different pathological states to compare the result found with data from the literature and validate the performance of the circuit before testing the VAD. The circuit, presented in Figure 3.7, is characterized by simulating the pulsatile function

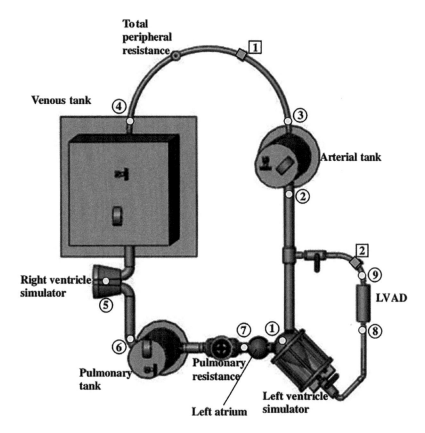

FIGURE 3.7 Simulation circuit presented by Ref. [13]. The numbered circles represent pressure measurement points, and the numbered squares are flow measurement points by an ultrasound flowmeter [Ref. 13].

of the left and right ventricles, the arterial, venous, and pulmonary complacency, and the vein resistance.

A silicone diaphragm mounted in a sealed transparent chamber forms the pumping chamber of the cardiac simulators. Two valves, positioned in the left ventricular simulator, simulate the mitral and aortic valves. The air pressure inside the heart simulator chamber is pulsatile and pneumatically controlled by a system that alternately compresses or expands the diaphragm. Three sealed tanks are used to simulate systemic arterial, venous, and pulmonary compliance with volumes of 4.9, 43.6, and 5.6 L, respectively. In the upper part of each tank, there is a valve to adjust the volume of air inside each chamber according to the pressure measured by a transducer. The adjustment of the peripheral resistance is done by tourniquet in a segment of the tube.

In Ref. [14], a simulator built to replicate the characteristics of the pulmonary and systemic circulatory system including right and left pulsatile ventricles driven pneumatically and connected to complacencies and resistances is presented. The equipment allows the evaluation of the hemodynamic effects of uni- or biventricular

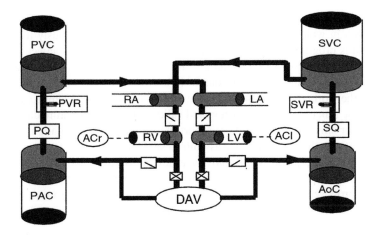

FIGURE 3.8 Simulator scheme (TIMMS et al., 2005): ACl is the left air compressor; ACr is the right air compressor; AoC represents the aortic compliance; LA is the left atrium; LV is the left ventricle; PAC represents the pulmonary arterial compliance; PQ is the pulmonary flow; PVC is the pulmonary venous compliance; PVR is the pulmonary vascular resistance; RA is the right atrium; RV is the right ventricle; SVC represents the venous compliance.

devices for circulatory assistance. This pneumatically actuated equipment follows the Frank–Starling law and simulates the self-regulatory mechanisms of the cardiovascular system in response to changes in the cardiac situation and drug therapy. Figure 3.8 details the system constructed.

Gwak et al. [15] proposed a device called fluidic operational amplifier formed by a high-gain current amplifier and a DC motor coupled to a closed-loop controlled gear system, Figure 3.9a. The proposal was to build the circulatory system with three amplifiers, Figure 3.9b: one for left ventricle simulation; another simulating the combined effects of the right ventricle and left atrium compliance; and a third combining the effects of aortic compliance, systemic resistance, and inertance. The objective of

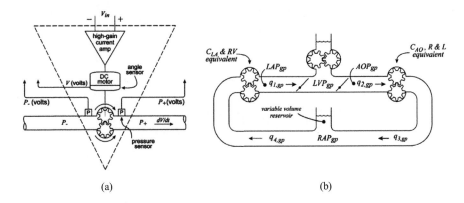

(a)   (b)

FIGURE 3.9 (a) Fluidic operational amplifier and (b) simulation circuit [Ref. 15].

this assembly is to replace the active and passive elements of a conventional simulation bench in which the pump formed by gears behaves analogously to a current source and is programmed to reproduce the dynamic relationship between pressure and flow desired. According to the authors, the use of this system allows repeatability of results, which is not possible to obtain in a system formed only by passive elements. In the work, the authors present simulation results in computer to prove conceptually the functioning of the system and validate it against literature data. Besides the computer simulation, the authors report the experimental evaluation in which a prototype of this fluidic amplifier was built to simulate only the left ventricle or the systemic resistance, in which the control was done by MATLAB/Simulink® software through a data acquisition board. Although the experimental results show the viability of the proposed concept, they reveal system limitations: open mesh operation; drive capacitance due to magnetic coupling; high friction; undulation due to "gear teeth," and bearing eccentricity.

The simulator presented by Ref. [16] is a hybrid assembly to evaluate the assistance provided by an intra-aortic balloon inserted in the hydraulic segment composed of a hydraulic model of the arterial tree—physical section, connected to the numerical model of the circulation developed in LabVIEW®—computational section, formed by the compartments: systemic venous circulation; right heart; pulmonary arterial circulation; pulmonary venous circulation; and left heart, Figure 3.10.

The interaction between the physical and numerical sections of the simulator is done by the flow signals: Q_{lo}—left ventricle outflow and Q_{as}—flow in the systemic artery, Figure 3.10. However, instead of using flow sensors, the desired flow is obtained in the numerical section by the following relationships:

$$Q_{lo}(t) = \frac{P_{lv}(t) - P_a(t)}{R_{lo}} \tag{3.1}$$

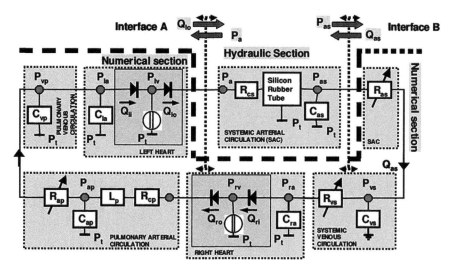

FIGURE 3.10 Hybrid model of circulation to concentrated parameters. The dashed line shows the hydraulic section [Ref. 16].

$$Q_{as}(t) = \frac{P_{as}(t) - P_{vs}(t)}{R_{as}} \tag{3.2}$$

where $Q_{lo}(t)$ and $Q_{as}(t)$ represent the left ventricle outflow and systemic artery flow, respectively; $P_{lv}(t)$ is the left intraventricular pressure; $P_a(t)$ is the blood pressure; $P_{as}(t)$ is the systemic blood pressure; $P_{vs}(t)$ is the systemic venous pressure; and R_{lo} and R_{as} are the left ventricle outflow and peripheral systemic resistance, respectively.

The pressures P_a and P_{as} are the variables measured in the hydraulic circuit, and the calculated flows are applied to the physical section using flow generators obtained from two "gear pumps," similar to the one presented in Ref. [15].

The behavior of the simulator was verified by the reproduction of physiological and pathological conditions—obtained by reducing the maximum elastance of the left ventricle and increasing the residual volume of the ventricle. The assistance provided by an intra-aortic balloon was evaluated by its insertion in the physical section (arterial segment).

The work presented by Ref. [17] is a hybrid simulator to evaluate the performance of dynamic cardiac compression (DCC). The numerical section of this simulator, formed by a numerical model of the cardiovascular system coupled with a position control algorithm to adjust the diameter of the simulated heart, was implemented in LabVIEW® and through a data acquisition board communicates with the physical section formed by a "heart simulator," Figure 3.11—an apparatus composed of mechanical arms activated electromagnetically, via computer, by the numerical section of the equipment, and which mimics the contractile movement of the ventricle. The prototype of the DCC assistance device is formed by several contractile belts that are installed around both ventricles of the heart to form a contractile blanket. The circumference described by these flexible belts is controlled by miniaturized DC motors.

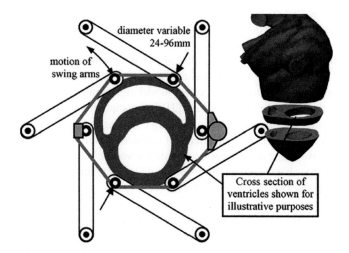

FIGURE 3.11 Heart simulator [Ref. 17].

In Ref. [18], the numerical and experimental validation of a modified elastance model for the activation of physically modeled piston pumped ventricles is presented. The apparatus constructed is a hybrid simulator in which only the vascular structures of the atrium and left ventricle, arterial and systemic circuit were considered.

The classic model of elastance presented by Sagawa [19], Equation 3.3, was modified to contemplate a nonlinear term for the variation of elastance in time and resistive and inductive terms present in the cardiac cycle, Equation 3.4.

$$P_{LV}(t) = P_0 + E(t) \tag{3.3}$$

$$P_{LV}(t) = P_0 + \varphi\left[V_{LV}(t), t\right] + R_i(t)\dot{V}_{LV}(t) + L_i\ddot{V}_{LV}(t) \tag{3.4}$$

where t is the time; P_{LV} and V_{LV} are, respectively, the left ventricle pressure and volume; P_0 and V_0 are, respectively, the ventricular pressure and volume at the point that is the root of the elastance function $E(t)$; $R_i(t)$ is the internal ventricular resistance acting during the ejection phase; $\varphi[V_{LV}(t), t]$ describes the nonlinear relationship between pressure and volume of the ventricle.

An application built in Simulink® is powered with the internal pressure signal from the pumping chamber using a transducer mounted in the chamber and a data acquisition board. Within the application, a numerical model of the cardiovascular system calculates the instantaneous volume that should be inside the chamber. This information is used to control the piston pump—left ventricle. Downstream of the pumping chamber was connected to a chamber to simulate the systemic arterial complacency, a tourniquet to adjust the systemic arterial resistance, a chamber to simulate the systemic venous complacency, and another tourniquet simulating the systemic venous resistance. The set was connected to a reservoir—passive left atrium model.

In the work presented by Ref. [20], a hybrid simulator of the cardiovascular system including the baroreflex effect was evaluated. The physical section of the simulator is formed by two complacency chambers—representing the left atrium and the systemic artery, a proportional valve as variable resistance mimicking the systemic vascular resistance, and a centrifugal pump simulating the pumping of the heart. This section is computer-controlled, via LabVIEW® program that through the measurement of systemic arterial pressure adjusts the pump speed and the proportional valve opening, according to the baroreflex model algorithm.

Although the work presented by Ref. [21] is a computer simulation of the cardiovascular system, a proposal similar to that implemented by Ref. [4] is made in which the actuation of a closed-loop controller over a system powered by a speaker manages to create the wave shape of the pressure inside the ventricle simulated from the internal volume of this chamber as a reference variable. A rotating VAD was inserted into the simulation, and the pressure waveforms presented were compatible with cardiac function in the presence of an assistive device.

In Ref. [22], the improvement of the performance of a pneumatic physical simulator from numerical models for building the chamber of variable compliance is presented. Initially, a mathematical model was built to represent the initial simulator in a MATLAB/Simulink environment contemplating adjustment variables such as resistance, complacency, and fluid inertia. This model was validated by adjusting the physical properties and comparing the pressure and flow curves obtained in the simulator and in the computational simulation. Then, a chamber with variable compliance was designed to reproduce parameters determined by the mathematical model, in which the variability function was obtained by controlling the pressure exerted on the pump diaphragm to alter the compliance of the simulated ventricle. This improvement allowed obtaining pressure and arterial flow pulses compatible with those seen in the literature.

In Ref. [23], the project of a left circulation simulator (systemic) to replicate the physiological environment to evaluate an intra-aortic balloon is presented. Unlike most simulators found in the literature, this one has resistances and complacencies distributed along the circuit, and the resistances were implemented by capillary tubes of different diameters and the complacencies by syringes with variable air volume. The artificial ventricle propulsion system was formed by a pneumatic and pulsatile VAD. The advantage of using such a distributed assembly lies in the possibility of studying the flow distribution in specific segments.

The work of [24] is the sequence of the work presented in 2006 by the same author, described above. In this work, the experimental verification of the viability of a cardiovascular impedance simulator in which the "gear pump" or operational fluidic amplifier, as described in the previous work, is used to reproduce the effects of systemic vascular impedance (resistance, compliance, and inertance), using a piston pump to simulate the left ventricle, Figure 3.12a. The activation of the impedance simulator is done in a closed loop according to a reference input, Figure 3.12b.

In Ref. [25], a compact simulator for "in vitro" VAD evaluation is presented. This tool is a physical system, in which the construction of the simulator was done based on parameters obtained from a mathematical model of a computational simulator of the cardiovascular system. This information was used to adjust resistance, complacency, and fluid inertia, as well as to adjust ventricular contractility, heart rate, and vascular volume. The hemodynamic data of pressure (arterial, venous, atrial, and ventricular), flow (systemic, branchial, and pulmonary), and volume (ventricular and ejected) are analyzed in real time.

In Ref. [26], an analysis of the effects of the left ventricle discharge, in some degrees of insufficiency, is presented when assistance is made by VAD. This evaluation was performed using the physical simulator developed at Penn State University [3,26]. The conclusion presented in the study is that for the same speed imposed on the VAD, the volumetric discharge of the ventricle is higher, in higher degrees of heart failure. This means that it is necessary to adjust the speed of the VAD as a function of the device's application time due to the ventricle's progressive recovery.

The work presented by Ref. [27] discusses the simulation of different degrees of cardiac pathologies due to variations in left ventricular elastance for a hybrid simulator of the cardiovascular system through the evaluation of the pressure × volume curve. In addition, a preliminary test with a pulsatile VAD was made to verify the interaction with the hybrid simulator.

Physical simulators have advantage in connecting real devices under evaluation; however, if system modifications are necessary, sometimes, it needs to be entirely disassembled. Also, it demands high cost. Numeric simulator is of low cost, has high

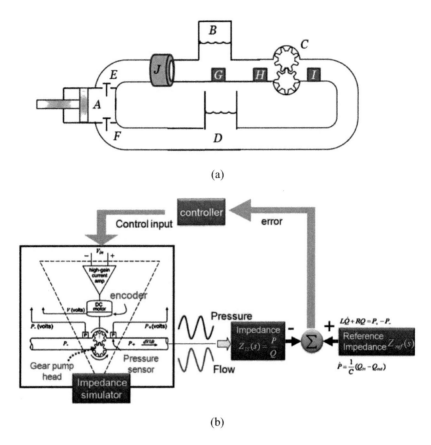

(a)

(b)

FIGURE 3.12 (a) Schematic diagram of the simulator: A—piston pump (left ventricle); B—compliance chamber; C—impedance simulator; D—reservoir; E-F—aortic and mitral valves; G—aortic pressure sensor; H-I—pressure sensors; J—flow sensor. (b) Working principle of the impedance simulator [Ref. 24].

flexibility to allow modifications, and also is possible to evaluate various physiological signals. However, it is not possible to connect a real assist device. A hybrid system combines the positive characteristics of two cardiovascular simulators. The Hybrid Cardiovascular Simulator (HCS) provides a flexible system where it is possible to connect a LVAD evaluating its control and performance. HCS is composed of two sections such as (i) *physical section*: left ventricle (LV), aorta compliance, systemic vascular resistance; and (ii) *numeric model section* concentrates lumped parameters of right heart, pulmonary circulation, and systemic circulation (Figure 3.13). Also, in numeric section, the coronary circulation and brachial shunt are modeled.

The HCS is a mock loop automatically controlled by computer, using a Virtual Instrument (LabVIEW®, National Instruments, Austin, TX), being able to model the human cardiovascular system. Also, the HCS is assembled in a Real-Time Solution (cRIO-9035, National Instruments, Austin, TX) (Figure 3.14).

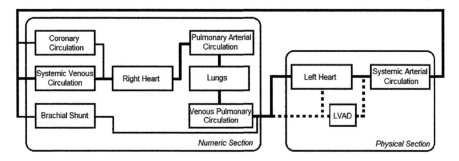

FIGURE 3.13 Hybrid cardiovascular simulator diagram.

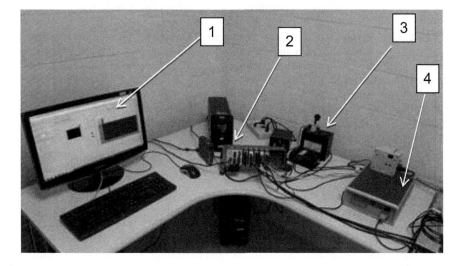

FIGURE 3.14 Hybrid cardiovascular simulator. [1] PC with LabVIEW®; [2] NI Compact RIO® cRIO-9035; [3] power supply; [4] ultrasound flowmeter (HT-110, Transonic, Ithaca, NY).

The physical section of HCS is composed of four modules: an electromechanical pump as LV, two prosthetic valves, an adjustable compliance chamber, and a proportional hydraulic resistance (EPV-375B, Hass Manufacturing Co., New York). In order to pump the working fluid, a brushless direct current motor has been used, driving a planetary roller screw that changes the motor rotation into linear displacement of a diaphragm (Figure 3.15).

All events are synchronized by computer through numerical section. Left ventricle elastance profile can be modified by numerical section controlling the motor speed. Instant left chamber volume was obtained using linear variable differential transformer (LVDT) (DC-SE, Schaevitz Sensors, Hampton, VA), by measuring the diaphragm displacement. The baroreflex was accomplished by numerical section measuring the arterial mean pressure and actuating in the motor speed and in the systemic vascular resistance, according to a table, controlling the heart rate.

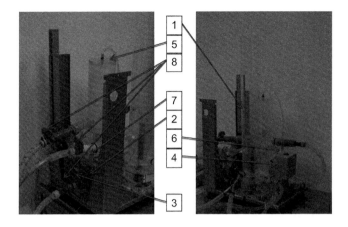

FIGURE 3.15 Hybrid cardiovascular simulator. [1] Reservoir (left atrium); [2] pumping chamber (left ventricle); [3] pumping-chamber internal pressure probe; [4] systemic vascular resistance; [5] adjustable compliance chamber; [6] systemic pressure sensor; [7] mechanical valves; [8] LVAD cannulation sites.

Baroreflex is an important component for arterial pressure (AP) short-term control. It transmits signal to autonomic nervous system. This signal is modulated by arterial blood pressure fluctuations. According to that signal, central nervous system actuates in heart rate, in strength of ventricular contraction and peripheral vascular resistance.

3.3   HYBRID CARDIOVASCULAR SIMULATOR EVALUATION TESTS

Before using the hybrid simulation tool developed, it is necessary to carry out tests for its validation. Therefore, the results of tests performed with the hybrid simulator in three different situations: (i) validation of the tool through the verification of the Frank–Starling law, (ii) simulation of heart failure, and (iii) interaction between the simulator and the ventricular assistance, both with a continuous flow VAD connected in parallel and in series and with a pulsatile flow assistance pump also in the two ways of cannulation, are presented here.

Suga and Sagawa [28] verified, by means of experiments with dogs, the left ventricular $P \times V$ characteristics through changes in the ventricular preload, afterload, and elastance.

According to Ref. [15], for a cardiovascular system simulator to be physiologically valid, the following conditions must be met:

- The Frank–Starling law must be obeyed; that is, the system must respond to changes in preload;
- The work done by the ventricle must remain unchanged for changes in the afterload;
- Consistency of E_{MAX} (elastance at the end of systole) considering changes in preload and afterload, that is, varying the preload or afterload, the elastance at the end of systole (E_{MAX}) should remain the same.

3.3.1 HYBRID CARDIOVASCULAR SIMULATOR PARAMETERS

As the main objective of the experimental tests was the hybrid simulator validation, it was made through direct comparison between the obtained results using a computational simulator previously validated and presented by Ref. [29].

The values applied for HCS configuration are compatible with those found in the literature [21,25,29,30–33].

Although the two models (computational and hybrid) have constructive differences, the comparison made here is valid, since in both cases, the ultimate goal is to model the behavior of the cardiovascular system.

The working fluid used in all tests is a solution composed of 1/3 of water, 1/3 of alcohol, and 1/3 of glycerin. According to Ref. [34], the properties presented by this solution at 25°C are compatible with those presented by blood at 38°C.

3.3.2 CHANGES IN LEFT VENTRICLE PRELOAD

In evaluation tests of system sensitivity for ventricular preload changes, the heart rate has been fixed at 75 bpm, the maximum ventricular elastance of the left ventricle was fixed at 3.8 mmHg/mL, and the systemic vascular resistance was fixed at 1.21 mmHg s/mL values compatible with the physiological value [21].

In these conditions, the $P \times V$ diagrams of the left ventricle (physical) were obtained for five chosen arbitrarily preload situations: 5.0, 7.0, 8.5, 10, and 12.5 mmHg.

It was also observed that although the left atrial pressure is physiologically pulsed, only its average value is used since the left atrium is modeled by a (passive) reservoir.

Figure 3.16 shows the test results for variations in ventricular preload.

The HCS validation was performed in two ways: model-by-model validation, using the computational simulation presented by Ref. [29], and model validation against the literature.

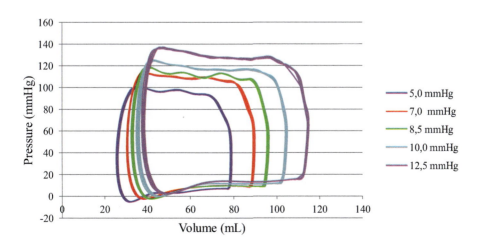

FIGURE 3.16 $P \times V$ loops for changes in LV preload.

The simulator presented by Ref. [29] is a complete model of the cardiovascular system implemented in PSpice® (MicroSim Co., Irvine, CA) that allows high flexibility in the choice of parameters. For evaluating the model, the author reproduced the experiments of Suga and Sagawa. Figure 3.17 reproduces the results found in the work.

By comparing Figure 3.16 with Figure 3.17, it is possible to observe that the increase in the preload of the left ventricle causes an increase in the final diastolic volume of the ventricle—the ventricle fills more, an increase in pressure at the end of systole, and an increase in final stroke volume. Thus, it is noticed that the behavior of the hybrid simulator follows the behavior of the computer simulation.

The $P \times V$ curves in Figure 3.18 show the results presented by Ref. [21] for changes in left ventricular preload.

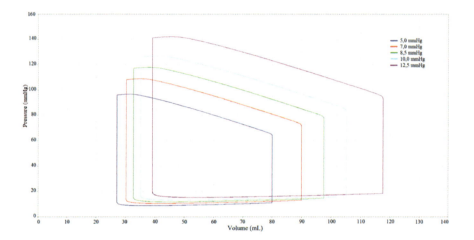

FIGURE 3.17 $P \times V$ loops for changes in LV preload (PSpice®).

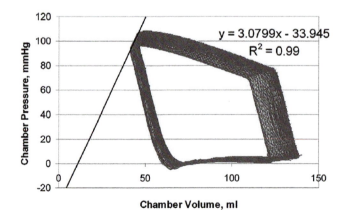

FIGURE 3.18   Work loops shifts ($P \times V$ loop) for changes in LV preload [Ref. 21].

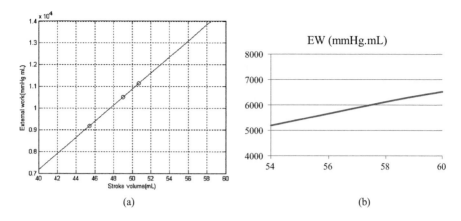

FIGURE 3.19 (a) Work performed by the left ventricle as a function of the ejected volume [Ref. 15]. (b) Obtained result with the left (physical) ventricle of the hybrid simulator.

TABLE 3.1

External Work Performed by the Left Ventricle as a Function of the Volume Ejected during Variations in the Preload.

Stroke Volume [SV] (mL)	External Work [EW] (mmHg mL)
53.61	5093.09
59.44	6419.67
63.80	7018.80
70.00	8120.08
77.48	9763.03

By comparison of Figures 3.16 and 3.18, it appears that both the ventricular end-diastolic volume and the final stroke volume increase with ventricular preload increasing.

Gwak et al. [15] verified the Frank–Starling law for validation of his simulator, which dissipates a curve that relates the work of the left ventricle "stroke work" or "external work" with the ejected volume "stroke volume," in which an increasing linear relationship between the variables was observed, Figure 3.19a. Table 3.1 shows the left ventricular work values for variations in the LV preload of the hybrid simulator, and Figure 3.19b shows the graph obtained from these values.

The linear characteristic of the work done by the ventricle as a function of the ejected volume (due to the variation of the preload) shown in Figure 3.19a is verified in the obtained result with the hybrid simulator in Figure 3.19b.

3.3.3 Changes in Left Ventricle Afterload

The test for behavioral verification of the simulated ventricles considering LV afterload changes was performed keeping the heart rate fixed at 75 bpm, the left ventricular preload fixed at 10 mmHg, the maximum ventricular elastance fixed at 3.8

mmHg/mL, and the arterial compliance set at 1.37 mL/mmHg, and the LV afterload changes have been made by changing the systemic vascular resistance, which causes an increase in the pressure against which the ventricle must pump.

Therefore, the values of 1.00, 1.21, 1.50, 1.75, and 2.00 mmHg s/mL for systemic vascular resistance adjustment were arbitrarily chosen.

Figure 3.20 presents the results found with these tests.

The simulation results for changes in the ventricular afterload in the PSpice® are those presented in Figure 3.21.

Figure 3.22 shows the results obtained by Ref. [15] for changes in left ventricular afterload.

Comparing the obtained results with the simulator, Figure 3.20, with the results presented by PSpice®, Figure 3.21, and with literature data, Figure 3.22, it is observed that with an increase in the afterload, there is both an increase in the

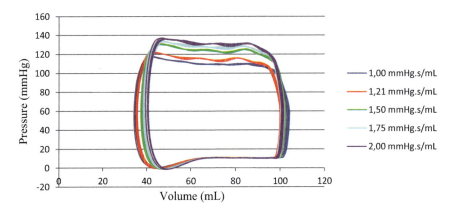

FIGURE 3.20 $P \times V$ loops for changes in left ventricular afterload.

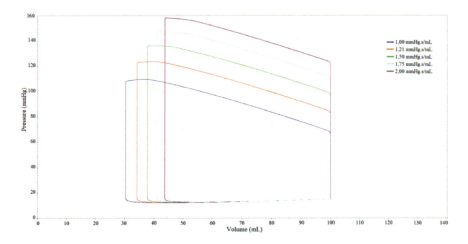

FIGURE 3.21 $P \times V$ loops for changes in left ventricular afterload (PSpice®).

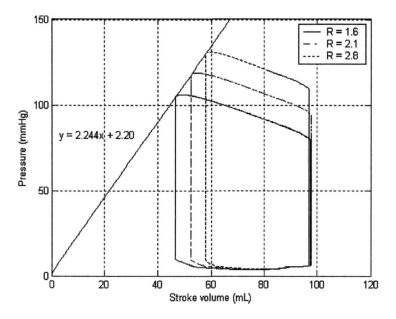

FIGURE 3.22   Shifts in the duty cycle ($P \times V$ loop) for changes in the afterload [Ref. 15].

final stroke volume (amount of fluid left in the ventricular chamber after systole) and an increase in left ventricular end-systolic pressure—the final diastolic volume remains unchanged.

The differences in pressure amplitude observed in the comparison between the tests in Figures 3.20 and 3.21 can be attributed to the regurgitation effect of the aortic valve.

3.3.4   CHANGES IN LEFT VENTRICLE ELASTANCE

In this test, the heart rate, arterial compliance, preload, and SVR parameters were set at 75 bpm, 1.37 mL/mmHg, 10 mmHg, and 1.21 mmHg s/mL, respectively. The values arbitrarily chosen for the maximum elastance of the left ventricle were 1.0, 1.8, 3.8 (physiological) 3.0 and 4.5 mmHg/mL.

Figure 3.23 shows the obtained results in the test.

The simulation in PSpice® for LV elastance changes is shown in Figure 3.24.

By comparison of Figures 3.23 and 3.24, it appears that the pressure at the end of the systole increases with the increase in ventricle elastance; however, the final stroke volume decreases, which means that the volume of ejected out fluid of the chamber during ventricular systole increases with the increase in ventricle elastance.

The results presented by Ref. [35] for variations in contractility of the physically simulated left ventricle are shown in Figure 3.25. It is possible to verify that the behavior obtained by the hybrid simulator presented in this work is adherent to that obtained by Ref. [35].

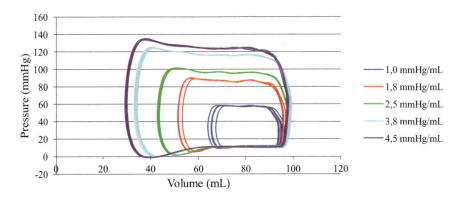

FIGURE 3.23 $P \times V$ loops for changes in left ventricular elastance.

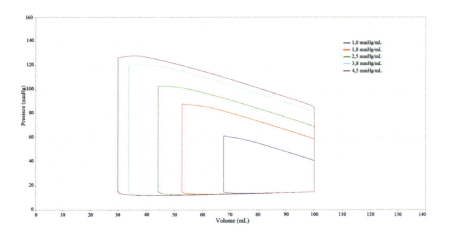

FIGURE 3.24 $P \times V$ loops for changes in left ventricular elastance (PSpice®).

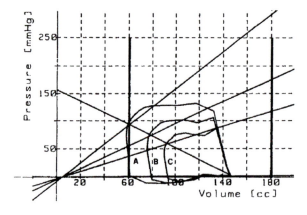

FIGURE 3.25 Work cycle shifts for three situations of cardiac contractility with fixed atrial pressure [Ref. 35].

3.4 DISCUSSION AND CONCLUSIONS

The works presented in this literature review were restricted to the physical and hybrid simulators of the cardiovascular system, as they allow the "physical" insertion of a circulatory assistance device, the central focus of this research.

Considering the aspects showed above and the importance to study the devices that have been developed in our research institution, a hybrid simulator of the cardiovascular system was constructed combining the characteristics mentioned in this chapter; once parameterized, it allows the study, for example, of the assistance provided by a VAD physically connected to the ventricle of the simulator in the apex-aortic position.

The assessment and validation of the hybrid simulator were carried out through tests to verify the simulator's ability to follow the Frank–Starling law, changing the preload, afterload, and left ventricular elastance.

The obtained results from these tests were compared with a computational model, already previously validated and implemented in an electrical simulator—PSpice®— and with literature data, which validated the developed hybrid tool.

Besides the characteristics mentioned above, the hybrid simulator considers the baroreceptor reflex effect.

Additionally, it is possible that the vascular compartments can be "switched"; that is, the physical ventricle can be either the left or the right, for example, by changing and parameterizing adequately the other compartments of the simulation, which significantly increases the field of study of the cardiovascular system.

REFERENCES

1. Pantalos, G. M. et al. Characterization of an adult mock circulation for testing cardiac support devices. *ASAIO J.*, v. 50, n. 1, pp. 37–46, 2004.
2. Kolff, W. J. Mock circulation to test pumps designed for permanent replacement of damaged hearts. *Cleve. Clin. Q.*, v. 26, pp. 223–226, 1959.
3. Rosenberg, G. et al. Design and evaluation of the Pennsylvania State University Mock circulatory system. *ASAIO J.*, v. 4, n. 2, pp. 41–49, 1981.
4. Borges, J. C. Contribuição ao Estudo de Sistemas de Controle de Corações Artificiais Implantáveis: Coração Artificial com Elastâncias Ventriculares Controladas. Master´s Thesis (Master in Electronic Engineering) – Technological Institute of Aeronautics, São José dos Campos, 1975.
5. Arabia, M.; Akutsu, T. A new test circulatory system for research in cardiovascular engineering. *Ann. Biomed. Eng.*, v. 12, n. 1, pp. 29–48, 1984.
6. Williams, J. et al. Load sensitive mock circulatory system for left ventricular assist device controller evaluation and development. *In Proceedings of the 16th Annual International Conference of the IEEE*, Baltimore, MD, v. 1, pp. 89–90, 1994.
7. Ferrari, G. et al. A hybrid mock circulatory system: Testing a prototype under physiologic and pathological conditions. *ASAIO J.*, v. 48, n. 5, pp. 487–494, 2002.
8. Pantalos, G. M. et al. Mock circulatory system for testing cardiovascular devices. *In Proceedings of Second Joint EMBS/BMES Conference*, Houston, TX, pp. 1597–1598, 2002.
9. Patel, S. M. et al. Design and construction of a mock human circulatory system. *In Proceedings of 2003 Summer Bioengineering Conference*, Sonesta Beach Resort in Key Biscayne, FL, 2003.

10. Bustamante, J. et al. Modelo físico del sistema cardiovascular: Dynasim. *Rev. Col. Cardiol.*, v. 11, n. 3, pp. 150–156, 2004.
11. Koenig, S. C. et al. Hemodynamic and pressure-volume responses to continuous and pulsatile ventricular assist in an adult mock circulation. *ASAIO J.*, v. 50, n. 1, pp. 15–24, 2004.
12. Vandenberghe, S. Modeling the interaction between cardiac assist devices and the left ventricle. Thesis (Doctor in Applied Sciences) - Ghent University, Ghent, 309 p., 2004.
13. Liu, Y. et al. Design and initial testing of a mock human circulatory loop for left ventricular assist device performance testing. *Artif. Organs*, v. 29, n. 4, pp. 341–345, 2005.
14. Timms, D. L. et al. A complete mock circulation loop for the evaluation of left, right, and biventricular assist devices. *Artif. Organs*, v. 29, n. 7, pp. 564–572, 2005.
15. Gwak, K. W. et al. Fluidic operational amplifier for mock circulatory systems. *IEEE Trans. Control Syst. Technol.*, v. 14, n. 4, pp. 602–612, 2006.
16. Ferrari, G. et al. Hybrid (numerical-physical) circulatory models: Description and possible applications. *The First IEEE/RAS-EMBS International Conference on Biomedical Robotics and Biomechatronics, BIOROB 2006*, Piscataway, NJ, IEEE, pp. 249–253.
17. Hanson, B. M. et al. Hardware-in-the-loop-simulation of the cardiovascular system, with assist device testing application. *Med. Eng. Phys.*, v. 29, n. 3, pp. 367–374, 2007.
18. Colacino, F. M. et al. A modified elastance model to control mock ventricles in real-time: Numerical and experimental validation. *ASAIO J.*, v. 54, n. 6, pp. 563–573, 2008.
19. Sagawa, K. The end-systolic pressure-volume relation of the ventricle: Definition, modifications and clinical use. *Circulation*, v. 63, n. 6, pp. 1223–1227, 1981.
20. Mushi, S.; Yu, Y. Control of a mock circulatory system to simulate the short-term Baroreflex. *In Proceedings of American Control Conference 2008*, Westin Seattle Hotel, Seattle, Washington, pp. 844–849, 2008.
21. Yu, Y. C.; Gopalakrishnan, S. Elastance control of a mock circulatory system for ventricular assist device test. *In Proceedings of American Control Conference 2009*, Hyatt Regency Riverfront, St. Louis, pp. 119–1014, 2009.
22. Gregory, S. D. Simulation and development of a mock circulation loop with variable compliance. Thesis (Master in Engineering), Queensland University Technology, Brisbane, 155 p., 2009.
23. Kolyva, C. et al. A mock circulatory system with physiological distribution of terminal resistance and compliance: Application for testing the intra-aortic balloon pump. *Artif. Organs*, v. 36, n. 3, pp. E62–E70, 2012.
24. Gwak, K. W. et al. Experimental verification of the feasibility of the cardiovascular impedance simulator. *IEEE Trans. Biomed. Eng.*, v. 57, n. 5, pp. 1176–1183, 2010.
25. Timms, D. L. et al. A compact mock circulation loop for the in vitro testing of cardiovascular devices. *Artif. Organs*, v. 35, n. 4, pp. 384–391, 2011.
26. Jhun, C. S.; Reibson, J. D.; Cysyk, J. P. Effective ventricular unloading by left ventricular assist device varies with stage of heart failure: Cardiac simulator study. *ASAIO J.*, v. 57, n. 5, pp. 407–413, 2011.
27. Fonseca, J.; Andrade, A.; Nicolosi, D. E. C.; Biscegli, J. F., Leme, J.; Legendre, D.; Bock, E.; Lucchi, J. C. Cardiovascular simulator improvement: Pressure versus volume loop assessment. *Artif. Organs*, v. 35, n. 5, pp. 454–458. doi: 10.1111/j.1525-1594.2011.01266.x
28. Suga, H.; Sagawa, K.; Demer, L. Determinants of instantaneous pressure in canine left ventricle: Time and volume specification. *Circulation*, v. 46, pp. 256–263, 1980.
29. Lucchi, J. C. Simulação Elétrica Aplicada à Investigação Hemodinâmica Da Assistência Ventricular. Thesis (Doctor in Sciences), Technological Institute of Aeronautics, São José dos Campos, 1999.
30. Baloa, L. A.; Boston, J. R.; Antaki, J. F. Elastance-based control of a mock circulatory system. *Ann. Biomed. Eng.*, v. 29, pp. 244–251, 2001.

31. Ferrari, G. et al. Hybrid model analysis of intra-aortic balloon pump performance as a function of ventricular and circulatory parameters. *Artif. Organs*, v. 35, n. 9, pp. 902–911, 2011.
32. Guyton, A. C.; Hall, J. E. *Textbook of Medical Physiology*, 11th ed. Philadelphia, PA: Elsevier Saunders Co., 1116 p., 2006.
33. Simaan, M. A. et al. A dynamical state space representation and performance analysis of a feedback-controlled rotary left ventricular assist device. *IEEE Trans. Control Syst. Technol.*, v. 17, n. 1, pp. 15–28, 2009.
34. Legendre, D. F.; Andrade, A. et al. Estudo de comportamento de fluxo através de modelo físico e computacional de aneurisma de aorta infra-renal obtido por tomografia. Thesis (Doctor in Mechanical Engineering) – Polytechnique School of University of Sao Paulo, São Paulo, 2009.
35. Ferrari, G. et al. Mock circulatory system for in vitro reproduction of the left ventricle, the arterial tree and their interaction with a left ventricular assist device. *J. Med. Eng. Technol.*, v. 18, n. 3, pp. 87–95, 1994.

4 Control Systems

Bruno Jesus dos Santos and Tarcísio F. Leão
Instituto Federal de São Paulo

CONTENTS

4.1 INTRODUCTION

Initial efforts in developing ventricular assist devices (VADs) focused on critical problems related to the effectiveness and robustness of the device, such as (i) component qualification, (ii) optimization of fluid flow dynamics, and (iii) patient selection for implants. In this initial scenario, less attention was focused on the problem of controlling these devices to respond to the changing demands of patients in dynamic evolution of the clinical status (Antaki et al., 2003). But in view of the difficulty of treatment aiming at reducing the dependence on clinical monitoring and allowing the patient to return home, with the consequent improvement in the quality of life, it is necessary to improve the control of these devices due to the complex interaction between the physiological system and the VAD (Alomari et al., 2012; Devore et al., 2017).

The limitations of open-loop control become evident as patients are rehabilitated and seek to adopt an active lifestyle within a productive daily life. The inability of the devices to respond automatically to changes in demand can drastically affect the quality of life of these patients (Kim et al., 1999). For long-term implants, the need for constant monitoring of the human operator in the functioning of the device must be eliminated (Antaki et al., 2003; Alomari et al., 2012).

With the increase in the duration of the VAD support, attention is changing to improve the quality of life of the patient. An important step is the optimization of the assistance provided with the VAD, which depends on the complex interaction between the individual physiopathology of the patient and the characteristics of the pump (Uriel et al., 2016).

DOI: 10.1201/9781003138358-5

4.2   ADVERSE EVENTS OF PATIENTS IMPLANTED
BY VENTRICULAR ASSIST DEVICES

The eighth annual report of the Interagency Registry for Mechanically Assisted Circulatory Support (INTERMACS) (Kirklin et al., 2017) brought a special focus on the impact of adverse events associated with mechanical circulatory support, with the survival rate among the 22,866 patients implanted between 2006 and 2016 being 81% in the first 12 months (for total artificial heart, 373 implants, the survival rate is <60%) and 70% in the first 24 months, with little variation since 2008 and essentially no change since 2013, of which 83% are left VAD (LVAD) and 90% are continuous flow devices. The hazard analysis on the number of deaths identified three distinct phases: (i) early hazard (EH), which rapidly drops, (ii) constant hazard (CH), which has a constant rate since approximately the first 3 months, and (iii) late hazard (LH), which gradually increases until in month 84 it exceeds the CH. Figure 4.1 shows the death risk rates associated with mechanical circulatory support (Kirklin et al., 2017).

The main risk rates for early death after implantation are multiple organ failure, right heart failure, and stroke (ischemic or bleeding). Already between 6 months and 4 years, the predominant risk rate of death is stroke (Kirklin et al., 2017). Figure 4.2 shows the main causes of death and the cumulative risk of death rate.

Within the risk factors for mortality, age (>60 years) represents the highest risk of both early and late mortality, and female gender is an important risk factor for early mortality. The type of flow of the device (axial or centrifugal) does not represent an early or late mortality factor. And critically ill patients increase the risk of early mortality. The interaction between the INTERMACS profile and age is so important that patients over 65 years of age are at particularly high risk when their circulatory state is deteriorating rapidly (profiles 1 and 2). Patients who receive an implant as a

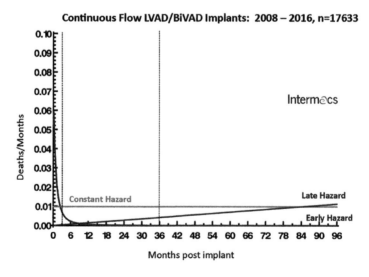

FIGURE 4.1   The hazard of death rates associated with mechanical circulatory support. (Supplementary data from INTERMACS, 2017.)

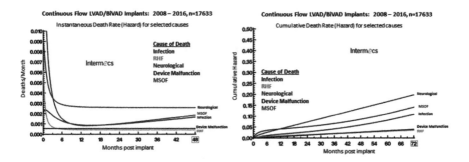

FIGURE 4.2 The risk of death rates associated with mechanical circulatory support (INTERMACS, 2017).

long-term support strategy (destination therapy; DT) continue to have worse survival than patients considered for heart transplantation. Bleeding as an adverse event is predominantly reflected in early-stage surgical bleeding and gastrointestinal bleeding after the first 3 months. After bleeding, infection is the most frequent adverse event during the first 3 months and the most common to occur after that time. The risk of stroke persists as a major adverse event throughout the first year after implantation. Table 4.1 presents the impact on mortality of major pre-implant adverse events (Kirklin et al., 2017).

The adverse events associated with mechanical circulatory support profoundly affect the quality of life and often the survival of the implanted patient. In addition to the preoperative variables examined in Table 4.1, the INTERMACS study (2017) included the main adverse events that occurred in the first 3 months, as well as the indicators of quality of life at 3 months; compared to the risk factors identified in the pre-implant model (Table 4.1), only four were retained in the three-month model, which included post-implant adverse events. A constant risk phase was identified, in which the presence of ascites, the need for continuous inotropic support, and the number of strokes during the first 3 months presented the highest risk rate for subsequent mortality of the implanted patient, and when multiple major adverse events occur, the effect is particularly severe (Kirklin et al., 2017).

VADs have a higher patient survival rate than transplants in the initial phase of treatment because they represent a lower aggression to the physiological system than an intruder organ, but as time goes by, the balance between artificial care and the physiological system deteriorates and the survival rate becomes lower and lower, when reaching the five-year care range, implants become less efficient than transplants (Abto, 2018; Kirklin et al., 2017). Patients with LVAD have high readmission rates due to multiple complications, including HF and adverse events related to hemocompatibility (Uriel et al., 2017). Figure 4.3 shows the comparison between the survival charts of the patient with heart failure (HF) who received heart transplantation and VAD implantation.

According to Uriel et al. (2020) although it is well established that LVADs significantly improve longevity and quality of life in patients with advanced HF, only a small percentage of potentially eligible HF patients receive a LVAD, and it is believed

TABLE 4.1
Impact on Mortality of Major Pre-Implant Adverse Events

	Continuous Flow LVAD/BiVAD Implants: 2008–2016, $n=17,633$ Adverse Event Rates (Events/100 Patient Months)					
	1st 3 Months Post		3–12 Months Post		1st 3 Months vs 3–12 Months	
Adverse Event	Events	Rate	Events	Rate	Ratio	p-value
Bleeding	7,810	16.24	4,205	4.08	4	<0.0001
Cardiac/vascular						
Myocardial infarction	54	0.11	31	0.03	3.74	<0.0001
Cardiac arrhythmia	5,026	10.45	1,359	1.32	7.94	<0.0001
Pericardial drainage	858	1.79	17	0.02	108.30	<0.0001
Arterial non-CNS thrombosis	162	0.34	52	0.05	6.69	<0.0001
Venous thrombotic event	663	1.38	80	0.08	17.78	<0.0001
Infection	6,552	13.63	4,692	4.55	3.00	<0.0001
Stroke	1,162	2.42	1,154	1.12	2.16	<0.0001
Neurological: non-stroke	640	1.33	332	0.32	4.14	<0.0001
Renal dysfunction	1,687	3.51	495	0.48	7.31	<0.0001
Hepatic dysfunction	453	0.94	167	0.16	5.82	<0.0001
Respiratory failure	3,212	6.68	567	0.55	12.16	<0.0001
Wound dehiscence	194	0.40	58	0.06	7.18	<0.0001
Psychiatric episode	751	1.56	279	0.27	5.78	<0.0001
Other SAE	5,340	11.11	2,170	2.10	5.28	<0.0001
Total burden	34,564	71.89	15,658	15.19	201.28	<0.0001

Source: Supplementary data from INTERMACS (2017).

CNS, central nervous system; VAD, ventricular assist device; BiVAD, biventricular assist device; SAE, Serious Advent Event.

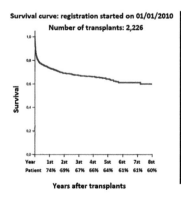
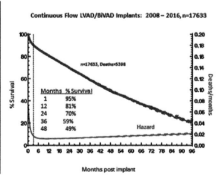

FIGURE 4.3 Comparison between the survival of patients with heart failure transplanted in Brazil and implanted by an LVAD in the United States. (Adapted from ABTO (2018) and Kirklin et al. (2017).)

that this is mainly due to high rate of complications and readmissions that limit the acceptance of this form of therapy between patients and referring physicians.

In the recent study of the most modern VAD on the market MOMENTUM 3 (Multicenter Study of MagLev Technology in Patients Undergoing Mechanical Circulatory Support Therapy With HeartMate® 3), there were 2.1 hospitalizations per patient-year, with a 10% incidence of stroke, 27% incidence of gastrointestinal bleeding, 24% incidence of ventricular arrhythmias, and 24% incidence of driveline infections (Mehra & Goldstein, 2018; Mehra et al., 2018a,b; Uriel et al., 2020).

4.3 LVAD PHYSIOLOGICAL CONTROLLERS

To improve the flow optimization capability of the LVAD, an active flow adjustment scheme is required that can automatically adapt and adjust the pump speed based on demand without requiring manual inputs (Tchantchaleishvili et al., 2017). This requires the identification of a measurable control variable that can be used to ensure optimal perfusion. This strategy may allow the development of a Frank–Starling-type controller capable of a true physiological adjustment of the flow of LVADs (Tchantchaleishvili et al., 2017).

The characteristic response of a centrifugal LVAD to changes in the hydrodynamic charge is precisely the opposite of the body's requirement: Its pressure generation decreases with flow, while the body requires an increased flow to increase pressure. Therefore, the pump speed must respond dynamically to changes in preload and afterload to meet infusion demand, avoiding the risk of exceeding the available blood flow capacity. The consequences of both insufficient and excessive extraction will limit the quality of life and can pose serious risks to the patient's health. Insufficient pumping may cause blood to regurgitate from the aorta to the left ventricle through the pump (reflux) and even pulmonary congestion, while excessive pumping may cause heart and vessel collapse (Gwak, 2007).

The physiological controllers of LVAD can be subdivided into five main categories (Ochsner et al., 2014): (i) preload-based; (ii) afterload-based; (iii) heart rate-based; (iv) multi-objective; and (v) hemodynamic controllers.

4.4 STRATEGIES FOR PRELOAD-BASED PHYSIOLOGICAL CONTROLLERS OF LVADs

In many patients, the native heart continues to provide residual contractility during LVAD support, even if the amount of blood flow produced by the heart is not sufficient to sustain the patient, it is sufficient to vary the pump load, in these cases the hemodynamic signals such as aortic pressure, left ventricular pressure, and aortic blood flow will exhibit various degrees of pulsatility when the pump is used. Because of the pulsating load conditions presented to the pump, the pump flow and motor drive current are also pulsating. This phenomenon is commonly used in strategies based on controlling preload variation to specify the operating point for the pump speed using only (electrical) pump input signals, eliminating the need for blood pressure or flow transducers (Choi et al., 2001).

The objective of Endo et al. (2000) was to investigate *in vivo* (five male piglets; mean 38.9 kg; recovered from global ischemia) a strategy for the control of biventricular assist device (BiVAD) composed in two stages sequentially according to cardiac recovery and based on the detection of ventricular collapse. In this strategy, no sensors were used to detect ventricular collapse, so the current amplitude index (CAI) was calculated from the current waveform of each BiVAD motor and its simultaneous mean value. The CAI formula is as follows:

$$\frac{\left(l_{max} - l_{min}\right)}{l_{med}} \tag{4.1}$$

The work of Choi et al. (2007) describes a LVAD control strategy in which the speed setting value is defined by a fuzzy logic algorithm in order to obtain the pulsatility ratio for the LVAD that provides an adequate perfusion according to the physiological demands of the patient, avoiding adverse conditions. The use of fuzzy logic is indicated for systems that are complex and show uncertainty values in their parameters. The pulsatility control index is based on the cyclical variation of the hemodynamic load placed on the LVAD by the residual contractility of the native heart. As the pump speed increases and ventricular decompression occurs, the signal pulsatility decreases and reaches a minimum as the suction approaches. The operating point error, defined as the difference between the desired (reference) pulsatility and the actual pulsatility, and the changes in error are used as inputs for the fuzzy logic controller. The output of the fuzzy logic controller is the pump speed change.

The controller proposed by Choi et al. (2007) includes a flow estimator based on the electrical parameters of the LVAD motor, an extractor algorithm of pulsatility control index, and a fuzzy logic inference system to determine the required change in pump speed for a given flow pulsatility.

Figure 4.4 presents the schematic diagram of the proposed LVAD control strategy by Choi et al. (2007), and for this proposal, the results evaluated the control performance for afterload and preload sensitivity and influence of contractility.

Gwak's work (2007) describes a LVAD control strategy in which the demand-based speed setting value is defined by an extreme search control (ESC) algorithm that finds and tracks the optimum set point based only on estimated pump flow information. The typical LVAD support graph indicates a peak near the start of suction, which varies dynamically according to changes in blood availability (preload) or

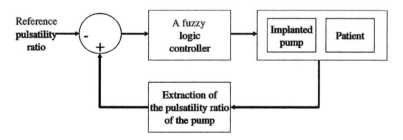

FIGURE 4.4 Schematic diagram of the LVAD control strategy proposed by Choi et al. (2007).

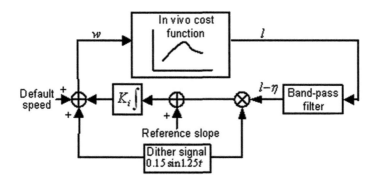

FIGURE 4.5   Schematic diagram of the LVAD control strategy proposed by Gwak (2007).

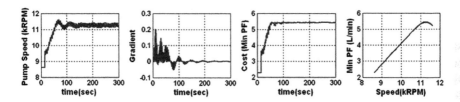

FIGURE 4.6   Results obtained by the LVAD control strategy proposed by Gwak (2007).

vascular resistance (afterload). ESC is a real-time optimization tool that can locate and track the mobile peak point (cost function) under dynamic conditions. The controller with ESC algorithm must regulate the pump speed so that the operating point remains at the peak of the flow curve that corresponds to the maximum cardiac output without risk of suction. Figure 4.5 presents the schematic diagram of the LVAD control strategy proposed by Gwak (2007).

Figure 4.6 shows the results obtained in an *in vivo* test by the LVAD control strategy proposed by Gwak (2007), where the initial operating point of the LVAD was set at 8.5 k rpm corresponding to 2.1 L/min minimum pump flow. When the ESC was started ($t = 15$ seconds), the controller drove the speed quickly to the optimum point. A degree of overpressure was observed indicating a suction hazard, but it was dampened in some periods of oscillation. The response obtained resembles that of a typical proportional–integral–derivative (PID) controller with an established set point, but with the advantage that the ideal operating point is not known *a priori,* but rather sought by the algorithm in consideration of system dynamics.

The work of Arndt et al. (2008) describes a LVAD control strategy in which the speed setting value is based on the regulation of the left ventricle (LV) filling pressure, or correspondingly, of the filling volume, which, because of the nonlinearities, is reflected by the differential pressure (dP) signal pulsatility index (PI) between the inlet and outlet of the LVAD for a given contractility (maximum elastance) and afterload (aortic pressure) of the patient. PI is related to the degree of LV filling. PI is deduced from the axial thrust measured by the pump's magnetic bearing. The PI

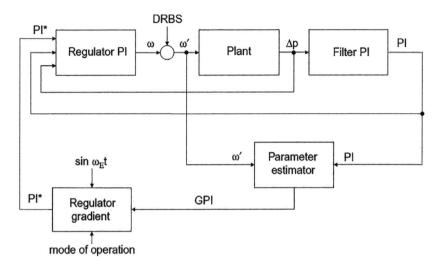

FIGURE 4.7 Schematic diagram of the LVAD control strategy proposed by Arndt et al. (2008).

gradient in relation to the pump speed (PIG) is estimated by identifying the dynamic system by *low-pass* filtering the magnitude (abs) of the *high-pass* filtered dP signal. The external cascade controller routine sets the PIG to a reference value that meets the selected control objective. The internal controller routine sets the PI to a reference value set by the external routine. Figure 4.7 shows the schematic diagram of the LVAD control strategy proposed by Arndt et al. (2008).

In the LVAD control strategy proposed by Arndt et al. (2008), there are two operational points: total assistance (TA), which is the maximum support with the aortic valve (AV) closed, but with enough safety margin to avoid suction; and partial assistance (PA), which is the moderate support in the transition region between the AV opening and a permanently closed AV with almost physiological LV volume, better LV decompression, and moderate LV load. In the work, simulations were performed for both modes of operation.

Figure 4.8a shows the transition from TA mode to PA mode to demonstrate the performance of the external routine to PIG control. PIG changes from −11 to the required −3 mmHg/min in 500 seconds. At the same time, PI increases from 12 to 22 mmHg, pump speed decreases from 7,700 to 6,400 rpm, and pump flow decreases from 5.0 to 3.5 L/min. Figure 4.8b shows the transition back to TA, PIG, and PI, and pump speed and flow are reverted to their original values. This transition takes about 1,000 seconds. In TA mode, the flow level of the pump was high enough to maintain the LV volume in a range where the LV pressure is well below the aortic pressure (Figure 4.8c). In PA mode, the LV pressure briefly reaches the level of the aortic pressure, which allows the AV to open (Figure 4.8d).

The work of Petrou et al. (2016) describes a LVAD control strategy in which the speed setting value is used to mimic the Frank–Starling mechanism based on the measurement of the pump inlet pressure (PIP) using the systolic pressure (SP) of the

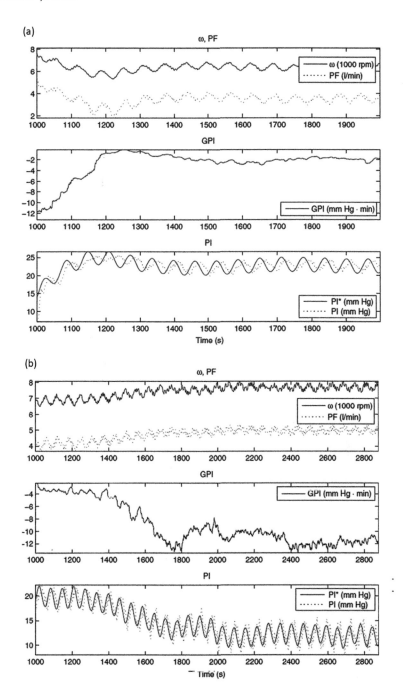

FIGURE 4.8 Results obtained by the LVAD control strategy proposed by Arndt et al. (2008). (a) Transition from TA mode to PA mode; (b) transition from PA mode to TA mode; (c) pressure waveform to TA mode; and (d) pressure waveform to PA mode.

(Continued)

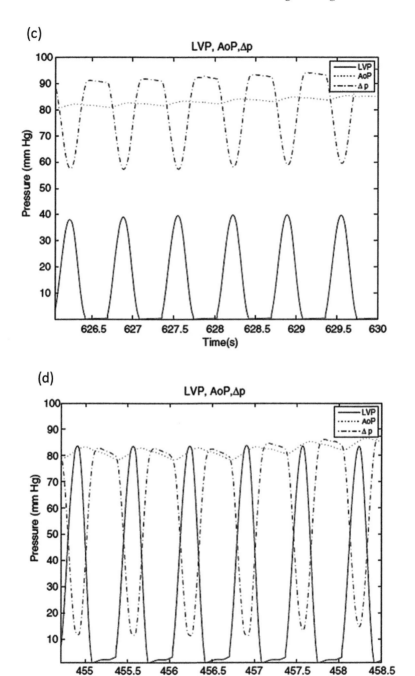

FIGURE 4.8 (*CONTINUED*)   Results obtained by the LVAD control strategy proposed by Arndt et al. (2008). (a) Transition from TA mode to PA mode; (b) transition from PA mode to TA mode; (c) pressure waveform to TA mode; and (d) pressure waveform to PA mode.

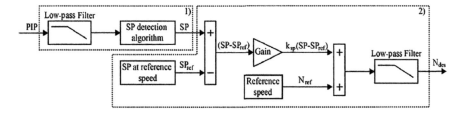

FIGURE 4.9 Schematic diagram of the LVAD control strategy proposed by Petrou et al. (2016).

LV. An increase in preload (increase in diastolic end-to-end volume or Vdf) results in an increase in systolic volume (SV) and correspondingly cardiac output (CO), resulting in an increase in aortic pressure (AoP) and consequently an increase in SP (Klabunde, 2011). A reduction in preload will have opposite effects, i.e., a decrease in SV, CO, AoP, and SP. The controller includes a pressure sensor in the inlet cannula (IC) of the LVAD, a *low-pass* filtering of the pressure (system inlet and outlet), a SP detection algorithm, and a system to determine the necessary change in pump speed for a given SP. Figure 4.9 shows the schematic diagram of the LVAD control strategy proposed by Petrou et al. (2016).

During afterload and preload increase, the heart is unable to increase its intraventricular pressure and the influence on SP is limited through the plateau area of the end-systolic pressure–volume relationship (ESPVR); in this case, as long as filling is below the plateau area, SP depends directly on LV filling and can therefore be seen as a preload measure (Klabunde, 2011) (Figure 4.10d, e, g, and h illustrates this limitation).

In the proposal of Petrou et al. (2016), it is associated with measurement of LV's SP as a physiological index for the LVAD controller keeping the LV pressure–volume loops below the plateau area of the ESPVR curve and above the suction area of the LVAD (as illustrated in Figure 4.10g and h). Figure 4.10a shows the afterload dependence of the SP, where the SP increases as the afterload increases and decreases as the afterload decreases, respectively. Figure 4.10b shows that pre-charge changes affect SP in a similar way to afterload changes. Figure 4.10c shows the dependence of SP on contractility. Figure 4.10d–f shows the pressure–volume loops of a pathological circulation where the contractility of the simulated heart was reduced, during the afterload, preload, and contractility variations. Figure 4.10g–i shows the same experiments of afterload, preload, and contractility variations conducted with a pathological circulation assisted by a LVAD adjusted at a constant speed, which provides 5 L/min at rest. Figure 4.10i shows that the LV contractility also influences the SP, which therefore cannot be seen as independent of the contractility.

Figure 4.11 shows the results obtained in an *in vitro* assay by the LVAD control strategy proposed by Petrou et al. (2016), where the resulting signals are shown for pump speed, cardiac output (CO), systolic pressure (SP), and end-diastolic pressure (EDP) during preload, afterload, and contractility variation experiments for a physiological circulation (C1), a pathological circulation assisted by a LVAD's constant speed (C2), and a pathological circulation assisted by a LVAD controlled by the SP controller (C3).

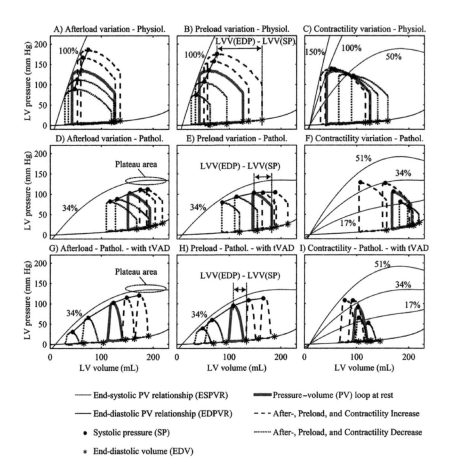

FIGURE 4.10 Associations between left ventricular systolic pressure and volume of the proposal by Petrou et al. (2016).

4.5 STRATEGIES FOR AFTERLOAD-BASED PHYSIOLOGICAL CONTROLLERS OF LVADs

Physiologic controllers based on afterload adapt the pump speed according to aortic pressure (AoP) or pump pressure. These controllers intend to keep the AoP (or the pressure gradient of the pump) constant, so that the cardiac output (CO) is regulated by the vascular resistance (Ochsner et al., 2014).

The work of Waters et al. (1999) describes a LVAD control strategy in which the speed setting value is defined by a proportional–integral (PI) gain algorithm in order to maintain the reference differential pressure of the system even when changes in the natural heart occur. The load on the motor is the pump rotor and the load on the pump rotor is the blood, so there is a relationship between the motor current, voltage, and the counter electromotive force (emf) for the blood flow and pressure through the LVAD. The motor feedback method used in the proposal by Waters et al. (1999) explores this relationship to estimate the true left ventricle pressure and use it to

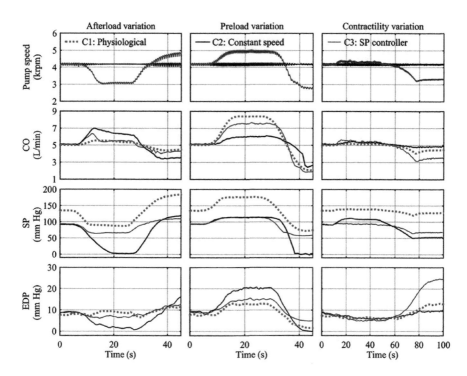

FIGURE 4.11   Results obtained by the LVAD control strategy proposed by Petrou et al. (2016).

control the speed of motor rotation of the LVAD. Figure 4.12 presents the schematic diagram of the LVAD control strategy proposed by Waters et al. (1999).

Figure 4.13 shows the results obtained in an *in vitro* assay by the LVAD control strategy proposed by Waters et al. (1999), where the resulting signals are shown for the closed-loop response with reference pressure = 110 mm Hg (Figure 4.13a), closed-loop response with reference pressure = 110 mm Hg and a step disturbance (Figure 4.13b), and closed-loop response with a sinusoidal disturbance (Figure 4.13c).

The work of Bullister et al. (2002) describes a LVAD control strategy in which the speed setting value is defined by a hierarchical algorithm using the PIP as the primary independent variable and the pump outlet pressure as the secondary dependent variable to maintain stable ventricular and arterial filling pressures. Monitoring algorithms based on pressure inputs are able to approximate the flow rate and hydraulic power of the pump and the left ventricle. The pressures were measured at the pump inlet and outlet using APEX pressure sensors (APSs) (APEX Medical Inc, Walpole, MA). The APSs are a patented long-term implant flow blood pressure sensor designed to control implantable heart pumps. The APS uses a pressure-sensing diaphragm that can be integrated into the wall of any titanium pump or IC (Bullister et al., 2002). Mounted on the pressure-sensing diaphragm is a molecular bound thin film strain gauge whose strain measurement elements are located at the highest stress and compression points. Figure 4.14 shows the schematic diagram of the LVAD control strategy proposed by Bullister et al. (2002).

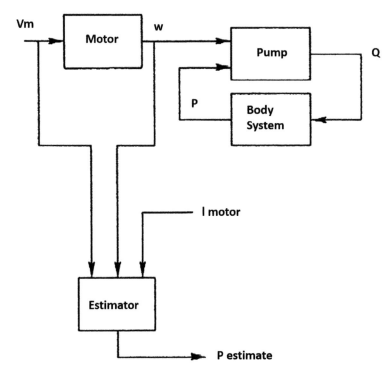

FIGURE 4.12   Schematic diagram of the LVAD control strategy proposed by Waters et al. (1999).

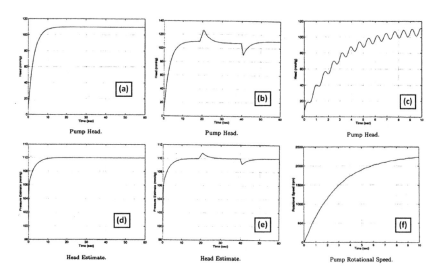

FIGURE 4.13   Results obtained by the LVAD control strategy proposed by Waters et al. (1999) in different disturbance.

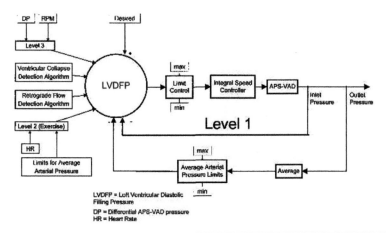

Goal	Level 1 control	Level 2 control
Primary	Keep LVDFP within limits	Keep LVDFP within limits
Secondary	Keep arterial pressure within limits	Control to variable arterial pressure set point (based on bpm)
Tertiary	Control to LVDFP set point	

LVDFP: left ventricular diastolic filling pressure, bpm: beats per minute.

FIGURE 4.14 Schematic diagram of the LVAD control strategy proposed by Bullister et al. (2002).

The controller proposed by Bullister et al. (2002) has two levels of control (Figure 4.17), which are as follows:

1. The main objective of Level 1 control was to keep the left ventricular end-diastolic pressure (LVEDP) filling, or filling pressure, within a range programmable by the physician. Thus, within the physician-programmed LVEDP range and the target range of mean arterial pressure (MAP), the overall goal is to have the left heart and the assisting rotating device pump all incoming blood incrementally from the left ventricle without allowing excessive blockage or suction that can lead to left ventricle collapse;
2. The objective of Level 2 control was to keep the mean pump outlet pressure (representative of MAP) at a target value during high levels of ventricular pulsation, such as during exercise. Level 2 uses heart rate as a physiological indicator based on the regulation of the sympathetic nervous system of the circulatory system during exercise or stress. The typical increase in mean blood pressure is ~30% during exercise; however, as the left ventricle is compromised, the patient cannot increase cardiac output in response to exercise. Therefore, the heart rate is used to increase the pump speed, resulting in higher MAPs.

Figure 4.15 shows the results obtained in an *in vitro* assay by the LVAD Level 1 control strategy proposed by Bullister et al. (2002).

The work of Giridharan and Skliar (2006) describes a LVAD control strategy in which the speed setting value is defined by an algorithm using the estimated differential

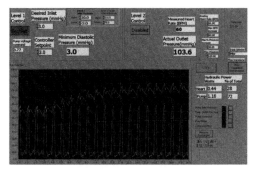

| | | Mean arterial | | |
| LVDFP | | pressure | LVAD flow rate | LVAD speed |
(mm Hg)		(mm Hg)	(L/min)	(rpm)
10.0		52	4.1	2,490
9.0		58	5.0	2,720
8.0		64	5.7	2,920
7.0		68	6.0	3,080
6.0		74	6.7	3,250
5.0		79	7.2	3,420
4.0		86	7.7	3,600
3.0		93	8.1	3,780
2.0		102	8.7	4,010
1.0		109	9.1	4,170
0.0		116	9.5	4,320
−1.0		124	9.8	4,490
−2.0		136	10.4	4,710

FIGURE 4.15 Results obtained by the LVAD control strategy proposed by Bullister et al. (2002).

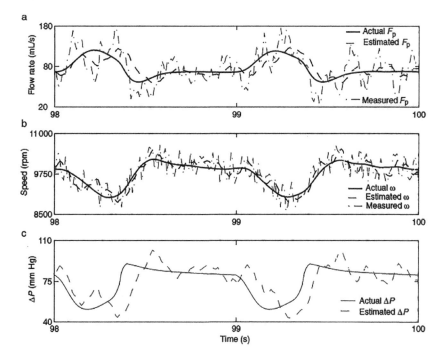

FIGURE 4.16 Results obtained by the LVAD control strategy proposed by Giridharan and Skliar (2006).

pressure (ΔP) of the pump inlet and outlet pressure. The estimator developed consisted of an extended Kalman filter in conjunction with the Golay–Savitzky filter. In the control approach of ΔP, the aim is to maintain a constant mean reference pressure difference between the left ventricle and the aorta by automatically manipulating the pump speed. The pump power input is changed by manipulating the motor current to adjust the speed so that the error between the actual and desired ΔP is reduced.

Figure 4.16 shows the results obtained in an *in vitro* assay by the LVAD control strategy proposed by Giridharan and Skliar (2006), where ΔP is estimated

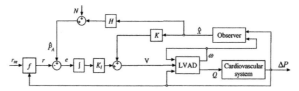

Physiological control system structure. r: reference pressure of aortic pressure. r_m: preset constant reference pressure. ΔP: pump head of the LVAD (human cardiovascular system output). e: tracking error of aortic pressure to r. $\hat{x}$: the estimated state of system x. P_A: the estimated aortic pressure. H: transformation matrix from x to $\hat{P}_A$. K_I, K: PI controller gains. V: the control output (the desired pump motor voltage).

FIGURE 4.17   Schematic diagram of the LVAD control strategy proposed by Wu et al. (2007).

on the basis of speed measurements only: (i) real, estimated, and measured flow rates; (ii) real, estimated, and measured pump speed; and (iii) real and estimated ΔP.

The work of Wu et al. (2007) describes a strategy of an optimal adaptive LVAD controller to control the estimated aortic pressure to track an updated reference signal by a nonlinear function of the pump pressure gradient to meet the physiological need of the patient. The proposed controller consists of three parts: (i) an adaptive parameter estimation algorithm to estimate total peripheral resistance; (ii) an adaptive state observer using the total peripheral resistance estimation; and (iii) an optimal PI controller also using the total peripheral resistance estimation for controller parameter selection. Figure 4.17 presents the schematic diagram of the LVAD control strategy proposed by Wu et al. (2007).

Figure 4.18 shows the results obtained in an *in vitro* assay by the LVAD control strategy proposed by Wu et al. (2007). During exercise, the control system was able to maintain aortic pressure and increase total peripheral flow by adjusting the controller gain and voltage.

4.6   STRATEGIES FOR HEART RATE-BASED PHYSIOLOGICAL CONTROLLERS OF LVADs

Rotary pumps are set to a constant speed level that can be increased when the patient has an increased venous return as a result of physical activity. The chosen constant speed setting should not result in excessive discharge that could cause suction, blood trauma, endothelial wall injury, or reduced right ventricular performance (Vollkron et al., 2005).

Heart frequency (HR)-based LVAD controllers detect the patient's HR and adapt the pump speed according to a predefined relationship between the HR and the desired pump flow.

The work of Ohuchi et al. (2001) describes a control strategy for determining the target pump rotation that provides the flow required by the body with fine-tuning of rotation to minimize deleterious effects such as ventricular suction and evaluation of ventricular function for successful weaning from LVADs. To determine the target pump rotation, the relationship between native HR and cardiac output (CO) and the relationship between pump rotation and centrifugal output were used. The native HR was continuously monitored by means of an electrocardiogram (ECG).

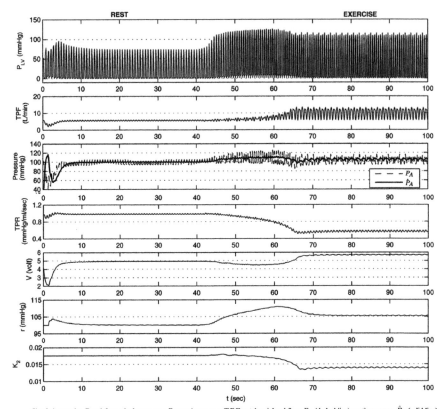

Simulation results. P_{LV}: left ventricular pressure. P_A: aortic pressure. TPF: total peripheral flow. P_A (dashed line): aortic pressure. $\hat{P}_A$ (solid line): estimated aortic pressure. TPR: total peripheral resistance. V: control input voltage. r: reference value. K_2: the second element of controller gain.

FIGURE 4.18   Results obtained by the LVAD control strategy proposed by Wu et al. (2007).

The desired level of CO was obtained from the relationship between predetermined HR and CO.

In the LVAD control strategy proposed by Ohuchi et al. (2001) for the fine adjustment of pump rotation, the motor current waveform was used. With the occurrence of suction or regurgitation, the flow and therefore the waveform of the motor current become distorted. To quantify the level of deformation of the waveform, the waveform strain index (WSI) of the motor current waveform was calculated by means of the fast Fourier transform. The power spectral density (PSD) of the fundamental motor current waveform corresponds to the native frequency of the heart. Therefore, the ratio of the sum of the PSD components above the fundamental frequency to the fundamental PSD implies the degree of deformation of the waveform. The WSI was calculated using the following equation: (PSD higher order harmonics)/(PSD of the fundamental frequency). When this ratio was greater than approximately 0.2, it was assumed that there would be a suction effect in the ventricle. For the evaluation of ventricular function, the amplitude of the motor current waveform was used.

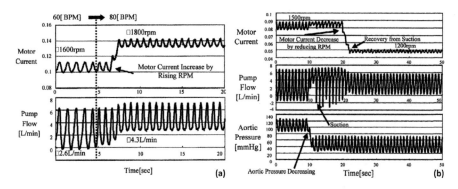

FIGURE 4.19 Results obtained by the LVAD control strategy proposed by Ohuchi et al. (2001) with changes in heart rate and occurrence of suction.

Figure 4.19 shows the results obtained in an *in vitro* assay by the LVAD control strategy proposed by Ohuchi et al. (2001), where in Figure 4.19a, the response of the system to changes in heart rate is shown, and in Figure 4.19b, the response of the system to the occurrence of suction is shown.

The work of Vollkron et al. (2005) describes a LVAD control strategy that analyzes pump performance based on available flow, HR, and short-term performance history. The system consists of two modules: The first monitors the venous return and determines the maximum blood flow that can be withdrawn from the right ventricle, while the second compares the available return with the level of perfusion required to establish the desired flow.

The clinician defines the levels of "desired flow" at rest and during exercise, depending on the HR. This desired flow level may depend on the patient's own HR, which usually correlates well with his or her level of activity. The flow dependency on HR can be chosen by the clinician to coincide with the particular purpose of pump support (e.g., maximum support, exercise dependent support, ventricular weaning training) (Vollkron et al., 2005).

The actual and appropriate level of venous return is derived from the flow pulsatility, which reflects the remaining function of the patient's own left ventricle. Even a severely damaged ventricle produces minimal contractions if its filling by the right heart is physiologically sufficient. These contractions are sufficient to provide filling information. The left ventricular filling for sufficient physiological volume levels also protects the right heart. In order to achieve the limited venous return discharge, the system maintains the flow signal pulsatility at a target value of 1.5–2 L/min. The pulsatility is defined as the difference between the maximum and minimum pump flow rate in one heart cycle (P2P flow value) (Vollkron et al., 2005).

At the work of Vollkron et al. (2005), a specialist system continuously checks the flow signal for any indication of suction. The periodic speed variations adapt the pump performance to the patient's conditions. As ineffective speed increases would degrade performance, the system also evaluates the effectiveness of speed changes in changing pump flow, energy consumption, and pulsatility (imposing and assessing speed variations periodically). If this desired flow cannot be maintained due

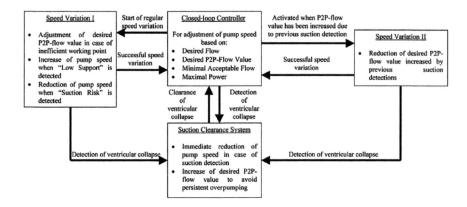

FIGURE 4.20   Schematic diagram of the LVAD control strategy proposed by Vollkron et al. (2005).

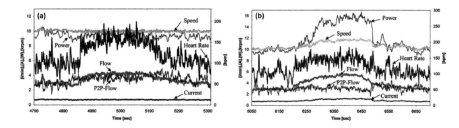

FIGURE 4.21   Results obtained in an *in vivo* assay by the LVAD control strategy proposed by Vollkron et al. (2005).

to limited venous return, the maximum available flow level is determined from an analysis of the actual pump data (flow, speed, and power consumption) (Figure 4.20).

The automatic speed control system of the LVAD control strategy proposed by Vollkron et al. (2005) consists of four interaction units, where the schematic diagram is presented in Figure 4.20.

Figure 4.21 shows the results obtained in an *in vivo* assay by the LVAD control strategy proposed by Vollkron et al. (2005), where in Figure 4.21a, the cycling exercise of a patient with a LVAD at a constant speed of 10,000 rpm is shown, and in Figure 4.21b, the cycling exercise of a patient with a LVAD with automatic speed control is shown. During cycling exercise with automatic speed control, in Figure 4.21b, the heart rate is lower, with greater flow and greater rotation, as a consequence of greater VAD power (minor cardiac work), when compared to constant control.

4.7   STRATEGIES FOR MULTI-OBJECTIVE-BASED PHYSIOLOGICAL CONTROLLERS OF LVADs

When using an assistive device to support a patient with heart failure, clinicians are concerned about more than just cardiac output. Since their goals can be conflicting, clinicians often describe them as restrictions. Based on discussions with several physicians at the University of Pittsburgh's Artificial Heart Program, the work of Boston et al. (2003) identified the following common restrictions for ventricular assist:

1. Cardiac output should be above the minimum value, usually between 3 and 6 L/min, needed to support the patient's level of activity;
2. Left atrial pressure should be kept below approximately 10–15 mmHg to avoid pulmonary edema and above ~0 mmHg to avoid sucking; and
3. Systolic blood pressure should be kept between the patient's specific limits to limit afterload sensitivity.

The complex multi-objective physiological controllers of LVAD attempt to estimate the state of the cardiovascular system and adapt the pump speed to meet various constraints simultaneously. Multi-objective optimization provides the most satisfactory approach to specify the pump speed as it considers all criteria of interest to clinicians.

The work of Boston et al. (2003) describes a LVAD control strategy in which the reference speed is determined by one of several algorithms (ideal, heuristic, or standard), depending on the patient's physical condition, the status of the device, and the confidence that precise measurements or estimates of hemodynamic variables are available. Each algorithm has a larger amount of information than the algorithm presented in the next paragraph in the structure and provides better performance if the information is accurate.

The controller includes a system identification module that attempts to identify a model of the patient's cardiovascular system using the measurements that are available. Suction rates can be combined using fuzzy logic detection (possibly combined with Bayesian or majority voting decision) to determine a reference pump speed as well as reliability for the algorithms. Finally, the standard control mode can be used in the event of extensive sensor failure, software failure, or uncertainty as to the reliability of the control actions or operation of the auxiliary device itself. The standard mode provides a constant pump speed, which is low enough in most cases to avoid suction while still providing a nominal flow output. This mode attempts to provide safe device operation without requiring any sensory information, state variables, or model parameter estimates. However, it generates low cardiac output without the ability to respond to changes in demand required and can result in adverse regurgitant flow through the pump circuit (Boston et al., 2003).

The intelligent control supervisor performs several tasks (Boston et al., 2003):

1. It determines the level of patient activity and therefore the demand for blood flow;
2. It calculates pressure setting points using systemic impedance;
3. It monitors the estimated parameters of the model and determines whether they are within acceptable ranges and whether the rates of parameter change are reasonable;
4. It selects the control algorithm to be used, based on available measurements, the reliability of the patient model being estimated, and the patient's previous history; and

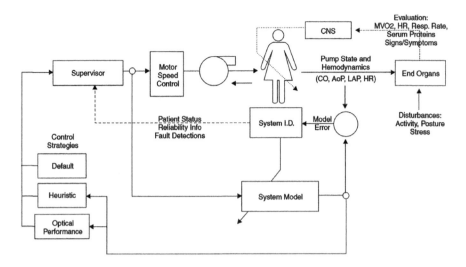

FIGURE 4.22   Schematic diagram of the LVAD control strategy proposed by Boston et al.
(2003).

5. It compares the model and pump parameters with previous system history
   to detect hardware failures or changes in the patient that would prevent the
   assistive device from providing adequate output.

Figure 4.22 presents the schematic diagram of the LVAD control strategy proposed
by Boston et al. (2003).

The work of Petrou et al. (2017) describes a new multi-objective physiological
control system that depends on the PIP. In this new study, an advanced control and
monitoring system is presented that uses the PIP to meet the following objectives:
(i) to adapt the pump flow to the physiological requirements of the pathological circulation supported by the LVAD, (ii) to increase the aortic pulse pressure, (iii) to
ensure an opening of the AV for a predefined period of time, (iv) to provide information about the preload and afterload conditions of the LV as well as the heart rate,
and (v) to ensure the safe operation of the control system so that no suction and LV
overload or backflow events of the pump occur. Figure 4.23 presents the schematic
diagram of the LVAD control strategy proposed by Petrou et al. (2017).

Figure 4.24 shows the results obtained in an *in vitro* assay by the LVAD control
strategy proposed by Petrou et al. (2017) during preload, afterload, and contractility
variations. The pump flow was physiologically adapted to the changes in preload,
while the aortic pulse pressure yielded a three-fold increase in relation to a constant
speed operation. The state of the AV was detected with an overall accuracy of 86%
and was controlled as desired. The proposed system has shown its potential for a
safe physiological response to the various perfusion requirements, which reduces the
risk of myocardial atrophy and provides important hemodynamic indices for patient
monitoring during LVAD therapy.

Leão et al. (2020) proposed the concept of a multi-objective physiological control
(MOPC) of VADs with harmonious adjustment of the assistance parameters with

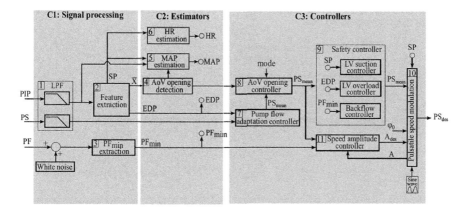

FIGURE 4.23   Schematic diagram of the LVAD control strategy proposed by Petrou et al. (2017).

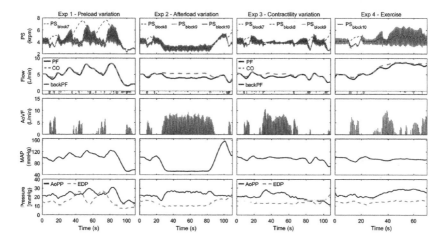

FIGURE 4.24   Results obtained by the LVAD control strategy proposed by Petrou et al. (2017).

the physiological system, aiming at the optimization of the interaction between the VAD and the body of the implant. The main interaction between the MOPC and the organism in which it acts is in the MAP regulation system (fundamental element of circulatory control).

The MOPC is composed of three layers: (i) proportional–integral control of the motor speed of the VAD; (ii) flow control based on estimated physiological parameters; and (iii) automatic control of the motor speed of the VAD by fuzzy logic, Figure 4.25.

MOPC had its operation validated in a device that emulates the physical connection of a VAD to the cardiovascular system, under physiological conditions considered normal or with alteration of some cardiovascular parameters to simulate HF as

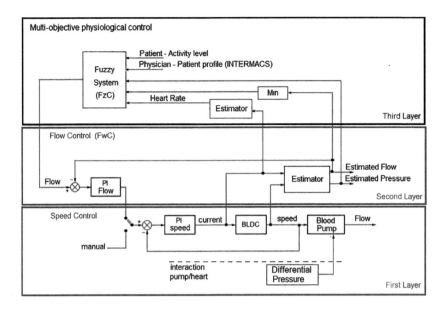

FIGURE 4.25   Multi-objective physiological control (MOPC) block diagram by Leão et al. (2020).

ejection fraction (EF) (15%–40%) and heart rate (HR) (50–110 bpm) (Leão et al., 2020). For the feasibility of the application of the MOPC concepts as a VAD controller solution, it is necessary that they are implemented in an embedded system.

Santos (2020) and Santos et al. (2019) proposed the design of strategies for implementing the multi-objective controller for VADs proposed by Leão et al. (2020) in an embedded system with characteristics of an intelligent system through the integration of real-time data processing, reconfigurable architecture, and communication protocols based on the concepts of Health 4.0. Due to the reconfigurable quality of the system, physiological control modules can be implemented and added to the existing control.

4.8   STRATEGIES FOR HEMODYNAMIC-BASED PHYSIOLOGICAL CONTROLLERS OF LVADs

The optimization of the patient's hemodynamic profile depends on the complex interaction between the patient's individual pathophysiology and the characteristics of the pump. On the patient's side, ventricular contractility and volume status, with pulmonary and systemic vascular properties, are important factors. On the other hand, the characteristics of the pump are quantified by pressure–flow relations dependent on speed (Uriel et al., 2016).

The *International Society for Heart and Lung Transplantation* (ISHLT) guidelines predominantly reflect expert opinion (Evidence C), and there is significant medical variability in the evaluation and treatment of patients implanted with LVAD (Feldman et al., 2013; Uriel et al., 2016).

The ISHLT (2013) has published guidelines for mechanical circulatory support where patients with hypertension and implanted with non-pulsatile LVADs should have an average blood pressure of ≤80 mmHg to avoid complications (recommendation class: IIb; level of evidence: C).

In the HeartWare ADVANCE (*Evaluation of the HeartWare Left Ventricular Assist Device for the Treatment of Advanced Heart Failure*), the hypothesis that higher blood pressure, increasing the afterload on the pump, reduces the flow of centrifugal pumps and increases the propensity for thrombi to be made by the device, which could manifest as embolic events or pump malfunction (Aaronson & Boyce, 2014; Najjar et al, 2014); therefore, centrifugal pumps are more sensitive to afterload (up to three times more sensitive compared to the heart) and have a greater reduction in pump flow in response to hypertension (Salamonsen et al., 2011), while axial pumps are more likely to cause hemolysis (artificial breakdown of blood red cells caused by VAD's rotor) and thrombosis (blood clotting zones within the device) due to their low volume and due to high motor speed (>10,000 rpm) (Burke et al., 2001; Bhamidipati et al., 2010; Cowger et al., 2014).

The work of Saeed et al. (2015) associates increased blood pressure (>80 mmHg) with adverse events such as intracranial hemorrhage, thromboembolic event, and progressive aortic insufficiency in patients implanted with VADs. In this study, 123 patients were implanted with HeartMate® II (111) and HeartWare® (12) between June 2006 and December 2013: (i) Thirty-one patients were in the "control" group (blood pressure <80 mmHg); (ii) 52 patients were in the "intermediate" group (blood pressure 80–90 mmHg); and (iii) 40 patients were in the "high" group (blood pressure ≥90 mmHg).

The results were as follows (Saeed et al., 2015): (i) 0% of the "control" group, 4% (2/52) of the "intermediate" group, and 15% (6/40) of the "tall" group developed intracranial hemorrhage and six patients died, and progression occurred early to implantation, with a mean time of 69 days after implantation (range, 31–226); (ii) 0% of the "control" group, 4% (2/52) of the "intermediate" group, and 10% (4/40) of the "high" group developed from moderate to severe aortic insufficiency, the progression occurring late, with a mean time of 347 days after implantation (interval, 102–513), emphasizing the importance of blood pressure control during all mechanical circulatory support; and (iii) 3.2% (1/32) of the "control" group, 5.8% (3/52) of the "intermediate" group, and 7.5% (3/40) of the "tall" group developed thromboembolic events.

The work of Lampert et al. (2014) aimed at mitigating the occurrence of adverse events associated with blood pressure elevation (>80 mmHg) by means of an effective antihypertensive medication regimen for patients with continuous flow LVAD. In this work, a clinical study was conducted with 96 patients implanted with HeartMate® II (59), VentrAssist® (Ventracor, Sydney, Australia) (22), HeartWare® (13), and Jarvik® 2000 (Jarvik Heart Inc, New York) (2), between January 2006 and October 2011. Outpatient blood pressure treatment was performed according to the institutional protocol (Figure 4.26).

Of the 74% who received antihypertensives, 54% needed 1 drug, 34% used 2, 10% used 3, and 3% used 4 or more. There was no difference between axial flow and centrifugal devices in the percentage of patients requiring antihypertensives. According to the protocol, angiotensin-converting enzyme (ACE) inhibitors or angiotensin II

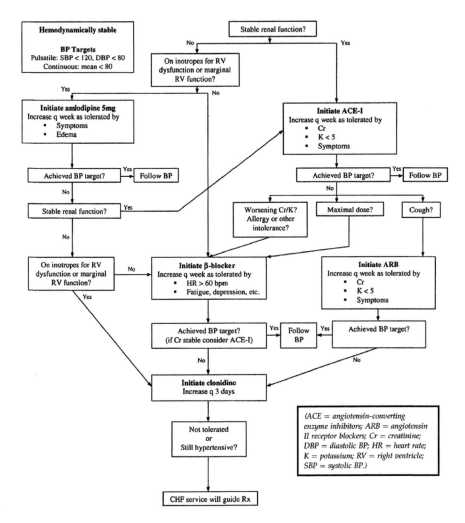

FIGURE 4.26 Blood pressure (BP) measurement algorithm in implanted patients proposed by Lampert et al. (2014).

receptor blockers were the most commonly prescribed drugs, used in 85% ($n = 60$) of patients in therapy. Lisinopril was the most commonly used ACE inhibitor ($n = 53$) with an average dose of 20 mg. Beta-blockers were used in 30% ($n = 21$) of patients, and carvedilol was used more frequently ($n = 20$) with an average daily dose of 27 mg. Calcium channel blockers were the most commonly used in 28% ($n = 20$) with amlodipine used in all patients except 1. Alpha-blockers were used in 21% ($n = 15$), all of which were clonidine (Lampert et al., 2014).

There were 31 neurological adverse events in 23 patients; 6 patients had 2 events and 1 patient had 3 events. Of these events, there were 20 strokes and 11 transient ischemic attacks. All events occurred within 12 months after implantation. Of the

20 strokes, 16 were ischemic and 4 hemorrhagic. In those patients who did not die during support, 87% needed at least 1 antihypertensive and more than 80% of those patients were treated with 1 or 2 medications (Lampert et al., 2014).

Good blood pressure control was achieved in patients who needed medical treatment. The cumulative rate of neurological events was higher in the population of patients who were not on antihypertensives; however, in those patients who needed antihypertensives, the number of drugs was not associated with an increase in the cumulative incidence of neurological events. The authors concluded that most patients with continuous flow LVADs require medical treatment of hypertension and that effective blood pressure control may affect the rate of adverse events, such as aortic insufficiency and neurological events (Lampert et al., 2014).

The work of Tank et al. (2012) tested the hypothesis that continuous flow VADs impair the control of the baroreflex of the sympathetic autonomic nervous system, further exacerbating sympathetic arousal, since the physiological dogma was that the cardiovascular autonomic homeostasis requires flow and pulsatile blood pressure. A clinical study was conducted with nine patients (age: 26–61 years; body mass index: 18.9–28.3 kg/m²) implanted with the LVAD HeartWare® and the control group was composed of 16 healthy men (age: 24–62 years; body mass index: 21–28.3 kg/m²), and measurements were recorded (measurements were taken in the morning after a night fast) the electrocardiogram (beaten blood pressure) (Finometer Midi, Finapres Medical Systems, Amsterdam, Netherlands), brachial systolic blood pressure (Doppler ultrasonography) and respiration (Niccomo, Medis GmbH, Ilmenau, Germany) and in addition, the muscle sympathetic nerve activity (MSNA) of the right fibular nerve (Nerve Traffic Analyzer 662C-3, Department of Biomedical Engineering, University of Iowa, Iowa) as described by Heusser et al. (2010).

The methodology used in the work of Tank et al. (2012) was as follows: After a rest period ≥15 minutes, baseline measurements were obtained for 10 minutes, followed by autonomic function tests, including deep breathing (respiratory rate of 6 per minute) and the Valsalva maneuver. After connecting the remote control to the LVAD, a second baseline was recorded. The speed of the LVAD was then gradually increased to a maximum of 3,200 rpm to further reduce the pulse pressure. A third baseline was recorded after returning to the LVAD baseline speed and disconnecting the remote control. For the last baseline, the head was tilted 15° up for 10 minutes to test the increase in sympathetic nervous traffic. The average speed of the LVAD was $2,860 \pm 37$ rpm. All patients were taking medicines for heart failure, including ACE inhibitors ($n=6$) or angiotensin II type 1 receptor blockers ($n=1$), adrenoreceptor blockers ($n=6$), loop diuretics ($n=3$), and oral anticoagulants ($n=9$).

The baroreflective regulation of MSNA has paradoxically been preserved. Furthermore, the sympathetic activity was surprisingly low in patients, considering the severity of the cardiac contractile dysfunction. Only 2 out of 8 patients exhibited MSNA measurements at rest close to the values reported in the literature for patients with severe heart failure (Floras, 2003). In general, only a trend of higher frequency of shots and higher median value of the normal distribution of the range of shots was observed in patients with LVAD compared to the control group. The incidence of firing and the area under firing were similar among the groups. The median of the normalized shooting range distribution (considered more informative than the shooting frequency alone) was similar in patients with LVAD and the control group (Tank et al., 2012).

The heart rate regulation by the baroreflex was intact, at least in part, in most patients, evidenced by the heart rate response during the Valsalva maneuver and the head's upward tilt. The mean values of heart rate variability and baroreflex sensitivity of the heart rate control were significantly reduced compared to the control group. However, abnormal spontaneous baroreflex sensitivities were recorded at ≤3 out of 8 patients, being an unexpected observation, as parasympathetic heart rate control is severely impaired in patients with heart failure (Floras, 2001). The patients presented reduced but preserved parasympathetic heart rate control evaluated by autonomic reflex tests and spectral analysis, similar to another study in patients implanted with a HeartMate® (Kim et al., 1996). Heart rate variability may improve with LVAD treatment (Kim et al., 1996), but for proof measures of heart rate variability before and after LVAD treatment are necessary (Tank et al., 2012).

The authors concluded that the low level of pulse pressure in patients implanted with continuous flow LVADs is sufficient to maintain cardiovascular control by baroreflexes, and given the central role of these mechanisms in adjusting heart rate and vascular tone to the demands of daily life, including regular standing, this is a relevant factor for performance and quality of life in implanted patients (Tank et al., 2012).

Optimization of the hemodynamic profile of a patient with continuous flow LVAD requires a detailed understanding of ventricular–vascular–LVAD interactions (Burkhoff & Naidu, 2012). The ISHLT guideline (2013) recommends that the revolutions per minute (rpm) value of the LVAD motor be adjusted to allow adequate left ventricular decompression, keeping the interventricular septum in the midline and minimizing mitral regurgitation (recommendation class: I; level of evidence: C). It is also recommended that the rpm value be low enough to allow the intermittent AV to open (ISHLT, 2013; recommendation class: IIb; level of evidence: B). Diuretics, ACE inhibitors, angiotensin receptor blockers, beta-blockers, and mineralocorticoids are considered useful for managing the volume status, blood pressure, arrhythmias, and myocardial fibrosis of implanted patients (ISHLT, 2013; recommendation class: I; level of evidence: C). Traditionally, echocardiography has been used to adjust the rate of LVAD to obtain an adequate discharge, but recent studies suggest that measurement of hemodynamics may provide crucial additional information for clinicians to better optimize the function of LVAD and thus the symptoms of patients (Uriel et al., 2016, 2020).

The work of Uriel et al. (2016) aimed at developing an evidence-based approach to the management of patients with continuous flow LVADs, based on the interaction between device function and patient hemodynamics. In this prospective study, 35 consecutive patients with continuous flow LVAD (14 with HeartWare® and 21 with HeartMate® II) were included and evaluated with a hemodynamic ramp test and echocardiography, and a standardized hemodynamic ramp protocol was applied in clinically stable continuous flow LVAD patients (in an outpatient setting, ideally between 1 and 3 months after LVAD implantation) to assess the impact of acute changes in the speed of continuous flow LVAD on hemodynamics and left ventricular decompression.

The patients were 58.5 ± 9.4 years old, and the majority were male (62.9%). Most patients were implanted for target therapy (71.4%). The mean time between ramp testing and device implantation was 321 days (range 13–1,954 days). The hemodynamic parameters recorded included initial Doppler arterial pressure (oD-AP) (Kato et al., 2014); central venous pressure (CVP); systolic, diastolic, and mean pulmonary artery pressures (PAP); and wedge pulmonary artery pressure (considered as capillary pressure) (PCWP). Cardiac output (CO) and cardiac index (CI) were calculated by Fick's indirect method. The hemodynamic parameters at baseline speeds ($9,094 \pm 417$ rpm for HeartMate® II and $2,704 \pm 147$ rpm for HeartWare®) were similar among the devices (Uriel et al., 2016).

In terms of ideal hemodynamics, 42.9% of the patients had CVP and PCWP in the defined normal range. The increases in device speed were associated with an increase in pulmonary artery oxygen saturation, indicating an increase in CO. In patients with HeartWare®, Fick CO averaged 4.2 L/min at 2,300 rpm and increased on average 0.09 L/min for each step of 100 rpm increase, so that in step 9 of rpm increase (ceiling), the flow was increased to 5.1 L/min. In patients with HeartMate® II, Fick DC averaged 3.7 L/min at 8,000 rpm and increased on average 0.21 L/min for each step of 400 rpm increase, so that in step 10 of increase of rpm (ceiling), the flow was increased to 5.2 L/min. In all patients and in both devices, the PCWP decreased with the increase of the device speed. On average, there was a 1.23 mmHg reduction in the PCWP at each rotation step (Uriel et al., 2016).

The authors pointed to three main results of the study (Uriel et al., 2016): (i) There was unexpectedly wide variability in baseline hemodynamics (i.e., pre-clamp testing) in our patients treated according to clinical standards; (ii) only 43% of patients had "normal" hemodynamic profiles at baseline speeds; this increased to 56% after speed adjustments based on test results; and (iii) axial and centrifugal VADs provided significant left ventricular discharge, manifested as decreases in the PCWP; these changes were flow-dependent, not device dependent.

The authors pointed out that an unexpectedly high proportion of patients with clinically stable and apparently well-compensated heart failure supported by LVAD had abnormal hemodynamic profiles, indicating that it is clinically challenging to assess the volume status and hemodynamic profile in LVAD patients based on routine clinical evaluation. And they concluded that patient outcomes and quality of life can be improved by periodic assessments of rpm value settings to achieve optimal hemodynamics for individual physiology and to guide a medical therapy, as there were limits to how much an abnormal hemodynamic profile could be "normalized" by modifying the rpm value settings, which reinforces the value of medical therapy optimization. These findings highlight the need to develop clinical tools to help physicians customize patient-specific management strategies, as the long-term effects associated with rpm value-dependent changes in renal perfusion, modulation of autonomic reflex activity, right heart function, and other factors are also likely to impact clinical outcomes (Uriel et al., 2016).

The hemodynamic ramp (HR) test is effective in guiding patient management to achieve more normal hemodynamic profiles, even in patients with apparently well-compensated and stable LVADs (Uriel et al., 2017), and furthermore, this hemodynamically guided management has been associated with a reduction in adverse events (Imamura et al., 2018, 2019).

RAMP-IT-UP was a prospective multicenter randomized pilot study, designed to assess the feasibility of implementing a standardized multicenter HR testing protocol, determine the impact on pump and medical management, and assess the impact on adverse events and quality of life (Uriel et al., 2020). The RAMP-IT-UP pilot study compared the results in patients with LVAD, using a HR-guided management strategy (HR group) versus a standard transthoracic echocardiographic management strategy (control group). Patients were enrolled and randomized 1–3 months after HeartWare® implantation and followed for 6 months. Twenty-two patients (57 ± 10 years, 73% male) were randomized to the HR group and 19 patients (51 ± 13 years, 63% male) to the control group (Uriel et al., 2020).

In the study, the data collection steps were as follows (Uriel et al., 2020): (i) With the initial HeartWare® speed from the patient's baseline, a complete set of hemodynamic data (CVP, PAP, PCWP, O_2 saturation in the pulmonary artery (SO_2 AP), cardiac index by thermodilution, sAPs, dAP, and mPA) and echocardiographic measurements were recorded; (ii) HeartWare® speed was reduced to 2,300 rpm with repeated collection of hemodynamic and echocardiographic data; and (iii) HeartWare® speed was increased in 100 rpm increments to a maximum of 3,200 rpm with repeated data collection at each interval.

Based on the results of the data collection, the speed of the LVAD was adjusted, and the speed could be increased, decreased, or left unchanged with the main objective of hemodynamic optimization, according to the following criteria (Uriel et al., 2020): *CVP <12 mmHg, PCWP <18 mmHg, and heart rate >2.2 L/min/m². If the PCWP was too low (<8 mmHg), the speed could be reduced to avoid suction events, and if the hemodynamic goals could not be achieved by rpm adjustments alone, adjustments in medical therapies (diuretics and neurohormonal blockade) would be made.*

Patients in the HR group had twice the number of changes in LVAD speed (1.68 versus 0.84 changes/patient, $P = 0.09$ with an incidence rate of 2.0, 95% CI, 0.9–4.7) with twice the magnitude of rpm (130 versus 60 rpm/patient, $P = 0.004$) during the study (Uriel et al., 2020). The authors of RAMP-IT-UP (2020) pointed to three main results of the pilot study: (i) The feasibility of conducting HR studies protocolled in several LVAD programs was demonstrated; this was important because these ramp studies were not a routine practice in three of the four centers involved in the study; (ii) despite the small sample size, it was shown that the availability of hemodynamics in the HR group was associated with a significantly higher number of changes in LVAD speed and drug dose adjustments for heart failure during the study period; and (iii) the analysis of clinical outcomes showed numerically lower rates of adverse events in the HR group, which were more apparent for heart failure and events related to hemocompatibility in general, although these differences were not statistically significant (Uriel et al., 2020).

Finally, the authors concluded that based on the results of the RAMP-IT-UP pilot trial, the HR test provides a safe and viable strategy for optimizing the speed of LVAD and pharmacological therapies and that a large randomized trial on the management of patients with HR-driven LVAD is required (Uriel et al., 2020).

4.9   COMPARISON BETWEEN LVADs'
PHYSIOLOGICAL CONTROL STRATEGIES

The work by Pauls et al. (2016) aimed to rigorously evaluate several physiological control strategies previously presented in the literature under identical conditions during *in vitro* simulations in a circulation simulation circuit (CSC). This study investigated the ability of each control system to improve LVAD's preload and afterload sensitivities, avoid ventricular suction, and prevent pulmonary congestion during vascular resistance and simulated postural changes. The eight physiological control strategies reported in the literature that were validated in this study are as follows:

1. Constant inlet pressure (CIP) controller, whose objective was to keep the LVEDP constant (Bullister et al., 2002);
2. Constant differential pressure controller (ΔP), whose objective was to maintain the mean pressure difference between the left ventricle and the aorta close to a specified reference differential pressure (ΔP_{ref}) (Giridharan & Skliar, 2003);
3. Controller of constant aortic pressure and differential pressure (AoP/ΔP), with two control objectives, whose main control objective was to keep the aortic pressure constant at a defined value, while the secondary control objective was to maintain the differential pressure of the pump ΔP constant in a defined value (Wu et al., 2004);
4. Constant flow controller (CQ), which aims to maintain the pump flow at a predefined reference flow rate (Casas et al., 2007);
5. Constant afterload impedance (CAI) controller, which used a linear relationship between LVEDP (a preload measurement) and the target flow of LVAD, to maintain a CAI, thus imitating the Starling relationship between flow and preload (Moscato et al., 2010);
6. Starling LVEDP (S-LVEDP) controller, which adjusts the speed of the LVAD pump to achieve a flow rate defined according to the preload (represented by LVEDP) (Stevens et al., 2014);
7. Starling pulsatility (SP) controller, which defines a target flow rate as a function of preload using LVAD flow pulsatility (difference between maximum and minimum flow rate during each cardiac cycle) as a substitute for preload (Gaddum et al., 2014); and
8. LVAD's IC compliance controller, this being a flexible section of tubing placed at the LVAD inlet to passively restrict the inner diameter as the preload decreases, and thereby increasing the resistance of the circuit and decreasing the flow of the LVAD to avoid ventricular suction (Gregory et al., 2012).

The work by Pauls et al. (2016) demonstrated that of the eight control strategies tested, four (IC compliance, CIP, CAI, and S-LVEDP) prevented ventricular suction events during all changes in pulmonary vascular resistance (PVR) and systemic vascular resistance (SVR) and during passive postural change, increasing the sensitivity of preload and decreasing the afterload sensitivity of LVAD. While IC compliance responded similarly to the constant speed mode during exercise simulations, active control systems capable of increasing the speed of the LVAD (CIP, CAI, and S-LVEDP) reduced the LV systolic work when compared to the other control systems and the pump running in constant speed mode. Of all the physiological control systems evaluated in this study, the three active control systems dependent on LVEDP as a substitute for preload (CIP, CAI, and S-LVEDP) performed better in all experiments. These results were later confirmed in the work by Petrou et al. (2018).

Pauls et al. (2016) pointed out in their study that despite the promising results found in physiological control, one of the limitations of the active control systems evaluated is the dependence on pressure and flow sensors. In the original works (AoP/ΔP, CQ, and CAI), flow and pressure estimation strategies were used based on the LVAD power variables (current, voltage) due to the good correlation between power and the torque of the motors used in this application (Wu et al., 2004; Casas et al., 2007; Moscato et al., 2010). However, estimators, particularly flow estimators used in clinics, have proved to be inaccurate in some cases (Slaughter et al., 2010), so estimators have been deliberately omitted and sensors have been used in the study by Pauls et al. (2016) to compare the merits of the control strategy alone, without the risk of errors introduced by inaccurate estimators. The need to develop sensors to provide physiological control of VAD was also pointed out in the literature review work by Tchantchaleishvili et al. (2017).

REFERENCES

Aaronson KD, Boyce SW. HVAD "Bridge to transplant ADVANCE trial investigators: An analysis of pump thrombus events in patients in the HeartWare ADVANCE bridge to transplant and continued access protocol trial". *The Journal of Heart and Lung Transplantation* 2014, 33:23–34.

ABTO – Associação Brasileira de Transplante de Órgãos, Registro Brasileiro de Transplantes, 2018, São Paulo, Ano XXIV, nº4, 2018. Disponível em: www.abto.org.br. Acesso em: 07 de janeiro de 2019.

Alomari A, Savkin A, Stevens M, Mason D, Timms D, Salamonsen R, Lovell N. "Developments in control systems for rotary left ventricular assist devices for heart failure patients: A review". *Physiological Measurement* 2012, 1:R1–R27.

Antaki J, Boston J, Simaan M. "Control of heart assist devices", *42nd IEEE International Conference on Decision and Control (IEEE Cat. No.03CH37475)*, Maui, HI, 2003, vol. 4, pp. 4084–4089.

Arndt A et al. "Physiological control of a rotary blood pump with selectable therapeutic options: Control of pulsatility gradient". *Artificial Organs* 2008, 32(10):761–771.

Bhamidipati CM et al. "Early thrombus in a HeartMate II™ left ventricular assist device: A potential cause of hemolysis and diagnostic dilemma". *The Journal of Thoracic and Cardiovascular Surgery* 2010, 140(1):e7.

Boston JR, Antaki JF, Simaan MA. "Hierarchical control of heart-assist devices". *IEEE Robotics & Automation Magazine* 2003, 10(1):54–64.

Bullister E, Reich S, Sluetz J. "Physiologic control algorithms for rotary blood pumps using pressure sensor input". *Artificial Organs* 2002, 26(11):931–938.

Burke DJ, Burke E, Parsaie F, Poirier V, Butler K, Thomas D, Taylor L, Maher T. "The HeartMate II: Design and development of a fully sealed axial flow left ventricular assist system". *Artificial Organs* 2001, 25:380–385.

Burkhoff D, Naidu SS. "The science behind percutaneous hemodynamic support: A review and comparison of support strategies". *Catheterization and Cardiovascular Interventions* 2012, 80:816–829.

Casas F, Ahmed N, and Reeves A. "Minimal sensor count approach to fuzzy logic rotary blood pump flow control". *ASAIO Journal* 2007,53:140–146.

Choi S, Boston JR, Antaki JF. "Hemodynamic controller for left ventricular assist device based on pulsatility ratio". *Artificial Organs* 2007, 31(2):114–125.

Choi, S. et al. "A sensorless approach to control of a turbodynamic left ventricular assist system". *IEEE Transactions on Control Systems Technology* 2001, 9(3):473–482.

Cowger JA et al. "Hemolysis: A harbinger of adverse outcome after left ventricular assist device implant". *The Journal of Heart and Lung Transplantation* 2014, 33(1):35–43.

Devore A, Patel P, Patel C. "Medical management of patients with a left ventricular assist device for the non-left ventricular assist device specialist". *JACC Heart Failure* 2017, 5(9):621–631.

Endo G. et al. "Control strategy for biventricular assistance with mixed-flow pumps". *Artificial Organs* 2000, 24(8):594–599.

Feldman D, Pamboukian SV, Teuteberg JJ et al. "The 2013 International Society for Heart and Lung Transplantation Guidelines for mechanical circulatory support: Executive summary". *The Journal of Heart and Lung Transplantation* 2013, 32:157–187.

Floras JS. "Arterial baroreceptor and cardiopulmonary reflex control of sympathetic outflow in human heart failure". *Annals of the New York Academy of Sciences* 2001, 940:500–513.

Floras JS. "Sympathetic activation in human heart failure: Diverse mechanisms, therapeutic opportunities". *Acta Physiologica Scandinavica* 2003, 177:391–398.

Gaddum NR et al. "Starling-like flow control of a left ventricular assist device: In vitro validation". *Artificial Organs* 2014, 38:E46–E56.

Giridharan GA, Skliar M. "Control strategy for maintaining physiological perfusion with rotary blood pumps". *Artificial Organs* 2003, 27:639–648.

Giridharan GA, Skliar M. "Physiological control of blood pumps using intrinsic pump parameters: A computer simulation study". *Artificial Organs* 2006, 30(4):301–307.

Gregory SD, Pearcy MJ, Timms D. "Passive control of a biventricular assist device with compliant inflow cannulae". *Artificial Organs* 2012, 36:683–690.

Gwak KW. "Application of extremum seeking control to turbodynamic blood pumps". *ASAIO Journal* 2007, 53(4):403–409.

Heusser K, Tank J, Engeli S, Diedrich A, Menne J, Eckert S, Peters T, Sweep FC, Haller H, Pichlmaier AM, Luft FC, Jordan J. "Carotid baroreceptor stimulation, sympathetic activity, baroreflex function, and blood pressure in hypertensive patients". *Hypertension* 2010;55:619–626.

Imamura T, Nguyen A, Kim G, Raikhelkar J, Sarswat N, Kalantari S, Smith B, Juricek C, Rodgers D, Ota T, Song T, Jeevanandam V, Sayer G, Uriel N. "Optimal haemodynamics during left ventricular assist device support are associated with reduced haemocompatibility-related adverse events. *European Journal of Heart Failure* 2018. doi: 10.1002/ejhf.1372.

Imamura T, Jeevanandam V, Kim G, Raikhelkar J, Sarswat N, Kalantari S, Smith B, Rodgers D, Besser S, Chung B, Nguyen A, Narang N, Ota T, Song T, Juricek C, Mehra M, Costanzo MR, Jorde UP, Burkhoff D, Sayer G, Uriel N. "Optimal hemodynamics during left ventricular assist device support are associated with reduced readmission rates". *Circulation: Heart Failure* 2019, 12:e005094.

INTERMACS - Interagency Registry for Mechanically Assisted Circulatory Support. Eighth annual INTERMACS report: Special focus on framing the impact of adverse events, 2017. Disponível em: https://www.jhltonline.org/article/S1053-2498(17)31896-X/pdf. Acesso em: 07 de Janeiro de 2018.

ISHLT - International Society for Heart and Lung Transplantation. The 2013 "International Society for Heart and Lung Transplantation Guidelines for mechanical circulatory support: Executive summary". *The Journal of Heart and Lung Transplantation* 2013, 32:157–187. doi:10.1016/j.healun.2012.09.013.

Kato TS et al. "Value of serial echo-guided ramp studies in a patient with suspicion of device thrombosis after left ventricular assist device implantation". *Echocardiography* 2014, 31: E5–E9.

Kim SY, Montoya A, Zbilut JP, Mawulawde K, Sullivan HJ, Lonchyna VA, Terrell MR, Pifarre R. "Effect of HeartMate left ventricular assist device on cardiac autonomic nervous activity". *The Annals of Thoracic Surgery* 1996, 61:591–593.

Kim HC, Khanwilkar PS, Bearnson GB, Olsen, DB. "Development of a microcontroller-based automatic control system for the electrohydraulic total artificial heart". *IEEE Transactions on Biomedical Engineering* 1999, 44:77–89.

Kirklin JK et al. "Eighth annual INTERMACS report: Special focus on framing the impact of adverse events". *The Journal of Heart and Lung Transplantation* 2017, 36(10):1080–1086.

Klabunde R *Cardiovascular Physiology Concepts*. Lippincott Williams & Wilkins: Philadelphia, Pennsylvania, 2011.

Lampert BC et al. "Blood pressure control in continuous flow left ventricular assist devices: Efficacy and impact on adverse events". *The Annals of Thoracic Surgery* 2014, 97(1):139–146.

Leão T, Utiyama B, Fonseca J, Bock E, Andrade A. "In vitro evaluation of multi-objective physiological control of the centrifugal blood pump". *Artificial Organs* 2020, 00:1–12.

Mehra MR, Goldstein DJ. "Magnetically levitated cardiac pump at 2 years". *The New England Journal of Medicine* 2018, 379:897.

Mehra MR, Goldstein DJ, Uriel N, Cleveland JCJR, Yuzefpolskaya M, Salerno C, Walsh MN, Milano CA, Patel CB, Ewald GA, Itoh A, Dean D, Krishnamoorthy A, Cotts WG, Tatooles AJ, Jorde UP, Bruckner BA, Estep JD, Jeevanandam V, Sayer G, Horstmanshof D, Long JW, Gulati S, Skipper ER, O'Connell JB, Heatley G, Sood P, Naka Y. "MOMENTUM 3 investigators: Two year outcomes with a magnetically levitated cardiac pump in heart failure". *The New England Journal of Medicine* 2018a, 378:1386–1395.

Mehra MR, Salerno C, Cleveland JC, Pinney S, Yuzefpolskaya M, Milano CA, Itoh A, Goldstein DJ, Uriel N, Gulati S, Pagani FD, John R, Adamson R, Bogaev R, Thohan V, Chuang J, Sood P, Goates S, Silvestry SC. "Healthcare resource use and cost implications in the MOMENTUM 3 long-term outcome study". *Circulation* 2018b, 138:1923–1934.

Moscato F et al. "Left ventricle afterload impedance control by an axial flow ventricular assist device: A potential tool for ventricular recovery". *Artificial Organs* 2010, 34:736–744.

Najjar SS, Slaughter MS, Pagani FD, Starling RC, Mcgee EC, Eckman P, Tatooles AJ, Moazami N, Kormos RL, Hathaway DR, Najarian KB, Bhat G, Aaronson KD, Boyce SW. "HVAD bridge to transplant ADVANCE trial investigators: An analysis of pump thrombus events in patients in the HeartWare ADVANCE bridge to transplant and continued access protocol trial". *The Journal of Heart and Lung Transplantation* 2014, 33: 23–34.

Ochsner G. et al. "A physiological controller for turbodynamic ventricular assist devices based on a measurement of the left ventricular volume". *Artificial Organs* 2014, 38(7):527–538.

Ohuchi K et al. "Control strategy for rotary blood pumps". *Artificial Organs* 2001, 25(5):366–370.

Pauls JP et al. "Evaluation of physiological control systems for rotary left ventricular assist devices: An in-vitro study". *Annals of Biomedical Engineering* 2016, 44(8):2377–2387.

Petrou A et al. "A physiological controller for turbodynamic ventricular assist devices based on left ventricular systolic pressure". *Artificial Organs* 2016, 40(9):842–855.

Petrou A et al. "A novel multi-objective physiological control system for rotary left ventricular assist devices". *Annals of Biomedical Engineering* 2017, 45(12):2899–2910.

Petrou A et al. "Standardized comparison of selected physiological controllers for rotary blood pumps: In vitro study". *Artificial Organs* 2018, 42(3):E29–E42.

Saeed O et al. "Blood pressure and adverse events during continuous flow left ventricular assist device support". *Circulation: Heart Failure* 2015, 8(3):551–556.

Salamonsen RF, Mason DG, Ayre PJ. "Response of rotary blood pumps to changes in preload and afterload at a fixed speed setting are unphysiological when compared with the natural heart". *Artificial Organs* 2011, 35:E47–E53.

Santos B. "Controle inteligente embarcado para dispositivos de assistência ventricular", Dissertação de Mestrado - Instituto Federal de Educação, Ciência e Tecnologia São Paulo, campus São Paulo, 2020. doi: 10.13140/RG.2.2.22462.43841.

Santos B, Leão T, Bock, E. "Intelligent control based on Fuzzy logic embedded in FPGA applied in Ventricular Assist Devices (VADs)". *In Proceedings of the 2019 4th International Conference on Robotics, Control and Automation*, New York, 2019, pp. 138–143.

Slaughter MS et al. "Clinical management of continuous- flow left ventricular assist devices in advanced heart failure". *The Journal of Heart and Lung Transplantation* 2010, 29:S1–S39.

Stevens M et al. "Physiological control of dual rotary pumps as a biventricular assist device using a master/slave approach". *Artificial Organs* 2014, 38:766–774.

Tank J et al. "Patients with continuous-flow left ventricular assist devices provide insight in human baroreflex physiology". *Hypertension* 2012, 60 (3): 849–855.

Tchantchaleishvili V et al. "Clinical implications of physiologic flow adjustment in continuous-flow left ventricular assist devices". *ASAIO Journal* 2017, 63(3):241–250.

Uriel N et al. "Development of a novel echocardiography ramp test for speed optimization and diagnosis of device thrombosis in continuous-flow left ventricular assist devices: The Columbia ramp study". *Journal of the American College of Cardiology* 2012, 60:1764–1775.

Uriel N, Sayer G, Addetia K, Fedson S, Kim GH, Rodgers D, Kruse E, Collins K, Adatya S, Sarswat N, Jorde UP, Juricek C, Ota T, Jeevanandam V, Burkhoff D, Lang RM. "Hemodynamic ramp tests in patients with left ventricular assist devices". *JACC: Heart Failure* 2016,4: 208–217.

Uriel N, Colombo PC, Cleveland JC, Long JW, Salerno C, Goldstein DJ, Patel CB, Ewald GA, Tatooles AJ, Silvestry SC, John R, Caldeira C, Jeevanandam V, Boyle AJ, Sundareswaran KS, Sood P, Mehra MR. "Hemocompatibility- related outcomes in the MOMENTUM 3 trial at 6 months: A randomized controlled study of a fully magnetically levitated pump in advanced heart failure". *Circulation* 2017, 135:2003–2012.

Uriel N et al. "Impact of hemodynamic ramp test-guided HVAD speed and medication adjustments on clinical outcomes: The RAMP-IT-UP multicenter study". *Circulation: Heart Failure* 2020, 12(4):e006067.

Vollkron M, et al. "Development of a reliable automatic speed control system for rotary blood pumps". *The Journal of Heart and Lung Transplantation* 2005, 24(11):1878–1885.

Waters T et al. "Motor feedback physiological control for a continuous flow ventricular assist device". *Artificial Organs* 1999, 23(6): 480–486.

Wu Y et al. "A bridge from short-term to long-term left ventricular assist device: Experimental verification of a physiological controller". *Artificial Organs* 2004, 28:927–932.

Wu Y et al. "Modeling, estimation, and control of human circulatory system with a left ventricular assist device". *IEEE Transactions on Control Systems Technology* 2007, 15(4):754–767.

5 Supervisory and Intelligent Systems

Marcelo Barboza, José Ricardo de Sousa Sobrinho,
Jonatas Dias, and Diolino José dos Santos Filho
Polytechnic School of the University of São Paulo

CONTENTS

5.1 INTRODUCTION: BACKGROUND AND DRIVING FORCES

Different implantable biosensors and actuators (e.g., ventricular pressure sensors, left and right VAD, implantable cardioverter defibrillators, and pacemakers) emerge to help therapies in patients with advanced heart failure. Hence, there is a possibility of increased life expectancy and quality through a new concept of customized treatment with integration and collaboration between these devices. A problem arises with that opportunity: integrating these devices into an autonomous and collaborative control system. There are standards for integrating systems in the industry. This chapter will explore a way to build a supervisory system for the VAD control system that, in addition to integrating dispersed devices, can increase safety and even connect the multidisciplinary medical team better to their patients with networked devices.

This chapter is divided into this short introduction and a bibliographic review of the main concepts needed to develop the supervisory system proposed in Section 5.2.

DOI: 10.1201/9781003138358-6

Section 5.3 presents the architecture of a VAD, and Section 5.4 presents a framework for specifying a supervisory system for VAD in the context of Health 4.0. Furthermore, we close this chapter with the conclusion.

5.2 BIBLIOGRAPHIC REVIEW

The development of a supervisory system for VAD requires a review of several issues. In this section, there are reviews for control systems and supervisory systems theory. Furthermore, two new themes are shown: digital transformation and Health 4.0.

5.2.1 CONTROL SYSTEMS THEORY

Structural and behavioral models are the first steps to design a control system. The process of designing the structural model of a control system consists of specifying its parts according to Figure 5.1 (Miyagi 2011).

The behavioral model represents the relationship between the input variables, the variables associated with the internal global state, and the output variables. These behavioral models describe the dynamics of state changes and outputs that describe the desired behavior for a given system over time and may involve events. In a continuous-variable dynamic system (CVDS), the system's behavioral model is the transfer function of that system, exhaustively studied through techniques involving classic and modern control theory (Nise 2002). Nevertheless, in a discrete-event dynamic system (DEDS), there is a logic that establishes the control of these events, resulting in behavior that happens due to these events' occurrence, which can be indeterminate concerning time, as occurs in most cases.

A continuous signal, also called a continuous-time signal, describes phenomena in a continuous-time domain or continuous-time interval. For example, a sine function can represent the response of an ideal pendulum's dynamic behavior, which is described by a continuous signal that varies in amplitude over time and without discontinuities. Even though there are signs with discontinuities at isolated intervals, statistical models over time are used to analyze it (da Costa 2017).

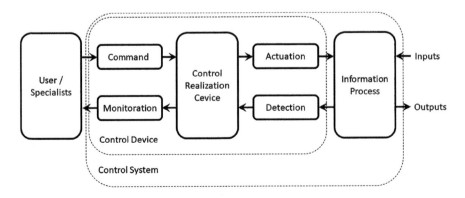

FIGURE 5.1   Structural model of a control system (see Miyagi 2011).

DEDS consists of discrete signals that assume amplitude values between a maximum value and a minimum value. The techniques used in DEDS models do not always depend on the time since the events can be temporal, timeless, or interpreted, from the external environment. Thus, event-driven processes happen with discontinuous signals. They are interpreted as logical signals and can be treated using computer systems. The occurrence of an event determines the change of state, for example, activation of a sensor or an actuator in a physical system (Cassandras and Lafortune 2010).

Based on the characteristics mentioned so far, we can highlight two different classes of systems: (i) CVDS in which all signals are modeled exclusively as continuous signals and (ii) DEDS in which the signals are modeled exclusively as discrete binary or M-ary signals.

A VAD has different subsystems, and each of them can be classified as a Continuous Variable Systems (CVS). Since there is an interaction between these subsystems, a VAD may be classified as a hybrid system, a class of systems that combines time-driven dynamics with event-driven dynamics (Cavalheiro et al. 2011).

The main control strategies used in supervisory systems are as follows: hierarchical, robust, adaptive, excellent, intelligent, among other techniques (Goodwin, Graebe, and Salgado 2001).

Hierarchical control systems carry out supervision through master–slave architectures, where collaboration between controllers at the same hierarchical level is not implemented. An example of a hierarchical control application is ISA'95 itself, shown in Section 5.2.2 (Boston, Antaki, and Simaan 2003).

Robust control is usually proposed to control systems to guarantee high-reliability levels and may have to model uncertainties. The most used technique is the infinite H that will not be covered in this chapter. One of the prominent applications controls loads in a smart grid electrical network (Sinitsyn, Kundu, and Backhaus 2013).

The difference from robust control to adaptive control is that in the latter, the plant changes a function over time and, therefore, the structural model changes too. For this reason, the control must adapt to these changes. It was used for the first time in aerospace applications (Åström 1983).

Optimal control uses numerical methods to minimize a cost function. An example of an application of optimal control is to find the path for a rocket to make its way toward the moon, consuming the least amount of fuel possible (Kirk 2004).

Intelligent control uses artificial intelligence techniques such as fuzzy logic, artificial neural networks, machine learning, or evolutionary computing to determine the control rules that are the most appropriate to promote the dynamic behavior of the system (Krijgsman, Verbruggen, and Rodd 1992).

Among the intelligent control techniques, fuzzy logic has gained popularity in the industry. Its great advantage is the ease of translation for the control system's behavior from the specialist's language through conditions and consequences (Krijgsman, Verbruggen, and Rodd 1992).

Another strategy used to model systems is to consider it an anthropocentric system. Anthropocentric systems are characterized by the intensive interaction between humans and machines (P. Miyagi, Santos Filho, and Arata 2000).

These strategies can be applied alone or together depending on the system's complexity under study and the desired solution.

In general, each subsystem of a VAD can be structured using different control theories. Some of these subsystems are considered dynamic, time-varying, or non-linear systems:

- Dynamic systems: The outputs depend on the input values. The response of the system varies depending on the values entered in the system input. An example is the actuator's speed control loop to deliver the blood pump's adjustment parameters depending on the demand for blood flow.
- Time-varying systems: The system's response is not always the same because, over time, the system's behavior changes. An example is a mechanical wear on the pump's propulsion assembly, or the electrical power supply system, the patient's clinical condition, among others.
- Nonlinear system: It is a system that involves nonlinear modeling or equation. An example is an interaction between the human body, VAD, and adverse events.[1]

5.2.2 Supervisory Control System Architecture

Supervisory systems are control systems used in the most diverse industrial applications to establish communication and supervision levels of the processes that occur in the control object. Industries generally use supervisory systems to (i) integrate local control systems; (ii) remotely control local control systems; (iii) store and concentrate information from lower layers; and (iv) maintain management, alarms, and other process indicators (Daneels and Salter 1999).

By definition, ANSI Standard C37.1 establishes that the supervisory control and data acquisition (SCADA) system has as its primary objective to provide the user with the ability to exercise control over a specific device and confirm its performance according to the targeted action and hierarchy levels. Figure 5.2 shows the functional hierarchy of a supervisory system in accordance with IEC 62264 and ISA'95 standards.

A supervisory hybrid control system is a global monitoring system that combines continuous variables over time and discrete events. According to Cassandras and Lafortune (2010), a hybrid monitoring and control system, according to Figure 5.3, represents the architecture of these systems (Cassandras and Lafortune 2010).

In the last years, the demand for faster and customized products pressured the classical theory of supervisory systems for collaboration between devices. The industry has undergone a transformation; as a result, old standards were revised and new models were created.

---

[1] Adverse events: The use of ventricular assist devices (VADs) to treat heart failure exposes the patient to adverse events (AEs) that can progress to severe complications and increase the patient's risk of death. According to the U.S. Food and Drug Administration, (FDA) an AE is any undesirable occurrence associated using a medical product on a patient (Food and Drug Administration 2016).

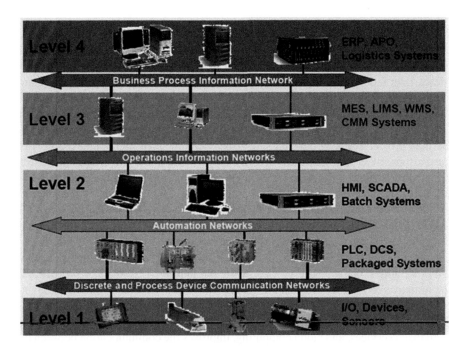

FIGURE 5.2   Reference for hierarchical integration architecture model of ISA'95 (see Nagorny, Colombo, and Schmidtmann 2012).

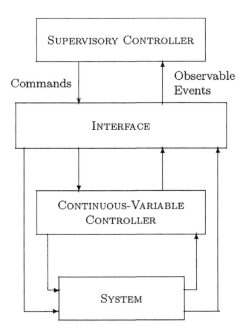

FIGURE 5.3   Conceptual architecture of the hybrid monitoring and control system (see Cassandras and Lafortune 2010).

5.2.3 DIGITAL TRANSFORMATION

Industry 4.0 (I4.0) refers to the fourth industrial revolution or the digital transformation in the industry. For the first time, it was used at the 2011 Hannover Messe International, an exhibition that takes place annually in Central Germany (Kagermann, Wahlster, and Helbig 2013).

In 2013, the German government created the *Plattform Industrie* 4.0 project. Germany's goal was to prepare its industry to lead the next phase of innovation. The German project seeks to develop small and medium-sized manufacturing companies, a robust German industrial sector. *Plattform Industrie* 4.0 creates standards, encourages tests, and funds academic research (Kagermann, Wahlster, and Helbig 2013).

Since then, institutions have created other initiatives all over the world. In the United States, the movement is called the industrial Internet of things. It differs from the German initiative. It was created by a consortium of companies, prioritizing commercial technologies and products and encompassing other applications such as aircraft engines, connected cars, and the health industry (Presher 2015). In Brazil, the initiative calls advanced manufacturing (Ministério da Ciência, Tecnologia and Ministério da Indústria 2016).

I4.0, using Internet of Things (IoT) technologies, cyber-physical systems (CPSs), virtualized services, and cloud computing, improves the communication between the resources present in the smart factory in order to meet the demands of consumers in an individual and personalized way (Pisching 2018).

With the use of CPS and IoT on the shop floor, companies will be able to deploy global networks in order to increase collaboration and integration between machines with the sharing of knowledge, skills, and competencies (Kagermann, Wahlster, and Helbig 2013).

In I4.0, connected machines make a collaborative community, which implies using computational tools to process data and transform it into information systematically. In this context, business models will also change. Today, the industry is predominantly product-oriented. This technological revolution will change the context for service orientation (Lee, Kao, and Yang 2014).

The second and third industrial revolutions sought efficiency and cost reduction, mainly through a sizeable standardized production. To meet consumer demands individually and in a customized way (Brettel et al. 2014), I4.0 needs to approach problems differently. Two critical paradigms that started in the fourth industrial revolution are autonomy and decision distribution (Pisching 2018).

This new approach in the production system forces products and equipment to have individual identifiers with information about their history, current situation, and alternative routes. Consequently, the resources of an assembly line and the products communicate during the manufacturing process. In this context, other manufacturing units, even in distant locations, exchange information about the purchasing, sales, logistics, inventory systems, and the production processes themselves. Thus, I4.0 will create collaborative service networks between companies, converging to a closer relationship between the real and the virtual world (Pisching 2018; Kagermann, Wahlster, and Helbig 2013).

To integrate different management systems, the International Society of Automation (ISA) developed, in 1990, the international standard ISA'95/IEC 62264 and proposed a reference architecture model. This standard aims to reduce risk, cost, and errors by implementing interfaces between management systems. ISA'95/IEC 62264 provides a hierarchical organization for the production system (Garcia et al. 2018; Nagorny, Colombo, and Schmidtmann 2012; Pessoa 2015).

With I4.0, the need for integration was much more significant, not only for management systems. Each device can have a different interface. Therefore, *Plattform Industrie* 4.0 proposed a new reference architecture model.

5.2.4 RAMI 4.0

RAMI 4.0 is a Reference Architecture Model for Industry 4.0. It was presented at Hannover Messe International in 2015 (Adolphs et al. 2015). *Plattform Industrie* 4.0 created the reference architecture RAMI 4.0, shown in Figure 5.4. This architecture has three axes (Pisching 2018):

1. Axis of hierarchical levels that goes from product to connected world.

    It is the axis on the right as shown in Figure 5.4. IEC 62264/ISA'95 hierarchy levels in the industry are based on this axis. It represents the sectors of the industry that need to integrate their control systems. It considers industrial processes, automation, and industry management. Four hierarchical levels taken from ISA'95 presented in Figure 5.2 are adopted: "company," "work center," "station," and "control device." Even so, three more

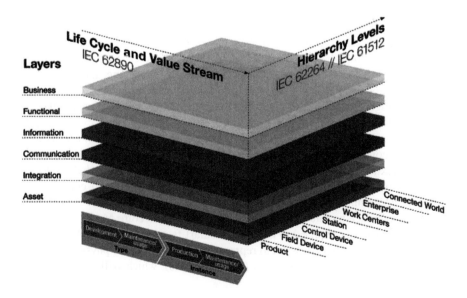

FIGURE 5.4   Reference Architecture Model Industrie 4.0 (RAMI 4.0) (see Adolphs et al. 2015).

hierarchical levels to support the digital transformation in the industry are as follows: "field device," "product," and "connected world."

2. Layers of information flow.

    This axis has six layers that describe the component from the information in the physical asset to its virtual representation. According to Figure 5.4, its layers are as follows: "technical asset," "integration," "communication," "information," "functional," and "business rule."

3. Life cycle axis and product value chain.

    The left axis of Figure 5.4 is used to manage the life cycle of entities. According to RAMI 4.0, entities can be parts, products, devices, machines, and even plants. This axis is based on the IEC 62890 standard.

5.2.5 HEALTH 4.0

Personalized health is the central concept of the European initiative Horizon 2020, which provides guidelines for research and funding (Comissão Europeia 2020). The heterogeneity of patients' reactions to diseases suggests that prevention and treatment strategies should be adapted or customized according to the biochemical, physiological, environmental, and behavioral profile unique to each individual (Goetz and Schork 2018). Health 4.0 appears to meet these requirements.

In order to increase the efficiency of health services, improve quality of life, increase patient survival, and develop new business models in the sector, some studies have used Health 4.0 technologies (Islam et al. 2015; Demiris 2016; El Saddik 2018; Cavallone and Palumbo 2020; Sharp, Jacks, and Hockfield 2016; Ilin, Iliyaschenko, and Konradi 2018).

Health 4.0 is a strategic health concept based on Industry 4.0 (I4.0). Since the main focus of I4.0 is to establish mass customization, this causes an affinity with Health 4.0 that seeks to meet each patient's nosological identity reliably. In this context, Health 4.0 aims to ensure the implementation of personalized medicine through technologies such as the IoT, the Internet of services, the capacity to process and use a large amount of data, cloud computing, machine learning, and blockchain. These technologies make it possible to develop artificial intelligence solutions to provide knowledge and analysis of many patients' medical data (Ilin, Iliyaschenko, and Konradi 2018).

A German institution called *Plattform Industrie* 4.0 promotes I4.0, and its focus is to serve a consumer who increasingly wants customized products in small batches. In this context, intelligent and integrated machines throughout the global production chain can autonomously exchange information, trigger actions, and control themselves (Kagermann, Wahlster, and Helbig 2013).

A new reference architecture model, Reference Architecture Model for Industry 4.0 (RAMI 4.0), was required to meet these smart factories' needs. RAMI 4.0 was created by *Plattform Industrie* 4.0 to represent, in addition to the physical structure, the digital structure of these systems (Pisching 2018), which will be presented in Section 5.2.4.

5.3   ARCHITECTURE OF A VAD CONTROL SYSTEM

The VAD can be partially implantable, which requires a connection between the internal environment and the external environment using a data and electrical power cable known as driveline, or fully implantable. The devices currently sold are partially implanted, and their configurations consist of (i) intracorporeal elements: blood pump, cannulas, and actuator; and (ii) extracorporeal elements: local controller and batteries (Han and Trumble 2019).

The motor, usually brushless direct current (BLDC) electric motor, is magnetically coupled to the blood pump rotor. The most basic control loop must ensure that the coupling occurs correctly and adjust the motor signal. The pump rotation remains at the reference speed, regardless of variations in the load (Stevens et al. 2018). In some VAD control systems, the device operates at a fixed rotation, and the multidisciplinary medical team is responsible for adjusting the reference rotation according to the patient's clinical conditions (Al Omari et al. 2013).

Some papers have studied the effect of the variation in VAD rotation. Jung et al., after a randomized study with 19 patients, suggest that the automatic increase in the rotation of the VAD during mild exercises may contribute to the increase in quality of life (Jung et al. 2017). Gross et al. concluded that VAD with fixed rotation provides, at best, sufficient cardiac output only for low-intensity activities (Gross et al. 2019). The same group, in another article, concluded that although we do not fully know the impacts of the increase of VAD rotation, doing so resulted in greater cardiac output, making evident the need to design a customized physiological control system for the specific needs of each patient (Gross et al. 2020).

A larger mesh, called physiological control, automatically adjusts the rotation reference. This control enables faster rotation changes in response to changes in the circulatory system's behavior. The purpose of this layer of the controller covers one or more controlled variables (parameters of the device or circulatory system) and their respective reference values to ensure adequate cardiac demand to the patient. Control engineering techniques are then used to keep the variables controlled according to the patient's specifications (which can be constant or vary over time), automatically adjusting the rotation reference (Stevens et al. 2018).

Physiological control requires implantable sensors or estimators to monitor hemodynamic quantities. Although many control system developers have avoided implantable sensors to avoid rejection and other problems, these have been widely studied, and some are already in clinical trials (Brancato et al. 2016; Dual et al. 2019, 2020; Hubbert et al. 2017; Neto et al. 2020; Staufert and Hierold 2016; Stephens et al. 2020; Veenis, Birim, and Brugts 2019). Some studies also present cases in which VADs were implanted in patients with pacemakers or implantable cardioverter defibrillators. Other devices with other control systems compete with each other and with the patient's native control systems (Harris et al. 2017; Kooij et al. 2019; Parker et al. 2020; Vakil et al. 2016).

Figure 5.5 presents the structural model of the local control system of a VAD, according to Stevens et al. (2018).

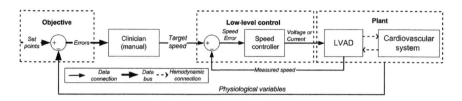

FIGURE 5.5 Structural model of a VAD control system (see Stevens et al. 2018).

The elements of this model are "objective," "physiological controller," "speed controller," and "VAD." The "objective" depends on the specification of the control system. To increase the patient's quality and life expectancy, customizing the control system is necessary. Hence, the objectives must be customized for each patient. The "physiological controller" is responsible for compensating the speed set point's value depending on the error of the variable or the objective physiological variables. The "speed controller" controls the engine speed of the "VAD," which interacts with the "cardiovascular system."

The need for remote monitoring by the multidisciplinary medical team and the opportunity for collaboration between dispersed devices are indicative of the need for a supervisory control system to integrate control systems. It has to provide an interface that monitors clinical parameters, operates the device, and sets adjustment commands for local control, database feeding, and the global control loop management.

Another application of a supervisory system for VAD can be used to treat and mitigate failures in the system. Cavalheiro (2013) proposed a hierarchical supervisory control system considering the VAD as a hybrid system for diagnosing and treating failures as shown in Figure 5.6.

In the supervisory system proposed by Cavalheiro (2013), the security control system is a layer of control that manages local control in case of failure. Cavalheiro created the behavioral model for the failures using risk analysis techniques that involved interviews with a multidisciplinary team.

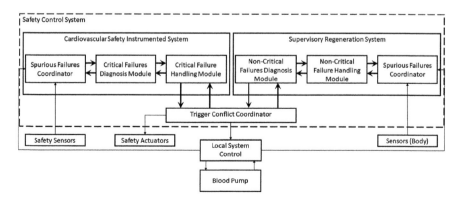

FIGURE 5.6 Architecture of the security control system for VAD (see Cavalheiro 2013).

5.3.1 CYBER-PHYSICAL VAD DEFINITION

Digitization, currently present in all economic, social, health, industry, and education, transforms the real world into a binary model of zeros and ones. Addressing the digital issue involves talking about numbers, as a considerable amount of data has been produced in recent years. Digital technology led to changes in the media at first, with a significant impact on information technology. Based on the idealization proposed by Norbert Wiener in 1948, when he coined the term cybernetics, combined with the creation of the ARPANET network in 1969, a precursor to the current Internet, digitization sowed a vast technological field such as IoT, big data, cloud computing, additive manufacturing, artificial intelligence, and advanced robotics. These technologies permeated all knowledge areas, causing multiple economic and social transformations (Meyer, Schaupp, and Seibt 2019).

The adhesion of digitalization to the productive environment resulted in the concept of Industry 4.0, about what would be called the fourth industrial revolution. This concept has become a new production paradigm, promoting the junction of the real and virtual world by creating CPSs, making it possible using several integrated technologies, which we can call 4.0 technologies. The impact of applying this concept to the industry goes beyond gains on the factory floor, as it allows for shortening production times, making production lines more flexible, as well as the cycle for launching new products on the market and allows companies to integrate into global value-adding chains (Auer and Kalyan 2020; Anand and Kumar 2020).

A great example of trade-off in the industry of yore was mass customization; a conflict between the scale of production and personalization; the materialization of this concept in the industry manages to unite this antagonism in a harmonic and common point, since the flexibility of the production lines allows high production with customization.

The term Industry 4.0 is also related to the integration of the production system with networks of suppliers in the supply chain and other industries. This concept is based on integrating dynamic value creation networks, supported by substructures supported by sensors, machines, workstations, and information technology that structure intelligent and communicative systems, supported by the Internet, also called CPSs (Auer and Kalyan 2020).

Therefore, a cyber-physical VAD consists of the hardware and software for control and supervision that are embedded or remote. A cyber-physical VAD is monitored, controlled, and simulated remotely. It also has a degree of autonomy to react with minor changes in the patient's hemodynamics or the environment. For this, the cyber-physical VAD uses IoT and Health 4.0 technologies and paradigms.

5.4 VAD SUPERVISORY SYSTEM

A proposal for the development of the architecture of the reconfigurable hybrid physiological control system framework must begin with the presentation of its structure model. Firstly, the structure model will first be presented using ISA'95/IEC 62264 as a reference to understand better. Finally, the model is translated to RAMI 4.0 standard in Section 5.4.2.

5.4.1 Architecture Model for Supervisory System for VAD

The Architecture Model of the Reconfigurable Hybrid Physiological Control System (AMRHPCS) of the patient with VAD consists of four interrelated layers. This model allows the multidisciplinary medical team to configure or reconfigure the customized system architecture to accommodate intrapatient or interpatient variations. AMRHPCS is presented in Figure 5.7.

The first layer is shown in Figure 5.8 and represents the patient. A model of the patient was considered in order to control his survival. This model must contain at least the elements "adverse events" and "implantable/virtual sensors." The "implantable/virtual sensors" are the monitors prescribed by the multidisciplinary medical team, implanted in the patient or estimated from their data, and will provide information to the rest of the control system. The "adverse events" represent the unwanted effects caused by the therapy that can change with the control system's reconfigurations. The patient's digital representation for storing all pre-implant information, digital medical records, and post-implant VAD data will be treated in Section 5.4.2.

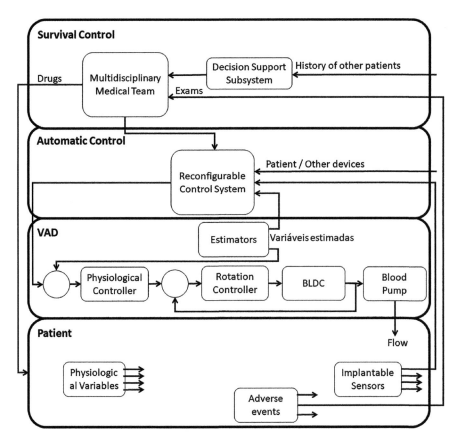

FIGURE 5.7 Reconfigurable hybrid physiological control system model for a patient with a VAD.

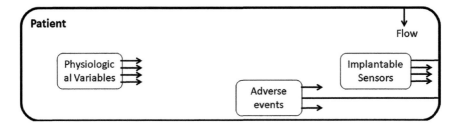

FIGURE 5.8 First layer of the reconfigurable hybrid physiological control system model, patient.

The multidisciplinary medical team considers the patient's diagnosis must specify the monitored and stored physiological variables.

The second layer represents the VAD prescribed by the multidisciplinary medical team. As a CVS (Miyagi 2011), the VAD structure was modeled as a CVS in Figure 5.9. Although this block is dependent on the VAD prescribed by the multidisciplinary medical team, the structure found in the most recent research has a blood pump, engine, speed controller, physiological controller, and estimators (Leao et al. 2020; Stevens et al. 2018).

The objective or multiple objectives and their respective references of the physiological controller depend on the multidisciplinary medical team's prescription, the device, and the patient. The elements of this layer are "physiological controller," "estimators," "speed controller," "BLDC," and "blood pump." The "physiological controller" is responsible for compensating the speed's set point value depending on the variable's error or physiological variables. The "estimators" are a set of calculations and formulas that estimate physiological variables such as flow, pressure, heart rate, the opening of the aortic valve, according to the current and rotation of the VAD motor. The "speed controller" controls the rotation of the "BLDC," which through a magnetic coupling rotates the "blood pump" rotor.

The requirements for automatic adjustment of the physiological controller set point, communication with other devices, and a reconfiguration interface with a multidisciplinary medical team create the third layer's need, as shown in Figure 5.10. The "automatic control" layer connects to the "VAD" layer. It has a digital representation to be accessed by the "multidisciplinary medical team" treated in Section 5.4.2. The "reconfigurable control system" is the element that defines the set point (s) of

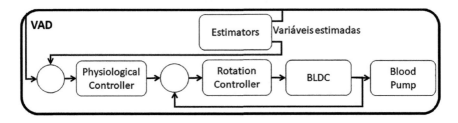

FIGURE 5.9 Second layer of the reconfigurable hybrid physiological control system model, VAD.

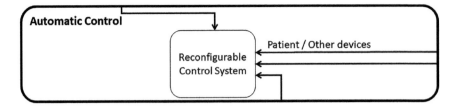

FIGURE 5.10   Third layer of the reconfigurable hybrid physiological control system model, automatic control.

the physiological variable (s) and receives information from "implantable/virtual sensors," "other devices," and "estimators." According to each patient's needs, the "reconfigurable control system" element is reconfigured by the multidisciplinary medical team, changing the control system's behavior (Figure 5.10).

This proposal values the interaction between the multidisciplinary medical team on VAD control systems to specify/prescribe a set of devices and behaviors that best suit the patient or remotely monitor the patient's evolution and the interaction between the device and patient. Subsequently, the system must be considered an anthropocentric system with the multidisciplinary medical team at the system's center.

The multidisciplinary medical team is dispersed. It is distant from the other layers of the control system and only connects when necessary. The element that represents the multidisciplinary medical team is the main element of the "survival control" layer. This layer, shown in Figure 5.11, is responsible for controlling the patient's survival. The "multidisciplinary medical team" can prescribe "drugs" based on data from "exams." The "multidisciplinary medical team" can also reconfigure the behavior of the reconfigurable hybrid physiological control system by modifying its association functions, as well as the heuristic rules of "automatic control," and can count on the help of a "decision support subsystem." Changing the behavioral model makes it possible to customize the control and validate the control system's behavior using the Bayesian inductive probability.

This model was built using the ISA'95/IEC 62264 architecture model and therefore inherits its limitations. One of the limitations is that the multidisciplinary medical team is dispersed, and this model does not adequately support this representation. The second limitation is integrating agents from different manufacturers, being in

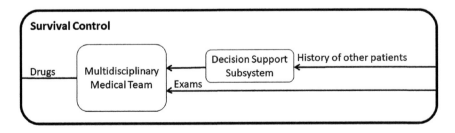

FIGURE 5.11   Fourth layer of the reconfigurable hybrid physiological control system model, survival control.

different locations, and using different technologies. Translate it into RAMI 4.0 going to meet these requirements.

5.4.2   RAMI 4.0 in the Health Context 4.0

As seen in Section 5.2.4, RAMI 4.0 was developed by *Plattform Industrie* 4.0 to digitally represent technical assets, manage its life cycle, and facilitate the integration of dispersed elements in the global manufacturing industry chain. These requirements are standard in the context of Health 4.0 and in the development of AMRHPCS.

As previously presented, the "patient" and "automatic control" layers must have digital representations. The patient's digital representation can be called a digital twin according to the I4.0/S4.0 nomenclature and must store pre-implant information, digital medical records, and post-implant VAD data. The "automatic control" layer must have a digital representation so that it is possible for the multidisciplinary medical team, which is a dispersed element, to assess the patient from a distance. The complete structural model of the reconfigurable hybrid physiological control system, as presented, does not have a digital representation of the layers yet. One of the tools used to achieve this representation is RAMI 4.0.

Figure 5.12 presents the structural model of the VAD + patient set of the architecture model of the hybrid control system of a VAD. The assets are the elements "patient" and "VAD." The layers of integration and communication are used to transfer information. In the information layer, there are three elements. "Patient data/

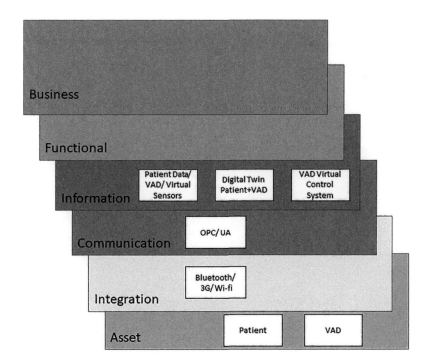

FIGURE 5.12   Structural model of the first part of AMRHPCS using RAMI 4.0.

VAD/implantable sensors/virtual sensors" is a database that stores the historical data of all these elements. "Digital twin of the patient-VAD" is an element responsible for storing pre-implant data and for formulating a model of patient behavior.

The "VAD virtual control system" is responsible for making reconfigurations in the technical asset "VAD." Behavioral changes, like a new heuristic rule. Structural changes, like routing an implantable sensor via Bluetooth.

The second part's structural model, or the second AMRHPCS administration shell using RAMI 4.0, is shown in Figure 5.13. This is the administration shell of the "implantable sensors" and the "virtual sensors."

The third AMRHPCS administration shell is necessary to integrate the multidisciplinary medical team with the control system. With the support of the "decision support subsystem" and through "automatic control," the "multidisciplinary medical team" can reconfigure the structure and behavior of the reconfigurable hybrid physiological control system and personalize it for the assisted patient (Figure 5.14).

The different administration shells can communicate through the "functional" layer or the "communication" layer. The "functional" layer must use communication between elements of this layer and route communications through the "communication" layer, via the Internet. The "communication" layer can be used for communication between "implantable sensors" and the VAD if this communication has already been routed previously. The flow of information between the information shells is shown in Figure 5.15.

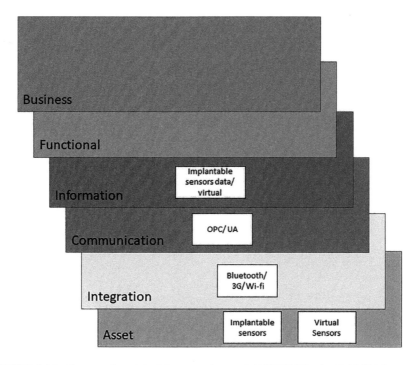

FIGURE 5.13   Structural model of the second part of AMRHPCS using RAMI 4.0.

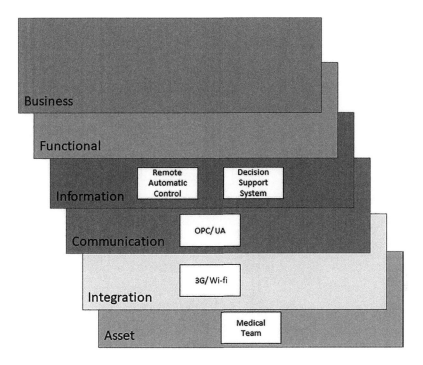

FIGURE 5.14   Structural model of the third part of AMRHPCS using RAMI 4.0.

5.4.3   The Behavioral Model of a VAD's Supervisory System

The system's behavioral model will be distributed in the local control systems and in "remote automatic control." Chapter 4 of this book covered the local control system's behavior, so the focus here will be on the programmed behavior into the "reconfigurable control system."

The multidisciplinary medical team needs to prescribe the system's behaviors through conditions and consequences. Therefore, "remote automatic control" must be programmable in fuzzy logic.

The "remote automatic control" must be remote. It must allow the multidisciplinary medical team to access it from anywhere and the system to work with the new behavior even from a distance.

The fuzzy logic can be hosted on the same hardware as the local control system. In this case, "remote automatic control" will be an interface that receives and stores data and transfers the fuzzy code to the local control system.

5.5   CONCLUSION

The new challenges in developing a VAD, such as remote telemetry, new biosensors, and other control systems working together with the VAD, and the need to customize the control system to better deal with adverse events place integration problems in the control system of the VAD.

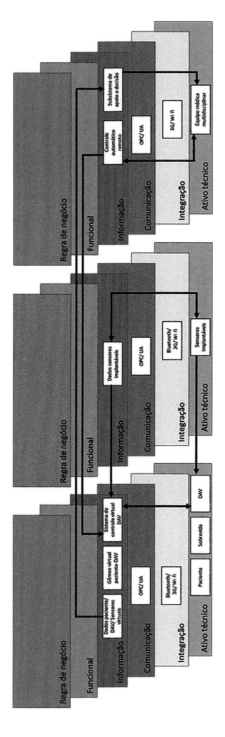

FIGURE 5.15   Information flow between AMRHPCS information shells.

Supervisory systems have been used in the industry for decades to integrate information at various levels. In the last years, with digital transformation, techniques have been developed to meet the new requirements.

In this chapter, the concept of Health 4.0 and a specification for a supervisory system to integrate the VAD control system were presented. The proposed supervisory system takes into account the patient and the multidisciplinary medical team that assists him. The proposal uses the concept of anthropocentric control to place the multidisciplinary medical team as responsible for specifying the monitoring and performance devices necessary for the best therapy of the patient, as well as specifying the behavior of the autonomous control system.

REFERENCES

Adolphs, Peter, Heinz Bedenbender, Dagmar Dirzus, Martin Ehlich, Ulrich Epple, Martin Hankel, Roland Heidel, et al. 2015. "Reference Architecture Model Industrie 4.0 (RAMI4.0)." Frankfurt am Main, Alemanha: ZVEI – German Electrical and Electronic. https://www.zvei.org/fileadmin/user_upload/Presse_und_Medien/Publikationen/2016/januar/GMA_Status_Report__Reference_Archtitecture_Model_Industrie_4.0__RAMI_4.0_/GMA-Status-Report-RAMI-40-July-2015.pdf.

Al Omari, Abdul-akeem H., Andrey V. Savkin, Michael Stevens, David G. Mason, Daniel L. Timms, Robert F. Salamonsen, and Nigel H. Lovell. 2013. "Developments in control systems for rotary left ventricular assist devices for heart failure patients: A review." *Physiological Measurement* 34 (1): R1–27. doi: 10.1088/0967-3334/34/1/R1.

Anand, Nayyar, and Akshi Kumar, eds. 2020. A Roadmap to Industry 4.0: Smart production, sharp business and sustainable development. In: *Advances in Science, Technology & Innovation.* Cham: Springer International Publishing. doi: 10.1007/978-3-030-14544-6.

Åström, Karl Johan. 1983. "Theory and applications of adaptive control-A survey." *Automatica* 19 (5): 471–86. doi: 10.1016/0005-1098(83)90002-X.

Auer, Michael E., and Ram B. Kalyan, eds. 2020. *Cyber-Physical Systems and Digital Twins,* Vol. 80. Lecture Notes in Networks and Systems. Cham: Springer International Publishing. doi: 10.1007/978-3-030-23162-0.

Boston, J. Robert, James F. Antaki, and Marwan A. Simaan. 2003. "Hierarchical control of heart-assist devices." *IEEE Robotics & Automation Magazine* 10 (1): 54–64. doi: 10.1109/MRA.2003.1191711.

Brancato, Luigi, Grim Keulemans, Tom Verbelen, Bart Meyns, and Robert Puers. 2016. "An implantable intravascular pressure sensor for a ventricular assist device." *Micromachines* 7 (8): 135. doi: 10.3390/mi7080135.

Brettel, Malte, Niklas Friederichsen, Michael Keller, and Marius Rosenberg. 2014. "How virtualization, decentralization and network building change the manufacturing landscape: An Industry 4.0 perspective." *International Journal of Information and Communication Engineering* 8 (1):37–44. doi:10.1999/1307-6892/9997144.

Cassandras, Christos G., and Stéphane Lafortune. 2010. Introduction to discrete-event simulation. *Introduction to Discrete Event Systems,* 2nd ed. Boston: Springer Science & Business Media. doi: 10.1007/978-0-387-68612-7_10.

Cavalheiro, André César Martins. 2013. "Sistema de controle para diagnóstico e tratamento de falhas em Dispositivos de Assistência Ventricular." São Paulo: Escola Politécnica da Universidade de São Paulo. https://teses.usp.br/teses/disponiveis/3/3152/tde-19092014-102819/pt-br.php.

Cavalheiro, André, Diolino José Santos Fo, Aron Andrade, José Roberto Cardoso, Osvaldo Horikawa, Eduardo Bock, and Jeison Fonseca. 2011. "Specification of supervisory control systems for ventricular assist devices." *Artificial Organs* 35 (5): 465–70. doi: 10.1111/j.1525-1594.2011.01267.x.

Cavallone, Mauro, and Rocco Palumbo. 2020. "Debunking the Myth of Industry 4.0 in health care: Insights from a systematic literature review." *The TQM Journal* (ahead-of-print). doi: 10.1108/TQM-10-2019-0245.

Comissão Europeia. 2020. "Horizon 2020 - Health, demographic change and wellbeing | horizon 2020." https://ec.europa.eu/programmes/horizon2020/en/h2020-section/health-demographic-change-and-wellbeing.

da Costa, Cesar. 2017. *Processamento de sinais para engenheiros: teoria e pratica*, 1ª Edição. Rio de Janeiro: Bonecker. https://www.travessa.com.br/processamento-de-sinais-para-engenheiros-teoria-e-pratica-1-ed-2017/artigo/8f59b998-ba3f-4a3e-976a-e28e17a52bac?pcd=041.

Daneels, A., and W. Salter. 1999. "What is scada?" *In International Conference on Accelerator and Large Experimental Physics Control Systems*, Trieste, Italy.

Demiris, George 2016. *Consumer Health Informatics: Past, Present, and Future of a Rapidly Evolving Domain*. doi: 10.15265/IYS-2016-s005.

Dual, Seraina Anne, Jan Michael Zimmermann, Jürg Neuenschwander, Nicholas Heinrich Cohrs, Natalia Solowjowa, Wendelin Jan Stark, Mirko Meboldt, and Marianne Schmid Daners. 2019. "Ultrasonic sensor concept to fit a ventricular assist device cannula evaluated using geometrically accurate heart phantoms." *Artificial Organs* 43(5): 467–77. doi: 10.1111/aor.13379.

Dual, Seraina, Byron Llerena Zambrano, Simon Sündermann, Nikola Cesarovic, Mareike Kron, Konstantinos Magkoutas, Julian Hengsteler, et al. 2020. "Continuous heart volume monitoring by fully implantable soft strain sensor." *Advanced Healthcare Materials*. doi: 10.1002/adhm.202000855.

Food and Drugs Administration. 2016. "What is a serious adverse event?" https://www.fda.gov/safety/reporting-serious-problems-fda/what-serious-adverse-event.

Garcia, Marcelo, Edurne Irisarri, Federico Perez, Marga Marcos, and Elisabet Estevez. 2018. "From ISA 88/95 meta-models to an OPC UA-based development tool for CPPS under IEC 61499." *In IEEE International Workshop on Factory Communication Systems: Proceedings, WFCS*, 2018 June 1–9. Institute of Electrical and Electronics Engineers Inc. doi: 10.1109/WFCS.2018.8402362.

Goetz, Laura., and Nicholas Schork. 2018. "Personalized medicine: Motivation, challenges, and progress." *Fertility and Sterility*, Elsevier Inc. doi: 10.1016/j.fertnstert.2018.05.006.

Goodwin, Graham Clifford, Stefan F. Graebe, and Mario E. Salgado. 2001. *Control System Design*. Michigan: Prentice Hall. https://books.google.com.br/books?hl=pt-BR&id=7dNSAAAAMAAJ&dq=Control+System+Design&focus=searchwithinvolume&q=intelligent.

Gross, Christoph, Christiane Marko, Johann Mikl, Johann Altenberger, Thomas Schlöglhofer, Heinrich Schima, Daniel Zimpfer, and Francesco Moscato. 2019. "LVAD pump flow does not adequately increase with exercise." *Artificial Organs* 43 (3): 222–28. doi: 10.1111/aor.13349.

Gross, Christoph, Heinrich Schima, Thomas Schlöglhofer, Kamen Dimitrov, Martin Maw, Julia Riebandt, Dominik Wiedemann, Daniel Zimpfer, and Francesco Moscato. 2020. "Continuous LVAD monitoring reveals high suction rates in clinically stable outpatients." *Artificial Organs* 44 (7): E251–62. doi: 10.1111/aor.13638.

Han, Jooli, and Dennis Trumble. 2019. "Cardiac assist devices: Early concepts, current technologies, and future innovations." *Bioengineering* 6 (1): 18. doi: 10.3390/bioengineering6010018.

Harris, Jill, Stephen Carlson, Aaron M. Wolfson, Leslie A. Saxon, and Rahul N. Doshi. 2017. "Pulmonary arterial pressure sensing in a patient with left ventricular assist device during ventricular arrhythmia." *HeartRhythm Case Reports* 3 (7): 348–51. doi: 10.1016/j.hrcr.2017.05.002.

Hubbert, Laila, Jacek Baranowski, Baz Delshad, and Henrik Ahn. 2017. "Left atrial pressure monitoring with an implantable wireless pressure sensor after implantation of a left ventricular assist device." *ASAIO Journal* 63 (5): e60–65. doi: 10.1097/MAT.0000000000000451.

Ilin, Igor, Oksana Iliyaschenko, and Alexandra Konradi. 2018. "Business model for smart hospital health organization." *SHS Web of Conferences* 44 (June): 00041. doi: 10.1051/shsconf/20184400041.

Islam, Riazul, Daehan Kwak, Humaun Kabir, Mahmud Hossain, and Kyung Sup Kwak. 2015. "The internet of things for health care: A comprehensive survey." *IEEE Access* 3 (June): 678–708. doi: 10.1109/ACCESS.2015.2437951.

Jung, Mette Holme, Brian Houston, Stuart D. Russell, and Finn Gustafsson. 2017. "Pump speed modulations and sub-maximal exercise tolerance in left ventricular assist device recipients: A double-blind, randomized trial." *The Journal of Heart and Lung Transplantation* 36 (1): 36–41. doi: 10.1016/J.HEALUN.2016.06.020.

Kagermann, Henning, Wolfgang Wahlster, and Johannes Helbig. 2013. "Recommendations for implementing the strategic initiative INDUSTRIE 4.0: Final report of the Industrie 4.0 working group." Berlin: Acatech. http://www.acatech.de/fileadmin/user_upload/Baumstruktur_nach_Website/Acatech/root/de/Material_fuer_Sonderseiten/Industrie_4.0/Final_report__Industrie_4.0_accessible.pdf.

Kirk, Donald. 2004. *Optimal Control Theory: An Introduction*. Mineola, New York: Englewood Cliffs. https://books.google.com.br/books?hl=pt-BR&lr=&id=fCh2SAtWIdwC&oi=fnd&pg=PA1&dq=control+theory&ots=xyeBYj33fY&sig=JTZf-EmTPcsaiXrJNQdFcmYyuhs#v=onepage&q=control+theory&f=false.

Kooij, Cezane, Yunus Yalcin, Dominic Theuns, Alina Constantinescu, Jasper Brugts, Olivier Manintveld, Sing-Chien. Yap, Tamas Szili-Torok, Ad Bogers, and Koray Caliskan. 2019. "Prevalence of electromagnetic interference from left ventricular assist devices in patients with implantable cardioverter defibrillator/pacemakers." *European Heart Journal* 40 (Supplement_1). doi: 10.1093/eurheartj/ehz746.0378.

Krijgsman, Ardjan, Henk Verbruggen, and Michael Rodd. 1992. "Intelligent control: Theory and applications." *IFAC Proceedings Volumes* 25 (6): 57–67. doi: 10.1016/s1474-6670(17)50881-2.

Leao, Tarcisio, Bruno Utiyama, Jeison Fonseca, Eduardo Bock, and Aron Andrade. 2020. "In vitro evaluation of multi-objective physiological control of the centrifugal blood pump." *Artificial Organs*. doi: 10.1111/aor.13639.

Lee, Jay, Hung-An Kao, and Shanhu Yang. 2014. "Service innovation and smart analytics for Industry 4.0 and big data environment." *Procedia CIRP* 16 (January): 3–8. doi: 10.1016/J.PROCIR.2014.02.001.

Meyer, Uli, Simon Schaupp, and David Seibt, eds. 2019. *Digitalization in Industry: Between Domination and Emancipation*. Switzerland: Palgrave Macmillan. https://www.amazon.com.br/Digitalization-Industry-Between-Domination-Emancipation-ebook/dp/B081KZBNL4.

Ministério da Ciência, Tecnologia, Inovações e Comunicações, and Comércio Exterior e Serviços Ministério da Indústria. 2016. "Perspectivas de Especialistas Brasileiros Sobre a Manufatura Avançada No Brasil: Um Relato de Workshops Realizados Em Sete Capitais Brasileiras Em Contraste Com as Experiências Internacionais." Brasilia, Brasil: Ministério da Ciência, Tecnologia, Inovações e Comunicações. http://www.abinee.org.br/informac/arquivos/maavmdic.pdf.

Miyagi, Paulo Eigi, D. J. Santos Filho, and W. M. Arata. 2000. "Design of deadlock avoidance compensators for anthropocentric production systems." *In IFIP - The International Federation for Information Processing IFIP*. Berlin, Germany. doi: 10.1007/978-0-387-35529-0.

Miyagi, Paulo Eigi. 2011. *Controle Programável*, 1ª Edição. São Paulo: Edgard Blucher.

Nagorny, Kevin, Armando Walter Colombo, and Uwe Schmidtmann. 2012. "A service- and multi-agent-oriented manufacturing automation architecture: An IEC 62264 level 2 compliant implementation." *Computers in Industry* 63 (8): 813–23. doi: 10.1016/j.compind.2012.08.003.

Neto, Silvestre Silva, José Ricardo Sousa Sobrinho, Cesar da Costa, Tarcisio Fernandes Leão, Sergio Augusto Senra, Eduardo Guy Perpétuo Bock, Givanildo Alves dos Santos, et al. 2020. "Investigation of MEMS as accelerometer sensor in an implantable centrifugal blood pump prototype." *Journal of the Brazilian Society of Mechanical Sciences and Engineering* 42 (9): 487. doi: 10.1007/s40430-020-02560-7.

Nise, Norman S. 2002. *Engenharia de Sistemas de Controle*, 3ª Edição. Rio de Janeiro, RJ: LTC Editora. https://www.amazon.com.br/Engenharia-Sistemas-Controle-Norman-Nise/dp/8521621353.

Parker, Alex M., Juan R. Vilaro, Juan M. Aranda, Mohammad Al-Ani, Phillip George, and Mustafa M. Ahmed. 2020. "Leadless pacemaker use in a patient with a durable left ventricular assist device." *Pacing and Clinical Electrophysiology* 43 (9): 13937. doi: 10.1111/pace.13937.

Pessoa, Marcosiris Amorim de Oliveira. 2015. *Arquitetura de Sistema de Planejamento e Controle Da Produção No Contexto de Empresa Virtual*. São Paulo: Biblioteca Digital de Teses e Dissertações da Universidade de São Paulo. doi: 10.11606/T.3.2015. tde-09092015-151246.

Pisching, Marcos André. 2018. *Arquitetura Para Descoberta de Equipamentos Em Processos de Manufatura Com Foco Na Indústria 4.0*. São Paulo: Biblioteca Digital de Teses e Dissertações da Universidade de São Paulo. http://www.teses.usp.br/teses/disponiveis/3/3152/tde-05032018-133720/pt-br.php.

Presher, A. L. 2015. "A look inside the industrial internet consortium: Delivering an industrial-strength internet will require new technology, reference architectures, security frameworks and, most of all, unparalleled collaboration." *Design News* 70 (3): 34–40. http://go.galegroup.com/ps/i.do?id=GALE%7CA419410248&v=2.1&u=capes&it=r&p=AONE&sw=w.

Saddik, Abdulmotaleb El. 2018. "Digital twins: The convergence of multimedia technologies." *IEEE Multimedia* 25 (2): 87–92. doi: 10.1109/MMUL.2018.023121167.

Sharp, Phillip, Tyler Jacks, and Susan Hockfield. 2016. *Convergence: The Future of Health*. Cambridge. http://www.convergencerevolution.net/2016-report/.

Sinitsyn, Nikolai A., Soumya Kundu, and Scott Backhaus. 2013. "Safe protocols for generating power pulses with heterogeneous populations of thermostatically controlled loads." *Energy Conversion and Management* 67 (March): 297–308. doi: 10.1016/j.enconman.2012.11.021.

Staufert, Silvan, and Christofer Hierold. 2016. "Novel sensor integration approach for blood pressure sensing in ventricular assist devices." *In Procedia Engineering* 168. doi: 10.1016/j.proeng.2016.11.150.

Stephens, Andrew F., Andrew Busch, Robert F. Salamonsen, Shaun D. Gregory, and Geoffrey D. Tansley. 2020. "Rotary ventricular assist device control with a fiber bragg grating pressure sensor." *IEEE Transactions on Control Systems Technology*. doi: 10.1109/TCST.2020.2989692.

Stevens, Michael C., Andrew Stephens, Abdul-Hakeem H. AlOmari, and Francesco Moscato. 2018. "Physiological control." In *Mechanical Circulatory and Respiratory Support*, 627–57. Amsterdam: Elsevier. doi: 10.1016/B978-0-12-810491-0.00020-5.

Vakil, Kairav, Felipe Kazmirczak, Neeraj Sathnur, Selcuk Adabag, Daniel J. Cantillon, Erich L. Kiehl, Ryan Koene, Rebecca Cogswell, Inderjit Anand, and Henri Roukoz. 2016. "Implantable cardioverter-defibrillator use in patients with left ventricular assist devices: A systematic review and meta-analysis." *JACC: Heart Failure* 4 (10): 772–79. doi: 10.1016/j.jchf.2016.05.003.

Veenis, Jesse F., Ozcan Birim, and Jasper J. Brugts. 2019. "Pulmonary artery pressure telemonitoring by cardioMEMS in a patient pre-and post-left ventricular assist device implantation." *European Journal of Cardio-Thoracic Surgery* 56 (4): 809–10. doi: 10.1093/ejcts/ezz041.

6 Safety and Security

André César Martins Cavalheiro
Fundação Santo André University Center

CONTENTS

6.1 INTRODUCTION

To trust a system, we need to know that it will be available when needed and will perform as expected. The system must be protected so that computers and data are not threatened. This means that issues relating to system trust and protection are often more important than the details of the system's functionality. Then, the first section of this chapter introduces the basics of safety and security and explains the fundamental principles of prevention, detection, and recovery to build reliable VAD control systems. Then, aspects related to requirements engineering, with the discussion of specific approaches to derive and specify system requirements for protection and trust, will be presented. So, a brief introduction to the use of formal specification will be approached, and tools that assist the VAD control system design will be presented. Threads are concerned with software engineering techniques for the development of reliable and protected systems and also discussed the importance of software architecture, current design guidelines, and programming techniques that help us achieve trust and protection. In addition, it explains why redundancy and diversity are important to ensure that systems can fail and also present the extremely important issue of survival or resilience, which allows systems to continue to provide essential services while their protection is being threatened. Finally, it deals with ensuring trust and

DOI: 10.1201/9781003138358-7

protection to explain the use of static analysis and model verification for system verification and fault detection (Sales et al., 2012; Mona et al., 2010). These techniques have been used successfully in critical system engineering and covered specific approaches to testing systems' trust and protection and explained why a trust case may be needed to convince an external regulator that a system is safe and secure.

6.2   SAFETY AND SECURITY CONCEPTS APPLIED ON VENTRICULAR ASSIST DEVICE CONTROL SYSTEM

Today, as computer systems are deeply rooted in our business and personal lives, the problems that result from systems and software failures are increasing. A failure of the server software in a company can cause a huge loss of revenue and even the loss of the company's customers. Infecting a company's PCs with malware can result in loss or damage to confidential information and requires costly cleaning operations to resolve the issue. A software error in a control system built into a VAD can lead to worsen health and in the worst case can be a factor of patient death (Dinkhuysen et al., 2007; Camp Sorrell, 2007; Andrade et al., 2008).

Because software-intensive systems are so important to the patient's life, it is essential that the software used is reliable. The software must be available when necessary and must function correctly and without undesirable side effects. The term "trust" was proposed by Lee and Seshia (2017) to cover systems related to attributes of availability, reliability, security, and protection.

Lately, the reliability of VAD systems is often more important than their detailed functionality. The reasons for this are as follows:

1. System failures affect the patient's health: Many systems include functions that are rarely used. If these functions are left out of the system, only a small number of users will be affected. System failures, which affect the availability of a system, in turn, potentially affect all its users.
2. Users often reject unreliable, insecure, or unprotected systems: If the user realizes that a system is unreliable or unprotected, he will refuse to use it. In addition, he may also refuse to buy or use other products from the same company that produced the untrustworthy system, as he believes that these products can also be unreliable or unprotected.
3. Costs of system failure can be huge or in the case of a VAD control system can cost the patient's life. In this case, the cost of system failure is greater than the cost of the control system.
4. Unreliable systems can cause loss of information: Data collection and maintenance are very expensive procedures; generally, on VAD control system, the data is worth much more than the system in which it is processed. The costs of recovering lost or corrupted data are often very high.

The VAD control system is always part of a larger system. It runs in an operating environment that includes the hardware on which the software runs, the users of the software, and the organizational or medical team in which the software is used. Therefore, when designing a reliable system, you need to consider (Ian, 2011):

1. Hardware failure: Failures in system hardware can occur due to errors in their design, faults in the manufacture of components, or because the components have reached the end of their natural life.
2. Software failure: The software system may fail due to errors in its specifications, design, or implementation.
3. Operational failure: Users may fail to attempt to use or operate the system correctly. As hardware and software have become more reliable, failures in operation are perhaps the biggest cause of system failures.

These failures are generally interrelated. A flawed hardware component can mean that system operators have to deal with an unexpected situation, in addition to additional workload. Such a situation creates stress, and stressed people often make mistakes. This can cause software failures, which means more work for operators, even more stress, and so on.

As a result, it is particularly important that designers of reliable software-intensive systems have a holistic view of systems and do not focus on a single aspect of them, such as software or hardware. If the hardware, software, and operating processes are designed separately, without taking into account the potential weaknesses of other parts of the system, then errors are more likely to occur at the interfaces between different parts of the system. In the case of VAD control systems that consider safety and security as control, the data and the interaction of the system with the external environment can be structured into three parts: control, data, and hardware (Cardoso & Valette, 1997; Leão et al., 2011) where (i) the control part describes all potential event and activity threads, (ii) the data part (which can also be called the operative part) describes, at the same time, the data structures internal to the system and the calculations that are made on this data, without specifying at what times they will be performed, and (iii) in addition to the internal data, in these calculations, the information from the outside intervenes and can be of two types:

- The conditions for performing the calculations;
- The treatments or actions resulting from the calculations.

The interpretation and modeling of this information specify the links between the control part on one side and the data and external environment part on the other side. Figure 6.1 describes this structuring.

Thus, it is interesting to use a modeling tool that allows the analysis and validation of the system considering the characteristics of interaction of a discrete and continuous nature of this type of system. In this sense, an Interpreted Petri has a mathematical formalism to ensure a security net and be able to model this class of system considering the information coming from abroad that can be of two types:

- The conditions for performing the calculations;
- The treatments or actions resulting from the calculations.

The interpretation of the Petri net specifies the connections between the control part on one side and the data and external environment part on the other side, and in this case, the Petri net marking provides the status of the control system.

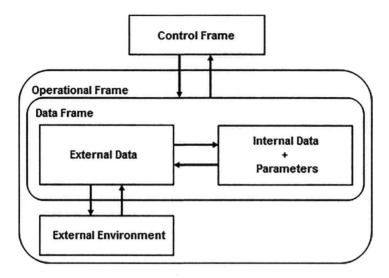

FIGURE 6.1 Interaction of a system with the external environment.

There are several systematization proposals for modeling Interpreted Petri net (Moraes et al., 2001; Cardoso & Valette, 1997; Miyagi, 1996; Santos Filho, 1998; Cavalheiro, 2004; Squillante, 2011). These methodologies make it possible to represent the dynamic behavior of systems that imply the representation of parallels, sequencing, and concurrency of events, resulting in the effective modeling for the formal representation and the realization of the discrete control of these systems.

6.3 CONTROL SYSTEM TOPOLOGY

According to (Dilts et al., 1991; ISA, 2000; Hernandez et al., 2005), the architecture of a system is defined as the structure and logical organization of the functioning of a system, where the interrelationships between the components of the system are determined and where each component has a specific control function. In this way, the systems can be classified into two groups according to the topology adopted to carry out the control, and they are as follows:

1. Centralized control system: These are systems that have a single controller, where all the control logic of the system is processed in this controller. This system is normally applied to small processes with fewer inputs and outputs. Figure 6.2a presents the schematic of a centralized control architecture;
2. Distributed control system: In this type of system, there are two or more controllers, involved in the execution of the control. In this context, controllers can be organized into three basic ways (Figure 6.2b–d):

- Distributed architecture of the hierarchical type;
- Distributed architecture of the modified hierarchical type; and
- Distributed architecture.

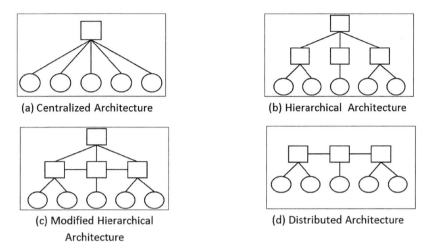

(a) Centralized Architecture

(b) Hierarchical Architecture

(c) Modified Hierarchical
Architecture

(d) Distributed Architecture

Obs.: ☐ Elements represent controllers and O Elements represent sensors and actuators

FIGURE 6.2   Basic forms of control architectures: centralized (a), hierarchical (b), modified hierarchical (c), and distributed (d).

According to Chapter 5, which shows the intelligent systems and architectures presented in Figure 6.2, it is consistent to conclude that the evolution of cyberphysical systems tends toward a distributed architecture. In this type of architecture, each component can control a local functionality of a global control. When a complex system like this is built in parts without considering a whole, the risk of failure increases. Therefore, a risk analysis carried out with strict criteria in this class of system is essential to increase security and develop a safety system.

6.4   RISK ANALYSIS APPLIED TO VAD CONTROL SYSTEMS

The term risk defines a metric to quantify a damage, damages or losses, in a correlated way, that is, the probability of the occurrence of a failure and the magnitude of the losses or losses resulting from this failure (Bell, 2008; ISO, 2007). Thus, the risk is measured in terms of the consequences for human life, damage to the environment, and loss of equipment. Still in this context, the concept of failure must be clarified. The term failure, according to IEC 61511 (IEC, 2003), is defined as an abnormal condition that can cause a reduction or loss of the capacity of a functional unit.

Certain established and standardized techniques can be used for risk analysis, such as failure tree analysis (FTA) (IEC, 2008), hazard and operability study (HAZOP) (IEC, 2001), and failure mode and effects analysis (FMEA) (IEC, 2006). These techniques are already used to identify failures and risks in different systems. Among the risk analysis techniques, one that stands out is the use of the HAZOP study, which is a systematic technique to identify dangers and operational problems as well as failures of elements of a system. This technique describes a detailed review of the process design and operation, focusing on deviations in the parameters involved, such as flow, pressure, temperature, vibration, among other parameters or elements that are associated with the occurrence of failures. In this technique, in addition to enabling the analysis of failures of an element, it is possible to perform the failure analysis of a set of elements as well as the analysis of actions and operations of devices in a system. Therefore, this technique addresses the needs for failure analysis in VAD (Cavalheiro et al., 2019).

In the HAZOP study, it is proposed to use guide words (e.g., more, less, none, and reverse) and to represent the deviations, and these are applied for each parameter. The consequences of deviations are evaluated, and, depending on the degree of severity, possible treatments are determined. The HAZOP study can be found in the IEC 61882 (2001) standard. Some adaptations are proposed to meet the multidisciplinarity and characteristics of a VAD (Bock et.al, 2011), since this tool was developed to be applied in critical industrial processes.

To use the HAZOP, the following steps are performed:

- Divide the system into parts;
- Choose a part and describe its expected behavior;
- Select a process parameter;
- Apply the guide words to the parameter and identify possible deviations;
- Determine the possible causes and consequences of deviation;
- Define the recommended action;
- Identify sensors and actuators that identify the deviation;
- Repeat the process for each element of each part of the system.

According to the IEC 61882 standard, data can be organized according to Table 6.1.

Applying the rules and following the HAZOP criteria, it is possible to complete table with the possible faults and diagnostics of VAD control system can present and thus increase a safety and security of the system with a safe and systematic form.

6.5 FAULT DIAGNOSIS

The diagnosis refers to the monitoring and interpretation of the sensors to assess and conclude a specific phenomenon, without interfering or modifying this phenomenon or the value of the generated signal. For the stages of diagnosis and treatment of failures, the structuring of information can be based on two approaches (Kurtoglu & Tumer, 2008):

- Analytical redundancy: It uses analytical mathematical models. In the analytical redundancy approach, you must have a sufficiently detailed model of the process, the quantities involved, and the degree of confidence of each variable. In this way, it is possible to detect, locate, and identify failures, comparing quantitative data collected with data obtained from the mathematical model of the system. To some extent, uncertainties and incomplete measures can be tolerated and, depending on the degree of these uncertainties, adaptive strategies or robust control can be used;
- Knowledge-based: It uses qualitative models. In the knowledge-based approach, artificial intelligence (AI) techniques should be applied that allow exploring the knowledge and accumulated experience regarding the system.

TABLE 6.1

Example of Documentation for a HAZOP Study

N	Element	Characteristic	Guide Word	Deviations (Effects)	Possible Causes	Consequences	Safeguards/ Maintenance	Comments	Actions	Action Allocated to
Number of element	Name of the element (element type)	Characteristic of the element	Word guide that defines the deviations of the element	Characteristic of the element + word guide and sensor (or situation) that detects the deviation	Failure associated with the deviation	Consequences of failure	What to do to avoid failure	Comments about failure	Action to treat the failure	Element responsible for the treatment of the failure

Source: IEC61882 (2001).

It is suitable especially in the case where the information provided by the sensors is insufficient and/or the models of the system are inaccurate. In many of these cases, techniques such as expert systems, genetic algorithms, neural networks, and fuzzy logic are being studied to solve the problem of controlling a VAD, but are not applied to the security systems of these devices (Spiegelhater, 1987; AIM, 2002; Kurtoglu, 2008).

Some modeling techniques using AI theory can be used to analyze uncertainties, such as neural networks, fuzzy logic, and Bayesian networks. These techniques are already used for the analysis of uncertainties and decision-making in several systems. Among the AI techniques, one that stands out is the Bayesian networks, which is a systematic and established technique for calculating uncertainties that can be used to identify dangers and operational problems as well as failures of elements of a system. This technique describes a detailed review.

According to Riascos and Miyagi (2010), the Bayesian network[1] is a graph that allows representing the combination of knowledge of a specialist, using the theory of probability for the construction of a diagnostic structure. Therefore, once the knowledge of the specialists on VAD has been obtained through the HAZOP study, it is possible, using the Bayesian network, to make a relationship between the faults and their effects to serve as a specification for the later construction of the VAD control functions.

To build a Bayesian network, it is necessary to calculate the conditional probabilities (numerical parameters) and identify the structure of the network, that is, identify variables and the dependence relationships of cause and effect, given by the arcs (HRUSCHKA JR, 2003). Therefore, the construction process is divided into two parts: learning the structure (relationships between variables) and learning of numerical parameters (conditional probability). Parts, structures, and parameters can be learned through an expert or through an inductive method (Squillante et al., 2011).

When the network is built by the learning method with specialists, it is understood that it will be responsible for defining and/or supervising the construction of the network based on their knowledge or the knowledge of others. Inductive learning, on the other hand, uses a database that contains the history of past operations, and based on this, the network is built automatically (Cooper; Herskovitz, 1992; Murphy, 2007).

In Darwiche (2010), it is mentioned that there are some methods for the construction of the Bayesian network, in an inductive way, from the learning of the network structure and from the numerical learning or the conditional probabilities between the variables. A method that is largely subjective and reflects human knowledge is used to capture the causal relationships between variables and represent them graphically through a Bayesian network.

However, it can also be observed that one of the advantages of using the Bayesian network is that it is an easy-to-understand tool and of great application in decision-making. Therefore, adopting the Bayesian network to obtain the decision-making models of the VAD control system being applied to the various possibilities and situations is an effective technique as presented in (Squilante et al, 2011).

6.6   FAILURE HANDLING IN VADs

A strategy for handling failures may depend on the level of control considered in the hierarchy of the control system. Based on the hierarchy presented in the VAD control architectures (Nakata et al., 1999; Oshikawa et al., 2000; Ayre, Lovell, Woodard, 2003; Al Omari, 2009; Giridharan & Skliar, 2006; Wu et al., 2005; Campomar, Silvestrini, D'attellis, 2005; Yi, 2007; Chang, Gao, Gu, 2011), some levels are defined for the analysis and failure treatment for this type of system:

- System level;
- Level of modules;
- Component level; and
- Operation level (of the user).

Operational failures are those that occur at the interface between the doctor or the patient and the VAD. These flaws are widely discussed in the literature (Camp Sorreli, 2007; Hill & Reinhartz, 2006; Park et al. 2009; Legendre, 2009; ISO, 2007; Yi, 2007). They correspond to operational failures that are not part of the scope of this work, as they would be specific issues related to the procedures that guide medical interventions in patients with VAD.

Therefore, one of the most important points in the treatment of failures is how, effectively, the repair will be carried out. In this context, there are two approaches to carry out repairs:

1. Adjustment of operating parameters: In this approach, adjustment of parameters is carried out without altering or reorganizing the logical structure of the equipment. This type of repair is carried out by reading the sensor signals and generating appropriate commands for the actuators, already in the system, to fully or partially recover the required functions. In the event of a failure, the system can continue to perform its functions, albeit with less performance, by changing some operating parameters. The system must collect the data from these components and determine whether it is necessary to make an adjustment to the operating parameters to keep the system in operation operating to an acceptable quality standard;
2. Use of redundant resources or elements: In this approach, the system must have mechanisms that make it possible to change its own logical and/or physical structure. That is, it is possible with the specification of additional components or redundant parts. This type of strategy, called functional redundancy, can involve costs, physical dimensions, performance, and complexity undesirable to VAD. Basically, in a safety system, through the adjustment of parameters, the same mechanical structure is preserved, but the idea is that with the introduction of some sensors and/or actuators, and some new considerations in the control, the system can acquire adequate tolerance.

In the case of treatment of critical failures, the IEC 61508 standard determines that a failure is defined based on the identification of an Instrumented Safety Function, called Safety Instrumented Function (SIF). Therefore, each SIF is associated with a fault that must be diagnosed and treated by the Safety Instrumented System (SIS), which, according to the IEC61508 standard, must be the safety system responsible for diagnosing and treating faults. An SIS performs its SIFs by (i) collecting process signals by one or more safety sensors, (ii) processing information by one or more control devices (electrical, electronic, or programmable electronic equipment), and (iii) sending signals to each of the safety actuators. In order to process and analyze the information, it is necessary to model the system so that it is possible to interpret the cause and effect relationships of the possible states that the system can reach.

The identification of the patient's condition and the failures that may occur (from the point of view of the safety of the patient with cardiovascular problems) are usually represented by events that inform the patient's condition.

In this context, depending on the nature of the failure, the control system can react according to the concepts defined below (Arakaki, 2004):

   a. Regeneration: It is the capacity that the system must have to recover, admitting new scenarios that can be increased through the doctor/patient/VAD interaction, and knowledge of the system;
   b. Degeneration: It is the loss of the original qualities or characteristics of the system that does not allow the recovery of its normal state of operation. In this context, the control system is limited to bringing the system to a safe state.

6.7   FAILURE RECOVERY METHODS

In a safe control system, in the case of regeneration due to the occurrence of a fault, a fault must be able to identify and correct it. According to Riascos and Miyagi (2010), there are four fundamental methods applied to recover from failures: (i) conditioned input method; (ii) alternative route method; (iii) direct recovery method and; and (iv) reverse recovery method. The methods mentioned are detailed below.

   1. Conditioned input method: In this case, when an abnormal state or a fault state is detected in a place p of the network, which represents a process or system state, it can return to the normal situation, if a corrective action is taken. Figure 6.3 outlines the failure recovery by this method, where Z represents the original Petri net and S' is an additional subnet, representing the failure recovery procedure presented in place p;
   2. Alternative route method: In this case, when an abnormal state is detected in the place p_j, it is about generating an alternative route from p_j to p_m through the subnet S', in which other states are generated that recover the system, thus avoiding the execution of activity S (Figure 6.4). This method is equivalent to performing the activity in an alternative way and can be applied when the equipment or the system changes state, for example, in the recovery of the patient, where the VAD must work with a different rotation or in the breaking of an VAD element where the process is executed by an alternative or redundant element;

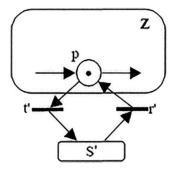

FIGURE 6.3 Recovery scheme using the conditioned entry method (see Riascos & Miyagi, 2010).

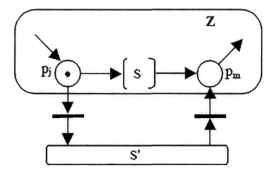

FIGURE 6.4 Recovery scheme using the alternative route method (see Riascos & Miyagi, 2010).

3. Inverse recovery method: In this method, when a failure is detected (in the p_m place) after the execution of activity S, this problem is treated with the execution of operations of a subnet S' that results in a re-execution activity S (Figure 6.5). This method is equivalent to the reprocessing of elements. For example, when there is a magnetic decoupling between the motor and

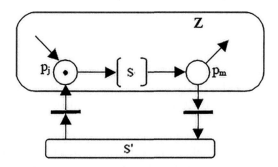

FIGURE 6.5 Reverse recovery scheme (see Riascos & Miyagi, 2010).

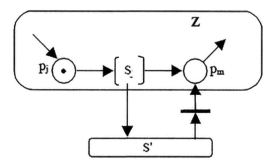

FIGURE 6.6   Direct recovery scheme (see Riascos & Miyagi, 2010).

the impeller of the VAD pump, it is necessary that the system performs a re-coupling routine;

4. Direct recovery method: In case of detection of a fault state in the S process, the system can return to a normal state by executing the S' subnet. This technique is used to recover from a failure that is detected only during the execution of the S process (Figure 6.6). For example, the closing command of the safety valve where it does not close due to a failure of activation implies the need for the VAD to assume a standard speed to prevent backflow.

The methods described above add nodes (places and transitions) in the original networks, which makes the model in Petri net with a greater number of elements to represent all possible processes (normal processes and abnormal situations). Thus, conflicts arise in places where the flow of brands is decided, that is, whether normal processes should continue (network Z) or the start of the execution of subnets to deal with abnormal situations (subnet S'). On the other hand, this approach guarantees the maintenance of the properties of the original model. A qualitative analysis of a Petri network includes the analysis of properties such as liveliness, security, restartability, among others.

6.8   METHOD FOR DEVELOPING THE SECURITY CONTROL SYSTEM FOR VADs

For the VADs, it is observed that there is a limitation of the proposals in the sense that this device works in parallel with the patient's ventricle, assisted by the control system that acts locally (White, 2009; Bolling, 2011; Morello, 2011; Ben Shalom, 2011a,b; Robert, 2009; Frazie et al., 2004; Schmidt et al., 2003; Muramatsu, Masuoka, Fujisawa, 2001; Snyder, Tsukui et al., 2007; Doi et al., 2004; El Banayosy et al., 2006; French, Andreas, Gifford III, 2006; Chen et al., 2002; Cotter & Bataille, 2010; Loree et al., 2001; Locke et al., 2003; Geertsma et al., 2007; Hill & Reinhartz, 2006; Coleman, Coleman, Neill, 2006; Dowling et al., 2004; Pacella et al., 2004). However, in terms of patient safety and, especially, in case of failures, the control systems should consider that the VAD is in series with the rest of the circulatory system, being able to strongly influence this and, consequently, the health status of the patient. In this context, VAD that is not fault-tolerant and does not show dynamic behavior according to the patient's situation becomes limited and can compromise the cardiovascular system if it presents an unsatisfactory performance.

Therefore, if the VAD fails, it compromises the patient's life causing a disturbance in the circulatory system. On the other hand, if the heart fails, the patient's life may be compromised, but due to the fact that VAD is in series with the circulatory system, it can provide survival.

Considering a new approach to address this problem, it is proposed to apply a mechatronic approach to this class of devices based on advanced instrumentation, control, and automation techniques. These techniques allow the treatment of certain limitations present in current solutions.

Thus, it is important to consider a control solution that considers the system variables globally, not only considering the heart locally, but considering it inserted in the cardiovascular system where the blood circulation is aided by a dynamic and safe VAD. For this, the control system must use the concepts of regeneration and degeneration considering the variables of the control system globally, not only including the variables associated with the sensing and actuation devices directly connected to the controller pump, but also considering physiological variables of the controller, patient's body through sensors using control models that make it possible to interpret these variables.

In this context, it is essential to specify a safety supervisory control system for a VAD that meets the following fundamental requirements:

- Allow to specify the logic for the pump speed control according to the dynamic behavior of the patient. Regenerative models are used in modeling the control system, and depending on the diagnosis and the dynamic state of the patient, the control system must react to adapt to the situation;
- Allow to specify the safety logic to address failures in the VAD that can cause risks to the patient. For this purpose, a fault survey is carried out based on the HAZOP technique. From this analysis, the Petri net is used to model the fault diagnosis and treatment system based on information obtained from the Bayesian network;
- Allow to verify and validate the mathematical model of the control system according to its interaction with a mathematical model of the human cardiovascular system (Abdolrazaghi, Navidbakhsh, Hassani, 2010; Sales, Santos Filho, Cavalheiro, 2010).

Thus, the safe control system can be specified and implemented to perform in vitro tests and in vivo tests in a consistent manner.

6.9   FAILURE SENSING AND SEVERITY

Considering the study carried out regarding the complexity of the failures that can occur during the operation of a VAD, it is possible to define a failure classification in two contexts:

1. Regarding severity:
   a. Critical failures: They are events associated with risks of an unaccept-able magnitude, that is, which must be prevented or mitigated, and can cause fatality and damage that lead the patient to death. In this context, the VAD control must degenerate the system in a controlled manner, by means of a specific security control system, to a safe state;
   b. Non-critical failures: They are events associated with risks of acceptable magnitude, that is, they can be recovered by the system (regeneration), or they can involve intervention by the doctor or the patient himself so that the abnormal condition situation can be regenerated and the system operates in a normal state.
2. As for the sensing resources (FRANK, 1992):
   a. Direct detection failures: They can be diagnosed directly by sensing the state of the system considering specific sensors. For example, to detect blood reflux in the VAD, a specific flow sensor can be used to check the status of this variable;
   b. Indirect detection failures: They require an interpretation (or logical procedure) of the system state in order to be able to deduce the type of fault. For example, to detect the failure of a heart valve to close, where there is no specific sensor that checks the state of this variable, a logical procedure is necessary to deduce this situation.

6.10   CONTROL SYSTEM ARCHITECTURE

As previously described, this chapter addresses the failures of system components that extend to the upper levels (modules and system). Thus, the diagnosis considered is that performed by components and its treatment is carried out at the appropriate level according to the strategy for its mitigation. The levels of failure analysis and treatment discussed in this work are detailed below.

a. Component level: At this level, the system must have a strategy that allows the detection of the failures of each component, if possible to recover the failing element automatically or through the intervention of an appropriate control module. To detect a failure, you must specify the characteristics of the components that perform the data acquisition of the relevant variables to recognize possible failure states. The fault diagnosis is performed by per-forming the "reasoning" to determine the causes of the failure and thus make decisions or corrective measures to recover the equipment;
b. Module level: This level considers the interaction that exists between the modules of a system. The fault must be dealt with through a control strat-egy that makes it possible to detect the faults of a module and, if possi-ble, recover the faulty module automatically or through the intervention of another appropriate control module. Some VADs, for example, have redundant battery charging modules (in the case of TET systems) that auto-matically change the power source, which allows these devices to directly address some failures. However, there are other modules that may not have

redundancy, for example, the local or supervisory control modules that need to be replaced in the event of a failure. Thus, for example, to avoid stopping the operations of a module that does not achieve its self-recovery, the treatment must be carried out by another module that must diagnose this failure and treat it in such a way that the system continues to function safely. The verification or reorganization of the control in the event of a failure can allow the system to continue performing its functions, albeit with a lower performance;

c. System level: This level considers the VAD control system as a whole (VAD plus human body). The status of each module considered at this level is of the type "module operating normally" or "module inoperative." In the case of a "module inoperative" (with faulty devices that cannot be treated), the system must be able to identify an output that guarantees a safe state, mitigating the fault until the inoperative module returns to its normal operating state.

At the component level, faults in the various sensors and actuators in the VAD control system are considered, for example, disruption in a circuit, decalibration of a sensor, failure of a sensor, and failure of the motor. For module and system levels, in some cases, it is not possible to directly detect the fault using a simple sensor. Therefore, reasoning is necessary to detect the failure. For this, as previously described, the following can be used: the Bayesian network and the Petri network, which are effective techniques for the development of systems considering the detection and treatment of failures and still allow the analysis of model properties, which is fundamental for the design and implementation of a secure control system.

Thus, in order to obtain a safe control system for a VAD in a structured way, Cavalheiro (2013) proposed a control system distributed in structured modules that have specific functionalities according to the architecture presented in Figure 6.7.

The diagnosis and treatment of critical failures are based on the concept of Instrumented Safety System (SIS), according to the IEC61508, and these safety control functions are implemented in the Cardiovascular Safety Instrumented System (SISC) module, which has the aim to degenerate the VAD to a safe state.

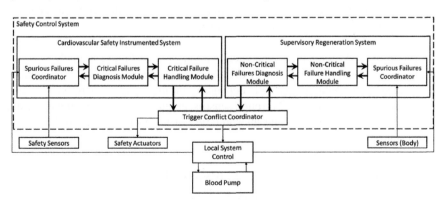

FIGURE 6.7   Safety control architecture for VAD proposed by Cavalheiro (2013).

The diagnosis and treatment of non-critical faults, on the other hand, are based on the concept of fault regeneration, and these control functions are implemented in the Supervisory Regeneration Control (SSR) module, which aims to regenerate the VAD to a new control state.

Each SCS module is divided into submodules, where each has its specific function and is needed for the correct functioning of the SCS. The following is a brief description of each module of the safety architecture.

1. Spurious fault coordinator module: This module has the function of filtering spurious faults from the system's sensors;
2. Fault diagnosis module: This module has the function of interpreting the state of the system sensors (effect) and diagnosing the occurrence of a fault (cause): If the fault is critical, then it will be diagnosed by the SISC, and if it is non-critical, then it will be diagnosed by the SSR;
3. Failure treatment module: This module has the function of generating treatment actions to mitigate a diagnosed failure, be it critical, which must be treated by the SISC, or non-critical, which must be treated by the SSR;
4. Triggering conflict coordinator module: This module has the function of checking the global state of the system and arbitrating which fault must be attended to when two or more faults occur simultaneously by activating the respective actuator according to the parameters specified from the Instrumented Safety Function Control (FISC);
5. Sensors and actuators: These are the physical elements responsible for detection and actuation. It is important to emphasize that whenever possible, specific sensors and actuators for the SISC should be used, even if this means having sensor redundancy. This distinction of sensors and actuators specific to the SISC occurs due to the severity of the failures and the way the SISC should act if they occur. The SISC must guarantee the integrity of the system, and, in case of failure, this module must cause the system to evolve to a safe state. Therefore, to ensure the safety of the system, the IEC61508 standard recommends the use of redundant sensors and actuators;
6. Local control module: It is a pump drive driver, where it has the function of guaranteeing the rotation of the pump according to the required speeds (set points) by the SISC and SSR controls.

For this proposed architecture, the specification of each failure is made from the identification of the FISCs. Thus, a FISC describes a failure that must be diagnosed and treated by the SISC or the SSR depending on its severity. Therefore, the SCS must be able to perform a FISC through sensors, actuators, and control devices using the control models that allow the interpretation of these elements according to the global state of the system.

6.11 METHOD FOR THE DEVELOPMENT OF THE SECURITY CONTROL SYSTEM

According to the modeling techniques presented, Cavalheiro (2013) proposed a method for developing the SCS of a VAD as shown in Figure 6.8.[2]

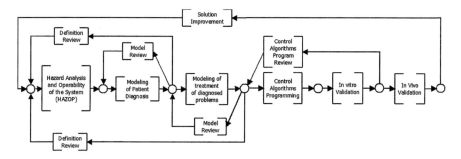

FIGURE 6.8 Method for developing the SCS proposed by Cavalheiro (2013).

In this method, a risk analysis is first performed and, together with the knowledge of the multidisciplinary team previously defined in the VAD design, the HAZOP study table is obtained as a result of this step of the method. Once the table has been obtained and the elements of the system and their possible failures have been defined, the next step is to generate the diagnostic models that are used in the control system to confirm and report the occurrence of a failure due to the overall behavior of the system. In this stage of the project, simulations and analyses are carried out using the diagnostic models obtained. In this step, if any non-compliance is verified, the elements or failure situations obtained in the HAZOP study can be reviewed. Depending on the non-conformity, changes can be made to the arrangement of the components or to the requirements considered in the models that do not meet the design situations, either due to the lack of sensor technology, or due to VAD characteristics, the patient or any other reason that influences the fidelity and validation of diagnostic models. Once the diagnostic models have been validated, the next step is the fault treatment part. At this point in the method, models are created that allow the treatment of a failure. These models can be degenerative, if the failure is considered critical, or regenerative, if the failure being treated is considered non-critical. Like the diagnostic models, the treatment models must also be simulated and analyzed and, if divergences are found, then these can be revised. Once the modeling part is finished, the implementation stage is reached. In this step, the models must be programmed considering the technology of the controller. In this way, control algorithms are designed in the programming language consistent with the controller. Once the system has been programmed and taking into account the technology considered in the project, the next step of the method foresees in vitro commissioning tests to verify whether the technology adopted together with the projected models meets the design requirements (Fonseca, 2012). If limitations are found in response time, signal processing, or any other shortcomings that could compromise VAD control, in this step, the adopted technology can be revised or even the control algorithm or system models reformulated so that their project specifications are met. In this step, computational and physical simulators can be used to assist in the commissioning and validation of the control system. The last step of the method is the in vivo validation of the VAD system. This step is essential for the VAD system to be approved by government agencies and for them to release the device to be implanted in human beings. In this stage, invasive tests and acute surgeries are performed and several protocols imposed by Organs responsible bodies are used for the device to be approved. Once the device has been approved by the responsible bodies and has passed all exhaustive tests, the device is ready to be implanted in human beings. At this stage, the method also provides feedback to the first stage of the method. This feedback is essential to create a knowledge base to feed inference algorithms with this information and thus allow the improvement and analysis of the HAZOP study, allowing for continuous improvement, increasing the intelligence of the system and the improvement of the control models.

6.12   FINAL CONCLUSIONS

In this chapter, a concrete way of representing a model of the security control system for a VAD is established, which is based on the concept of risk analysis, where we tried to specify the rules relevant to the behavior of the system due to possible failures that this one can present. Therefore, this information can be interpreted as a strong motivation in order to leverage future research in the area of safety and security systems for VADs that were not explored due to the complexity of the problem. In this way, it becomes a reality to research the impact of this new architecture on a series of themes that are being studied, for example, optimization of local control, autonomy of supervisory control, and improvement of fault-tolerant systems for these devices, among other matters that pass to be unveiled due to the initiation that this research provided with the new paradigm of application of discrete control using analysis of failures in the area of VADs control systems.

As a result, the application of a critical system control approach and risk analysis for control system projects for VADs was presented. To this end, a systematic approach was presented that provides a consistent solution for these systems to present a dynamic behavior that prevents the patient from suffering consequences in his health status due to the occurrence of critical failures of high severity that can put the patient's life at risk. In this way, the controlled device presents a level of improvement in terms of aspects related to its safety and reliability.

In this context, initially, concepts related to safety and security systems were presented, establishing an analogy between the main characteristics of the approaches inherent to them. Taking into account the aspects addressed, a succinct introduction about VAD control systems was made, establishing the main characteristics of the behavior presented by them and defining a set of important characteristics that should be considered in the set of properties of a tool capable of controlling these systems.

Subsequently, modeling tools were presented and fundamental attributes for modeling the VAD control were highlighted. In order to systematize and rationalize the task of modeling control functions and consider risk analysis as an essential procedure for the development of an autonomous and safety control, the Bayesian and Petri networks were presented as appropriate tools for learning and implementation control, respectively.

Once the functionalities of a VAD were defined, the next step considered was the definition of the fault handling functions and performance in the VAD control system. To specify the diagnosis and treatment strategies for control failures, an approach based on the performance of the system's risk analysis was considered. In this context, control architectures were presented with a study of factors that influence the performance of a VAD in relation to the patient's circulatory system and fault coordinators were shown to safely perform the regeneration or degeneration of the system considering treatment characteristics of spurious fails inherent to the components of this kind of systems. In order to design a VAD control system, the HAZOP study was adopted as a risk analysis tool, the Bayesian network as a learning tool, and the Interpreted Petri network as a tool for modeling the part corresponding to the device control, detailing, even, the modeling of the elementary control functions in a modular way.

In order to be able to explore the modeling capacity using these tools, a security control system (SCS) was presented through the application of a structured method for the modeling and implementation of elements that make up the VAD control architecture, capable of performing functions for device regeneration or degeneration depending on the overall analysis of the system and the nature of the failures involved.

Thus, this chapter describes a set of procedures and concepts that take a safety control system project to a VAD, considering the approach of discrete control systems and aspects of adaptability and security, providing autonomy to VADs in a safe manner. In this sense, activities related to each phase of the project were analyzed, proposing procedures and using appropriate tools to obtain an adequate specification. Through these procedures, techniques that have been proposed to design a safe and autonomous control system for VADs be introduced, highlighting the interfaces as well as the human element and its participation in decisions throughout its life cycle.

Thus, the application of the theory of control to discrete event systems (DES) for the modeling of the control architecture of a VAD stands out, contemplating (i) the modeling of the security functions and the relevant control algorithms; (ii) the diagnosis and treatment of non-critical failures for the regeneration of the device; (iii) the diagnosis and treatment of critical failures for the device to degenerate to a safe state; and (iv) the adequacy of a risk analysis technique for the VADs design associated with AI techniques such as the Bayesian network to provide a continuous improvement in failure control.

NOTES

1 The Bayesian network is represented through a directed and acyclic graph in which the nodes represent the variables of a domain and the arcs represent the conditional dependence between the variables of the system. This technique has been extensively applied for fault diagnosis (Chien, Chen; Lin, 2002; Lerner et al., 2002; Murphy, 2007).

2 The method was represented by a model based on Production Flow Schema that belongs to an unmarked Petri Canal - Agency network class (Miyagi, 1996).

REFERENCES

Abdolrazaghi, M.; Navidbakhsh, M.; Hassani, K. Mathematical modelling and electrical analog equivalent of the human cardiovascular system. *Cardiovascular Engineering*, v. 10, pp. 45–51, 2010.

AIM. Lessons learnt from bringing knowledge-based decision support into routine use. *AIM – Artificial Intelligence in Medicine*, v. 24, pp. 195–203, 2002.

Al Omari, A. H. H. et al. A dynamical model for pulsatile flowestimation in a left ventricular assist device. In: *International Conference on Bio-Inspired Systems and Signal Processing*, Porto, Springer, pp. 402–405, 2009.

Andrade, A. J. P. et al. Mock circulatory system for the evaluation of left ventricular assist device, endoluminal prothesis and vascular disease. *Artificial Organs*, v. 32, pp. 461–467, 2008.

Arakaki, J. Técnicas de degeneração no controle de sistemas produtivos. Tese (Doutorado) - Escola Politécnica, Universidade de São Paulo, São Paulo, 2004.

Ayre, P. J.; Lovell, N. H.; Woodard, J. C. Non-invasive flow estimation in an implantable rotary blood pump: A study considering non-pulsatile and pulsatile flows. *Physiological Measurement,* v. 24, n. 1, pp. 179–189, 2003.

Bell, R. Introduction to IEC 61508. *Artificial Organs*, v. 32, pp. 461–467, 2008.

Ben Shalom, Z. FlowMaker – Organ assist system and method. 7,988,614, 2011a.

Ben Shalom, Z. Impella Recover – Organ assist system and method. 7,988,614, 2011b.

Bock, E. et al. Design, manufacturing and tests of an implantable centrifugal blood pump. In: *IFIP Advances in Information and Communication Technology*, Lisboa, v. 349, pp. 410–417, 2011.

Bolling, S. F. Novacor – Implantable heart assist system and method of applying same. 7,993,260, 2011.

Camp Sorrell, D. Clinical dilemmas: Vascular acess devices. *Seminar in Oncology Nursing*, v. 23, n. 3, pp. 232–239, 2007.

Campomar, G.; Silvestrini, M.; D'attellis, C. An axial flow left ventricular assist device: Modelling and control. *Wseas Transactions on Biology and Biomedicine*, v. 2, n. 2, pp. 187–191, 2005.

Cardoso, J.; Valette, R. *Redes de Petri*. Florianópolis, SC: Editora da UFSC, 1997.

Cavalheiro, A. C. M. et al. Analysis and tests of supervisory control systems applied to a ventricular assist device. *ASAIO Journal*, v. 57, n. 1, p. 119, 2011.

Cavalheiro, A. C. M. Projeto de Sistemas de Controle Modulares e Distribuídos. Dissertação (Mestrado) - Escola Politécnica, Universidade de São Paulo, São Paulo 157 p., 2004.

Cavalheiro, A. C. M. Sistema de Controle para Diagnóstico e Tratamento de Falhas em Dispositivos de Assistência Ventricular. Tese (Doutorado) - Escola Politécnica, Universidade de São Paulo, São Paulo 213 p., 2013.

Cavalheiro, A. C. M. et al. A concept of safety embedded systems control applied to a 4.0 ventricular assist device. In: *ASAIO 65rd Annual Conference*, San Francisco, 2019.

Chang, Y.; Gao, B.; Gu, K. A model-free Adaptive control to a blood pump based on heart rate. *ASAIO Journal*, v. 57, n. 4, pp. 262–267, 2011.

Chen, C. et al. A magnetic suspension theory and its application to the heartquest ventricular assist device. *Artificial Organs*, v. 26, n. 11, pp. 947–951, 2002.

Chien, C. F.; Chen, S. L.; Lin, Y. S. Using Bayesian network for fault location on distribution feeder. *IEEE Transaction in Power Delivery*, v. 17, n. 3, pp. 785–793, 2002.

Coleman, E. J.; Coleman, G. T.; Neill, W. T. AbioCor: Implantable cardiac assist device. US 7,118,525, 2006.

Cooper, G. F.; Herskovits, E. A Bayesian method for the induction of probabilistic networks from data. *Machine Learning*, v. 9, pp. 309–347, 1992.

Cotter, C. J.; Bataille, O. C. HeartMate III: Heart pump connector. US 7,824,358, 2010.

Darwiche, A. What are Bayesian networks and why are their applications growing across all fields? *Communications of the ACM*, v. 53, pp. 80–90, 2010.

Dilts, D. M.; et al. The evolution of control architecture of automated manufacturing systems. *Journal of Manufacturing Systems*, v. 10, pp. 79–93, 1991.

Dinkhuysen, J. J. et al. Bomba sanguínea espiral: Concepção, desenvolvimento e aplicação clínica de projeto original. *Revista Brasileira de Cirurgia Cardiovascular*, v. 22, pp. 224–234, 2007.

Doi, K. et al. Preclinical readiness testing of the arrow international coraide left ventricular assist system. *The Annals of Thoracic Surgery*, v. 77, n. 6, pp. 2103–2110, 2004.

Dowling, R. D. et al. Initial experience with the abiocor implantable replacement heart system. *Journal of Thoracic Cardiovascular Surgery*, v. 127, pp. 131–141, 2004. doi: 10.1016/j.jtcvs.2003.07.023.

El Banayosy, A. et al. Initial results of a European multicenter clinical trial with the DuraHeart® mag-Lev centrifugal left ventricular assist device. *Heart Lung Transplant*, v. 25, n. 2, S145, 2006.

Fonseca, J. et al. Continuous versus pulsatile flow for left ventricle assist devices: Performance evaluation in a hybrid cardiovascular simulator. *ASAIO Journal*, v. 58. pp. 1–19. 2012.

Frank, P. M. Principles of model-based fault detection. In: *Proceedings of the Symposium on all in Real-Time Control,* Delft, pp. 363–370, 1992.

Frazie, O. H. et al. First clinical use of the redesigned HeartMate® II left ventricular assist system in the United States: A Case report. *Texas Heart Institute Journal,* v. 31, pp. 157–159, 2004.

French, R.; Andreas, B. H.; Gifford III, H. S. HeartQuest: Methods, systems and devices relating to implantable fluid pumps. US 7,037,253, 2006.

Geertsma, R. E. et al. New and emerging medical technologies a horizon scan of opportunities and risks. Netherland: Centre for Biological Medicines and Medical Technology; National Institute for Public Health and the Environment (Report 360020002), 116 p., 2007.

Giridharan, G. A.; Skliar M. Physiological control of blood pumps using intrinsic pump parameters: A computer simulation study. *Artificial Organs,* v. 30, n. 4, pp. 301–307, 2006.

Hernández, E. G. et al. Design strategy of discrete event controllers for automated manufacturing systems. In: *International Conference on Electrical and Electronics Engineering,* ICEEE, México, Piscataway, NJ, IEEE, 2005.

Hill, J. D.; Reinhartz, O. Clinical outcomes in pediatric patients implanted with thoratec ventricular assist device. *Pediatric Cardiac Surgery,* v. 9, n. 1, pp. 115–122, 2006.

Hruschka Jr, E. R. Imputação bayesiana no contexto da mineração dos dados. Tese de Doutorado (Doutorado) - Universidade Federal do Rio de Janeiro. Rio de Janeiro, 2003.

Ian, S. *Software Engineering.* London: Pearson Education, Prentice Hall, 9th edition, 2011.

IEC, International Electrotechnical Commission. IEC 61508: Functional safety of electrical/electronic: Programmable electronic safety-related systems, 1998.

IEC, International Electrotechnical Commission, Hazard and operability studies (Hazop studies): Application guide (IEC 61882), IEC, Geneva, Switzerland, 2001.

IEC, International Electrotechnical Commission. IEC 61511: Functional safety: Safety instrumented systems for the process industry sector, Geneva, Switzerland, 2003.

IEC, International Electrotechnical Commission. IEC 60812: Analysis techniques for system reliability: Procedures for failure mode and effectsanalysis (FMEA), 2006.

IEC, International Electrotechnical Commission. IEC 61025: Fault tree analysis (FTA), 2008.

ISA. ANSI/ISA-S95.1: Enterprise control system integration. 2000.

ISO International Standard. ISO14971: Medical devices: Application of risk management to medical, p. 82, 2007.

Kurtoglu, T.; Tumer, I. Y. A graph-based fault identification and propagation framework for functional design of complex systems. *Journal of Mechanical Design,* v. 130, n. 5, pp. 1–8, 2008.

Leão, T. F. et al. Modeling study of an implantable centrifugal blood pump actuator with redundant sensorless control. *IEEE Southeastern Symposium on System Theory,* Jacksonville, FL, v. 44, pp. 174–178, 2012.

Lee, E. A.; Seshia, S. A. *Introduction to Embedded Systems a Cyber-Physical Systems Approach.* Cambridge, MA: MIT Press, Second Edition, 2017.

Legendre, D. E. A. In vitro comparative analysis between in series and in parallel cannulations for ventricular assist device. *ASAIO Journal*, v. 55, n. 2, pp. 172, 2009.

Lerner, U. et al. Monitoring a complex physical system using a hybrid dynamic Bayes net. In: *Conference on Uncertainty in Ai(UAI)*, Edmonton, Canada. San Francisco: Morgan Kaufmann, pp. 301–310, 2002.

Locke, D. H. et al. Testing of a centrifugal blood pump with a high efficiency hybrid magnetic bearing. *ASAIO Journal*, v. 49, pp. 737–743, 2003.

Miyagi, P. E. *Controle Programável: Fundamentos do controle de sistemas a eventos discretos*. São Paulo: Edgard Blucher, 1996.

Mona, A.; Mahdi, N.; Kamran, H. Mathematical modelling and electrical analog equivalent of the human cardiovascular system. *Cardiovascular Engineering*, v. 10, pp. 45–51, 2010.

Moraes, M. C. J.; Moraes, D. J.; Bastos, E. S.; Murad, H. Circulação extracorpórea com desvio veno-arterial e e baixa pressão parcial de oxigênio. *Rev Bras Cir Cardiovasc*, v. 16, n. 3, pp. 251–261, 2001. ISSN 44205-554.

Morello, G. F. D. Blood pump system and method of operation. US 7,951,062, 2011.

Muramatsu, K.; Masuoka, T.; Fujisawa, A. In vitro evaluation of the heparin-coated Gyro C1E3 blood pump. *Artificial Organs*, v. 25, n. 7, pp. 585–590, 2001.

Murphy, K. Bayes net toolbox for MATLAB, 2007. Disponível em: http://code.google.com/p/bnt/, acesso em: 01/04/2013.

Nakata, K. et al. A new control method that estimates the backflow in a centrifugal pump. *Artificial Organs*, v. 23, n. 6, pp. 538–541, 1999.

Oshikawa, M. et al. Sensorless controlling method for a continuous flow left ventricular assist device. *Artificial Organs*, v. 24, n. 8, pp. 600–605, 2000.

Pacella, J. J. et al. AbioCor: Blood pump device and method of producing. US 6,808,482, 2004.

Park, J. W. et al. Estimation of native cardiac output of patients under ventricular assist device support using frequency analysis of arterial pressure waveform. *Artificial Organs*, v. 33, n. 5, 2009.

Riascos, L. A. M. and Miyagi, P. E. Fault tolerance in manufacturing systems: Applying Petri nets. VDM Verlag, 2010.

Robert, J. HeartMate II: Minimally invasive transvalvular ventricular assist device. US. 7,479,102, 2009.

Sales, T. P.; Cavalheiro, A. C. M.; Santos Filho, D. J. Mathematical modelling of the human cardiovascular system. In: *Simpósio Internacional de Iniciação Científica da Universidade de São Paulo*, São Paulo. SIICUSP: resumos. São Paulo: USP/Pró-Reitoria de Pesquisa, 2010.

Sales, T. P.; Passanesi, A. V. V.; Donomai, V.; Cavalheiro, A. C. M.; Miyagi, P. E.; Cardoso, J. R.; Andrade, A. P.; Fonseca, J. Hybrid availability control model for ventricular assist devices. In: *Colaob Congresso Latino Americano de Órgãos Artificiais e Biomateriais*, Anais Natal: COLAOB, 2012.

Santos Filho, D. J. Controle de Sistemas Antropocêntricos de Produção Baseado em Redes de Petri Interpretadas. Tese (Doutorado) - Escola Politécnica, Universidade de São Paulo. São Paulo, 1998.

Schmidt, T. et al. New experience with the paracardial right ventricular axial flow micropump impella elect 600. *European Journal of Cardio-Thoracic Surgery*, v. 24, pp. 307–308, 2003. doi: 10.1016/S1010-7940(03)00250-1.

Snyder, T. A. et al. Preclinical biocompatibility assessment of the Evaheart ventricular assist device: Coating comparison and platelet activation. *Journal of Biomedical Materials Research Part A*, v. 81, n. 1, pp. 85–92, 2007.

Spiegelhater, D. J. Probabilistic expert systems in Medicine. *Statistical Science*, v. 2, n. 1, pp. 3–44, 1987.

Squillante Jr, R. et al. Mathematical method for modeling and validating of safety instrumented system designed according to IEC 61508 and IEC 61511. *21st International Congress of Mechanical Engineering (COBEM)*, Natal, RN, 2011.

White, A. J. LionHeart: Internal organ support or sling, 2009.

Wu, Y. et al. Modeling, estimation and control of cardiovascular systems with a left ventricular assist device. In: *Proceedings of American Control Conference,* Portland, OR. Evanston, IL: American Automatic Control Council, 2005.

Yi, W. Physiological control of rotary left ventricular assist device. In: *Proceedings of 26th Chinese Control Conference*, Zhangjiajie, Hunan, China. Piscataway, NJ: IEEE Service Center, pp. 469–474, 2007.

Part II

---

*Biomaterials in Ventricular
Assist Devices*

7 Hemocompatibility, Hemolysis, Cell Viability, and Immunology

Wesley L. Fotoran
Butantan Institute

CONTENTS

7.1 INTRODUCTION: BIOCOMPATIBILITY IN MEDICINE AND SCIENCE

The biocompatibility is the most important issue arising in new technologies and medical assistance in devices and materials for medical application and ecological field. Biocompatibility is a general term for every necessity of use of inorganic or organic materials in translational science and medical care.[1] The urgent needs in different areas, e.g., vaccination,[2] transplant procedure,[3] bioengineering,[4] surgery, medical support, or drug delivery,[5] can lead to new researcher in different biocompatibility areas. To treat every biological aspect,[6] the term can be used for different aspects ranging from biodegradable cup for economic susceptibility,[7] passing by materials used in builds, and construction or in the natural spaces avoiding affect the climate.[8] In medicine, the term in general is used for the intersection between host/patient, material function, and material properties.[1,9]

DOI: 10.1201/9781003138358-9

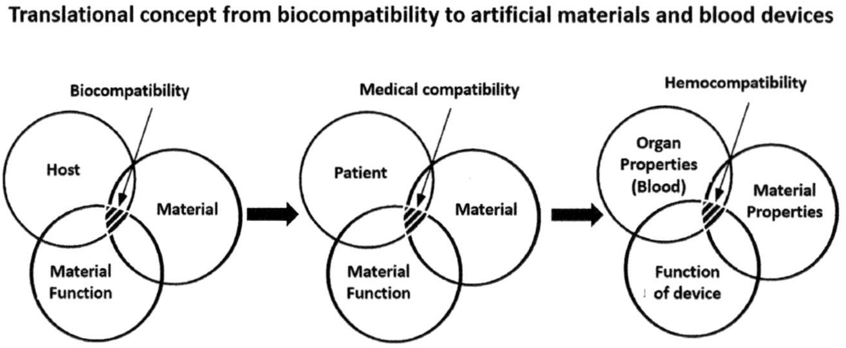

Translational concept from biocompatibility to artificial materials and blood devices

FIGURE 7.1 Concept of biocompatibility in the original definition to health care and science of devices designed to heart assistance.

Regarding the mammalian physiology, any organ can assume the role of host/patient creating new necessities for different aspects related to each organ or tissue. Virtually, thousands of goals can be hypothetically designed to each material to be used in medicine and bioengineering. For example, internal stitches should be biocompatible in resisting for an absorption without inflammation by the body of patient and immune system of the host. On the other hand, superficial stitches on the skin can be biologically inert to human body until the external remotion. In science and medicine, the diverse aspect has to be respected and became in many forms, for electrical stimulation; e.g., the need of biomaterial could stimulate one area for restoring the muscles movement[10] by electric stimulation. On the other hand, internally to central nervous system, the goal is to replace neuron populations with specific devices[11] or associated devices for stimulating and modulating heart beat.[12]

Exactly, the studies in biocompatibility are translational and associated with different knowledge using when possible, multidisciplinary professionals working together to reach the perfect combination for health care, science or medical procedures.[1,4,9] Herein, we will analyze the biocompatibility on the blood and the whole organ with different capacities and necessities. In this context, the biocompatibility adopts the term "hemocompatibility" being applied to devices and materials in direct contact with blood circulating cells and molecules, as shown in Figure 7.1.

7.2 HEMOCOMPATIBILITY AND A STANDARD PROTOCOL TO TEST TESTING MATERIAL CAPACITY TO BE BIOCOMPATIBLE (ISO 10993-4)

In translational studies of blood interaction, many different materials can be used with thousands of functionalities. Oxygenators (artificial lungs), dialyzer, catheters, vascular grafts, cardiac pacemaker, heart-supporting systems, stents, heart valves, nanoparticles and microparticles, and drug carriers are examples of different devices in direct blood contact with different functionality and with different design, interact with blood components. For correct use and propose, hemocompatibility studies provide guidance in development to drive studies and risks of using different materials. For this, guidelines created by International Organization for Standardization (ISO 10993-4)[13] use five principal aspects of blood to be observed, and if possible, all the aspects should be studied to achieve the best combination in hemocompatibility.

The hemocompatibility of different materials relies on five categories: (a) thrombosis; (b) coagulation; (c) platelets; (d) hematological and immunological interactions with complement system; and (e) leukocytes and inflammatory factors that have an intrinsic influence in all other aspects presented. All these five aspects will be analyzed in this chapter. Regarding the devices to be used in clinical contact with the blood, the ISO-10993-4 lead all analyses and divide devices into three major categories with blood contact. The first category is devices with indirect blood contact, defined as external communication devices, e.g., blood collection sets, cannulas, artificial lungs, and cell savers, and in general devices with a well-defined time of contact with blood and blood cells. The second class of devices is external communication devices with direct blood contact, e.g., guidewires, catheters hemodialysis equipment, and in general devices with direct contact and with possible longest time of interaction with blood components because the use depends on medical necessity. The last type of device is the implanted ones, e.g., heart valves, endovascular grafts and stents, devices designed for long time contact with blood and if possible, not needing be change and keeping contact permanently implanted.[14]

For each of these devices, different challenges in translational studies are required in the physiology propose, material, and mechanic engineering used. Due to that, the correct design has to be very carefully thought. For example, some characteristics of blood flow conditions such as static vs. dynamic or laminar flow vs. turbulent[15] can greatly influence the biological responses for all the five aspects standardized by the ISO-10933-4 in hemocompatibility. For devices with short time interaction with blood, e.g., catheters with noble metal alloy coating,[16] poly(2-dimethylamino-ethylmethacrylate) (PDMAEMA),[17] or DNA hydrogels,[18] the most important aspect to avoid is thrombosis and coagulation where the little time of blood contact, and the desired hemocompatibility oriented design should follow the aspect more relevant for this type of device. On the other hand, implantable devices have to be effective as long as possible, so different aspects beyond thrombosis and coagulation are required as well as platelets aggregation,[19] hemolysis, and an adequate immune interaction. Another aspects are produce the correct and desired cell growth with low inflammation and epithelial cell colonization to provide as longer as possible keeping the device implanted without side effects.[20] Therefore, it is essential to define the term "hemocompatibility," which is important to analyze this term to each device. Because it is more important to define the term related to the appropriate function, the use, for each medical device propose. Keeping these aspects in mind, we will analyze the principal aspects of hemocompatibility in the five principal biologic aspects from ISO 10933-4 and analyze the *in vitro* and *in vivo* aspects of hemocompatibility in different ways. Further, we will see two different proposes to overcome problems in the hemocompatibility based on hydrophobic materials and hydrophilic materials. Finally, we will conclude with the necessity of hemocompatibility for the cardiac devices, which is mostly explained and highlighted herein in this book.

7.3 FIVE COMPONENTS OF BLOOD FLOW NEVER WORKING ALONE

The blood is the single organ in the mammalian physiology, which has a contact with virtually all the other organs.[21] The definition of the organ is one tissue, denied by fixed cells and structure. Herein, we will deliberate the blood as an organ in flow with some particularities.[22] Due to this special characteristic, the blood does not have one special place to stay or produce its organic function, and it can be found in every place on the mammalian body in a flowing blood form. The blood has special tissues to create and replace their own different cell types (e.g., bone morrow and lymphoid tissues)[23] and protein components (e.g., liver[24] and kidney[25]), which together will compose the flow organ called the blood system. For fill its evolutionary role, the blood has different components, e.g., thrombotic proteins, adhesion factor, coagulating proteins, ghost-derived cells called platelets, transporting cells as erythrocytes, and immunologic proteins and cells to repair, protect, and fight against foreign materials encountered inside the mammalian body. These materials can be organic or inorganic materials, prokaryotic or eukaryotic cells, virus, or even foreign proteins alone. For our understanding and analyses, we, in general, study the components of blood, but it is crucial to remember as an organ, all the components work together in a living organism. Every ghost cell or full cell (e.g., epithelial cell wall, neutrophil, macrophage) will impact directly in a secondary process (e.g., thrombosis, coagulation, fibrin deposit, collagen remodeling) being indivisible in a complex system, in which a primary process (e.g., thrombosis, coagulation, fibrin deposit, collagen remodeling) can directly influence a secondary ghost cell or full cell (e.g., epithelial cell wall, neutrophil, macrophage) in a cyclic feedback positive or negative to the desire hemocompatibility process for different materials and devices. We divide this hemocompatibility aspect in the same aspect of ISO 10993-4: coagulation, thrombosis, platelets, hemolysis, and immune interactions in inflammatory processes.

7.4 COAGULATION

Coagulation is a blood process to stop bleeding, involved in tissue repair, and initiates the detection of damage or foreign material or cell.[26] In organisms that lack immunological adaptations to respond to bacteria and other pathogens that can pass thought innate immune responses, e.g., Arthropoda, in this type of animal de recognition of cells or material capable to be detect as non-self, it causes coagulation and it is useful to isolate the invasion and avoid parasitism or infections.[27] Coagulation starts in mammalian animals by solubilizing proteins in the blood and can be guided by the intrinsic pathway, which is activated by its contact with different materials or soluble molecules, and guided by the extrinsic pathway, which is activated by tissue damage or cell lysis.[28] The intrinsic pathway begins with plasma and surface proteins, as kallikrein serine proteases act on factor XII[29–33] in contact with artificial material, glass, silica, and dextran sulfate. This effect of serum proteins connected with material surface is called the Vroman effect.[34] Then, proteins from intrinsic pathway, which have more affinity for artificial materials, can promote the conversion of XII to the active form of XIIa, thereby initiating the coagulation cascade until the crucial conversion of X to active form Xa, which is responsible for the conversion of prothrombin (II) to thrombin (IIAa). The final step of the cascade is the conversion of fibrinogen to fibrin causing natural deposit in foreign material, turning possible the cross-linked fibrin clot by the action of the final enzyme XIIIa.[35]

In an extrinsic pathway, the trauma or tissue injury of different cell-type release proteins that start the conversion of VII factor to VIIa and the cascade finds the same crucial factor X to Xa and the final still the deposit of fibrin.[28,36] This is of crucial importance because *in vitro* and *in vivo* tests clearly point only fibrin deposition on materials, showing coagulation problems of the device or the material used.[37,38] Different kits or methodologies are used, but to find higher amount of fibrin demonstrates that one or both pathways are active and cause an undesirable protein deposit under the material used in hemocompatibility.[39] As coagulation depends on multiple proteins acting in the same place, the coagulation is higher in slow blood flow, or static flow, and it occurs in a longer time than processes where cells are not necessarily involved.[36] One example of the cascade connected with thrombosis is shown in Figure 7.2).[40]

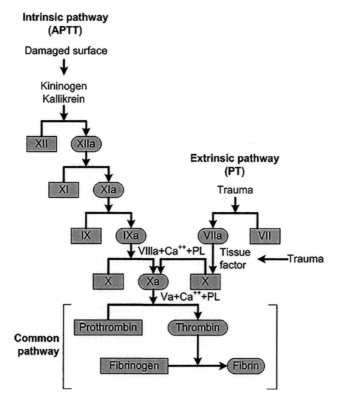

FIGURE 7.2   Connection of kallikrein–kinin system, coagulation cascade, and thrombosis system. These pathways, as described in the cascade model, are reflected in the laboratory analysis of coagulation, although as *in vitro* phenomena, with the intrinsic pathway reflected the measurement of the activated partial thromboplastin time (APTT) and the extrinsic pathway in the prothrombin time (PT).

7.5 THROMBOSIS

The effect named "thrombosis" rises from the thrombin (IIa), a plasma protein present in the cascade of coagulation, which can reinforce the coagulation process by conversion of the factor V to Va.[41,42] The activation factor Va converts prothrombin (II) to thrombin (IIa) in a cyclic positive feedback of reinforcement. In higher levels, thrombin (IIa) can activate thrombomodulin in the presence of protein C (one protein essential in inflammatory process and present in the cytoplasm of multiple cells ranging from epithelial, neutrophil, macrophage, and others) under the action of Protein S turning Protein C to Active Protein C.[43]

Active Protein C can inhibit the intrinsic pathway and thrombin (IIa) effect; in other words, under higher levels of thrombin (IIa), Active Protein C blocks the coagulation avoiding complete occlusion of venular or capillary artery protecting the circulation system to collapse.[44,45] It is important that the extrinsic pathway can maintain the process, where the cellular trauma is still under process or auxiliary cells are being destroyed locally like platelets,[46,47] erythrocytes, epithelial cell, or inflammatory/immune cells such as neutrophil, macrophages, and lymphocytes.[18,48–50] One example of coagulation and inflammation and thrombosis is shown in Figure 7.3.

Because thrombin (IIa) is present in the coagulation cascade, the most clear signal for thrombosis is the cellular presence of fibrin clot with hemolysis and other type of cells. In this scenario, if the process cause by one device in a place under slow flow the most probable process will be increase clots, that later, become fibrous tissue with encapsulation of the material or device turning the medical intervention useless and very danger.[51,52] The most common problem remain in piece's clot, which in the higher flow, can be release it and cause completely occlusion in capillary vessel distance of the implant turning possible strokes, heart attack or others occlusion problems.[44,45,53] *In vitro* or *in vivo* studies rely on finding this type of clot with different cell types forming fibrous tissue under, or not, flow studies.

7.6 PLATELETS

Platelets are ghost cells derived from megakaryocytes released from the bone marrow. These ghost cells are composed of cellular fractions with alpha granules (usually 60–80 in total) and dense granules (usually six to eight in total) along with procoagulant factors such as platelet factor $4^{36,54}$ (PF 4) and β-thromboglobulin (BT-G), which are used to verify the presence of platelet aggregation during *in vitro* assays.[55,56] Platelets can control the antithrombogenic effects forming nitric oxide (NO) to vasodilatation or releasing prostaglandin I_2 (PGI_2).[48,57,58] Prothrombogenic factors include ADP (adenosine diphosphate), ATP (adenosine triphosphate), divalent ions (Ca^{2+} and Mg^{2+}) histamine, and serotonin (5-hydroxytryptamine (5HT)).[59–61] Due to the minimal size (2–3 µm) in the blood flow, platelets are in general localized in the peripheral flux and do not interact with healthy endothelial cells.

Under damage or inflammation caused by rupture, endothelial cell secretes von Willebrand factor (vWF) together with fibronectin, exposes the subendothelial matrix, interacts with integrin receptor $\alpha_{IIb}\beta_3$ glycoprotein IIb/IIIa (GPIIb/IIIa) on the surface of platelets, and leads to the activation of them.[62] Positive

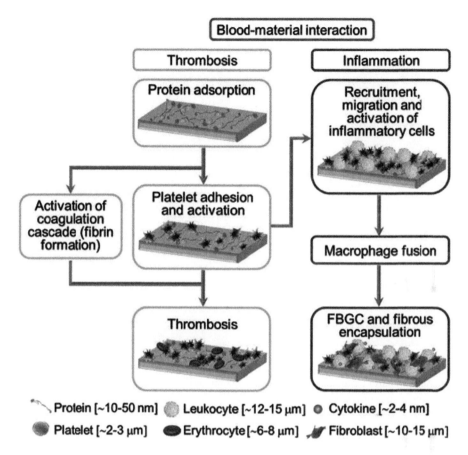

FIGURE 7.3 A schematic (not drawn to scale) illustrating the biological responses ensuing from blood–foreign material interaction.

electric charges of exposed material in response to charge and natural adhesion to these factor platelets starting an aggregate process to seal the damage tissue.[36] The platelets release the prothrombogenic molecules from the granulocytes, attracting more platelets to the damage tissue. Also, secreting PF 4 and TG-B platelets can recruit immunological cells such as leucocytes to the same prothrombotic sites. Releasing growth factors, e.g., VEGF, platelets, initiates the repair of the tissue, stimulate the division of endothelial cells, and can further active the coagulation factor XII by liberating diphosphates and by inhibiting the intrinsic pathway of coagulation.[63–65]

Because platelets present distinct effects at different times of coagulation process, which are possible to analyze, the form and shape of them verify the levels of activation. They can be found in four states of activation, as observed in Figure 7.4, namely, nonspread, discoid and early pseudopodal, spread, and dendritic or fully spread.[66]

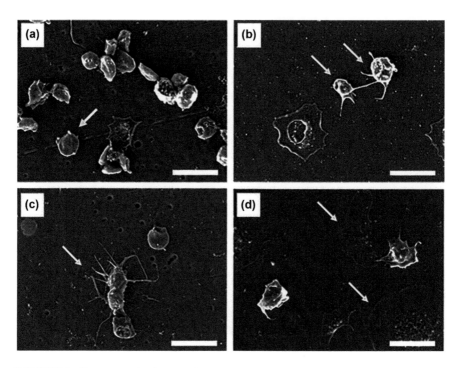

FIGURE 7.4   Representative images of platelets in varying states of activation: (a) nonspread, discoid and early pseudopodial, (b) and (c) spread and dendritic, (d) fully spread (scanning electron microscopy, scale bar = 5 m).

7.7   ERYTHROCYTES

For all the implanted devices static, or not, to maintain erythrocytes in intact condition is the mean goal. While coagulation and immunological reactions can be controlled by pharmacological drugs, process in which erythrocytes are not lysed is vital because the lyses of them can result in decreased oxygen transport and formation of free hemoglobin, leading to toxicity to kidney.[67,68] An illustration of hemolytic effects on coagulation and endothelial homeostasis is shown in Figure 7.5.[69] Erythrocytes are the major component of blood with $5-6 \times 10^6$ cells/μL, and their evolutionary function is transporting oxygen (O_2) from the lung to all tissues and cells and carbon dioxide (CO_2) from tissues back to the lung by osmosis in simple diffusion at different pressures of oxygen (PO_2).[70] Erythrocytes lack nuclear cell in mammalian, and because of that, they do not have metabolism; they are the most rigid cells in the blood, and are sensitive to rupture and hemolysis due to shear stress and changes in osmotic pressure.[71] Two methods can be used to verify hemolytic process or erythrocyte retention in thrombotic process. The first is direct count before and after the number of erythrocytes in hemocompatibility test of material or devices in direct contact with blood,[72] and the second is colorimetric assay measurement based on free hemoglobin by cyanmethemoglobin method (CMB).[73] Because erythrocyte has receptor on the surface similar to platelets, they can recognize vWF and fibrinogen, they can be entrapped in clot, and suffer from rupture lysis in flow devices, thus

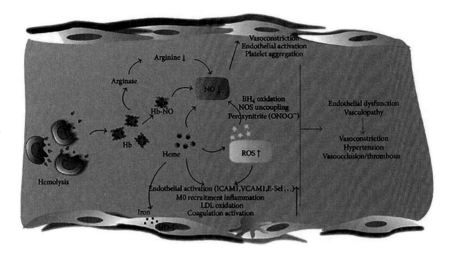

FIGURE 7.5 Hemolysis-driven endothelial toxicity. Free Hb/heme is responsible for reduced NO availability and ROS generation that contribute to endothelial dysfunction, leading to vasoconstriction, hypertension, and vasoocclusion.

leading to the liberation of ADP, serotonin, PF 4, and Ca^{2+} and increasing some thrombotic processes in course.[74]

The hemolysis is so important in hemocompatibility analysis that has a critical-level hemolysis of above 5%. The system for the standardization of hemolysis is: material resulting in over 5% hemolysis are classified hemolytic; between 5% and 2% as slightly hemolytic; and below 2% as nonhemolytic.[75]

7.8 IMMUNOLOGY AND INFLAMMATION

The immune role can be divided at least into two different ways to affect hemocompatibility assays. The first immune aspect is the innate reaction, which has an intrinsic contact with coagulation and thrombosis.[71] The second role of immune effect is regarding immune cells and sustaining of inflammatory process leading to persistent inflammation and rejection of implanted devices/materials.[76] As the other effects presented until here, both immunologic roles should be seen as interconnects and will be divide only for better clarification.

The Vroman effect is the most important event to initiate a strict innate immunologic role in hemocompatibility tests.[34] First, artificial materials are recovered by different plasma proteins such as albumin and fibronectin and others. After some time, by competition, soluble proteins with more lipophilic affinity assume the role in this coating as immunoglobulin, coagulating factors and mainly soluble proteins from innate immune response called complement system, specially C3 protein.[77] The complement system can be divided into three initiation cascades called classical, alternative, and mannose binding lectin (MBL) pathways.[78,79] The classical pathway is initialized by the deposition of antibodies, the alternative pathway is by C3 conversion, and the last one is by ligation with specific sugar groups from pathogen. Both classical and alternative pathways can be activated by the complement deposition on the artificial surface material, leading to C3 conversation into C3a and C3b with opsonizing effect and immune recruitment. The process continues until the formation of a complex of proteins named membrane attack complex (MAC) to destroy foreign cells. The cascade has one interesting intermediary product of cleavage C5, called C5a.[37,80,81] This molecule can increase the permeability of endothelial vessels and activate endothelial cells to expresses E-selectin, thus permitting the translocation of monocytes and neutrophil at the site of response.[82] Together with platelet activation which expresses another binder, as P-selectin find connection with P-selectin in neutrophil it leads to the neutrophil recruitment and activation.[83]

After the recruitment of activated immune cells, these cells start immunologic roles that culminated in the prolongation of inflammatory process.[84] Neutrophil recruitment will be culminating in the activation of these cells by tool like 4 to platelets and forming neutrophil extracellular nets (NET).[84,85] The formation of NET by itself can promote thrombosis, as demonstrated in animals.[86] Besides that, NET can be started by opsonization or by innate response by toll-like receptor, and the process consists in a burst of these cells liberating cytokines, resulting in the generation of ROS (superoxide anion ($O^{-2}O^{2-}$), hydrogen peroxide (H_2O_2), hydroxyl radical (HO), and singlet oxygen ($^-O_2$) and with nucleic material and proteins of the nucleic as histones one NET to entrap foreign cells.[78,87–89] This recruits more cells as other neutrophils, lymphocytes and macrophages.[90] In this environment, inflammation macrophages can become foam cells phagocytosing high levels of lipid vesicles as LDL (problem usually common in people needing ventricular assisting devices).[43,91,92] Macrophages can create a scenario of healing or still attracting immune cells and keep with the inflammatory process until clot formation turning the artificial material or device useless causing occlusion or more damage in the tissue.[91,93–95]

As hemolysis triggers the immune response it receive a strong importance because the process caused by the cell enrolled can rapidly progress to clots and systemic response causing shock syndrome known as cytokine storm.[96] According to ISO 10993-4, the complement activation can be analyzed by the detection of C3a, C5a, and the C5b-9 complex in the whole blood, as well as the 50% complement hemolytic activity (CH_{50}).[72] All these components working together with coagulation and thrombi formation are shown in Figure 7.6.

7.9 THE MAJOR TWO ALTERNATIVES TO AVOID PROBLEMS WITH HEMOCOMPATIBILITY: HYDROPHILIC MATERIALS AND HYDROPHOBICITY

Further in this book, alternatives to avoid problems of hemocompatibility will be discussed in detail in the optic of alternative materials, mechanic and physic properties of modified materials. So, herein, we will briefly discuss two opposite strategies: one classical and other recently becoming as an alternative for materials used in the devices which are direct contact with blood in static and flow scenario.

The classical alternative is materials with complete contact with blood and full hydrophilic profile. Metal and plastic formulation design designed for minimal interaction with components of the blood are the classical alternatives to produce devices for blood

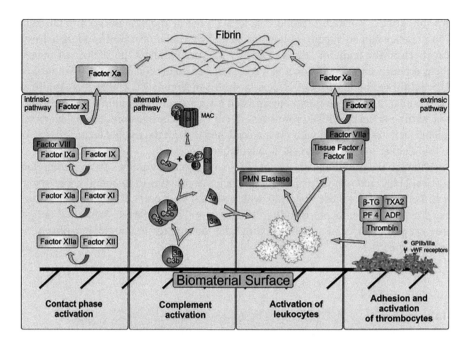

FIGURE 7.6 Schematic representation of major reactions in blood induced by biomaterial surface. Besides the complement system, intrinsic and extrinsic coagulation pathways can be activated. Coagulation activation results in the generation of a fibrin network. Furthermore, platelets can adhere and aggregate on the surface. The adhesion and activation of leukocytes can lead to the release of polymorphonuclear (PMN) elastase and tissue factor (TF) and result in the activation of extrinsic pathway. ADP, adenosine diphosphate; β-TG, β-thromboglobulin; GPIIb/IIIa, glycoprotein IIb/IIIa; MAC, membrane attack complex; PF4, platelet factor 4; TXA2, thromboxane A2; vWF, von Willebrand factor.

contact. Stents,[97,98] needles or catheters,[16] or even vascular system supports in general are made of rare metals or plastic compounds with low oxidative capacity or degradation by chemical conditions present in the blood.[99] Materials with these designs are produced, and they are resistant to variation in PH, oxidative stress, and their permeability (when necessary) and durability depend on their use.[100] For a long time, this research area was lead for coating simple material with noble metals for this propose.[101,102] This strategy increases the general cost of these products and in general still unable to produce long-term effect in hemocompatibility. In all the areas ranging from odontologist application to artificial hearts, this is the classical thinking in hemocompatibility. The new area on the hydrophilic alternative is the use of different materials that increase the attachment of cells in the materials used to create an artificial material to simulate the environment of the cells in the body,[103] where the device will be applied.[104,105] The basic new design is the use of materials that stimulate the colonization of epithelial cells[106] capable of regulating coagulation, thrombosis, hemolysis, and avoiding immune reaction.[38] Many examples are actually present in this field (see Chapter 9).

The opposite design is based on avoiding the complete contact with the all blood. Avoiding the contact with water, all the components of the blood are seal in the blood flow are almost isolated to blood contact with the artificial material around them. These tactics named super-repellent surfaces[56] were first observed in lotus leaves[107] and received the name of "lotus effect."[108] The design alters the surface of materials to produce the effect known as Cassie–Baxter state on a textured solid surface. A beautiful example of these effects is shown in Figure 7.7. Under this condition, the modifications on surface material keep air between the liquid phase, creating a non-wetting material with a promising effect.[109] These designs prevent the contact of soluble factor of the blood with the material, and turn all the soluble factors discussed in this chapter to interact and start coagulation process.

Although the promising effects *in vitro* conditions, few studies *in vivo* conditions are available[56] and in contrast, lipophilic factor as proteins from complement system is still able to affect these materials with potential start point of inflammation causing problems in hemocompatibility.[81] Whatsoever, in the future, both new designs are very promising and still an exciting area for studies in hemocompatibility for artificial materials.

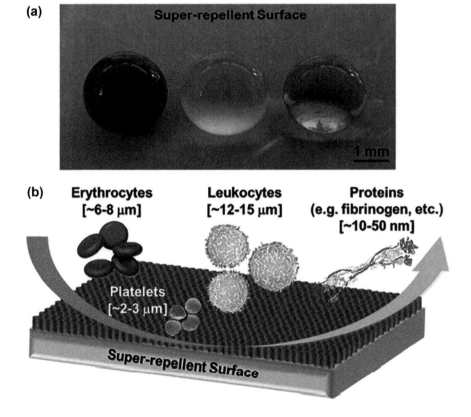

FIGURE 7.7 (a) Droplets of blood, plasma, and water beading up on a super-repellent surface. (b) Schematic (not drawn to scale) depicting the components of blood being "repelled" by a super-repellent surface due to the reduced blood–material contact area.

7.10 EVALUATION OF HEMOCOMPATIBILITY *IN VITRO* AND *IN VIVO*

To test the hemocompatibility of different materials, different aspects should be addressed. First of all, the type of assay has to be compatible for the use in clinical or science use. For example, for needles or suture stitches, simple static assays should be enough to predict the hemocompatibility. Regarding the same example, assays in flux condition are completely unnecessary, and in order to analyze *in vivo* experiments, biological assays with mice should bring the data necessary to evaluate the possible use in medical context.[110] The same scenario cannot be applied to other devices and in general requires more carefully studies for possible use, with significant differences in cost, scale, and methodology.[111] In general, for *in vitro* conditions, the deposition of proteins or cells can be direct assessment for visual experiments such as scanning electron microscopy (SEM) microscopy.[112–114] In some cases, the simple incubation of blood or cells with different materials in posterior evaluation of cell viability should be a good and less-expensive start.[115] In general, the direct visualization in a larger device, or more complex engineered, make all the surface of device unviable. One alternative is look for piece of the total material for this type of analyses. The critics for this approach are which the deposit of protein and cells can be different in the material used and not be homogenous. Systemic and multiple analyses for different randomized areas should be an alternative to problem.[116] For direct measurements, hemolysis can be evaluated by free hemoglobin or cell retention by the simple cell count.[117] ELISA [118] and flow cytometry can be very useful for analyzing the protein deposition and cell activation,[119] especially in immunology aspect. A summary of the test used for hemocompatibility can be seen in Table 7.1.

When the device is designed for flow conditions, the use of flow assays should be mandatory for a good clarification of hemocompatibility. This brings out the problem to another level.[120]

For ventricular devices for example, the flux conditions of human blood have to be recreated, even for *in vitro* assays. The most problem with this is to reproduce the veins and arterial conditions with the amount of blood for one person, proximately 5 L. In terms of supply, this is equivalent to 10 blood bags, which turn the *in vitro* experiment expansive.[121] As alternative, animal blood provided by slaughterhouse from porcine[122] or cattle[123] are used in many thrombotic od hemolytic assays. The most problem in these experiments is the quality of the blood, because they are not harvested with the appropriate attention for reproducible results. Commonly, the researchers found samples with hemolysis or cells with higher degeneration and deformation statuses.[124]

Medical devices in flow conditions find the most problem in *in vivo* assays. For this type of device, the *in vivo* assay is very important and demands higher cost. The experiment involves in general multiple professionals with a higher specialty in surgery, such as veterinarians and medical doctor. In general, an animal of huge size is connected to the device to analyze clots, thrombi or any problem do not simulate same *in vitro* conditions. The animal use is important because many different aspects regarding veins and arteries are almost impossible to be simulated in *in vitro* conditions.[125,126] In general, the requirements for hemocompatibility are higher when the device proposed is more complex or vital for the use in clinical area.[127] Due to this, many different controls part by part should be produced to a better control of the device as we have shown in chapters 4 and 6.

TABLE 7.1
Summary of Test Categories for the Hemocompatibility Analysis of Biomaterials

Test Category	Parameter	Test Principle
Complement system	C3a, C5a, Bb, C4d, C5b-9	ELISA
Coagulation	Factor XIIa, TAT, F1+a, free active thrombin, FPA, aPTT	ELISA, optical density, viscoelasticity
Fibrinolysis	D-Dimers	Immunoturbidimetry, LPIA, ELISA
Platelets	β-TG, PF4, number of platelets, P-selectin, activated GPIIb/IIIa	Elisa, cell counter, FACS
Hemolysis	Number of erythrocytes, hemoglobin	Cell counter
Leukocyte activation	PMN elastase, ROS detection, CD11b expression	Colorimetric assay, ELISA, fluorimetric or spectrophotometric methods, FACS, SEM, fluorescence microscopy
Surface analysis	Platelet adhesion, aggregation, leukocyte adhesion, plasma protein adsorption	ELISA, western blot

[a] PTT, activated partial thromboplastin time; β-TG, β-thromboglobulin; C3a, complement factor 3a; C5a, complement factor 5a; C4d, complement factor 4d; Bb, complement factor Bb; ELISA, enzyme-linked immunosorbent assay; FACS, fluorescence-activated cell sorting; FPA, fibrinopeptide A; F1 + 2, prothrombin fragment 1 + 2; LPIA, latex photometric immunoassay; PF4, platelet factor 4; TAT, thrombin–antithrombin III complex; PMN elastase, polymorphonuclear elastase; ROS, reactive oxygen species; SEM, scanning electron microscopy.

7.11   CONCLUSION FOR VAD DEVICES

As can be seen in Chapters 1, 3, 5, and 6, since the first steps of the VAD design, hemocompatibility is an essential requirement. More than this VAD are equipment which require approval in all the steps in ISO 10993-4 for hemocompatibility in all requirements in static and flow with real blood. The physiological parameters serve as basis for control, and there are several ways to pursue a more harmonious control system, which must be evaluated in simulators but is directly linked to the performance of blood. In Chapters 8, 9, and 12, we present several ways to computationally simulate the hemodynamics inside these pumps, biofunctional materials, and processes for obtaining surfaces and films developed to achieve this target.

REFERENCES

1. Materials biocompatibility: An overview | Science direct topics. https://www.sciencedirect.com/topics/chemistry/materials-biocompatibility.
2. van Riel, D. & de Wit, E. Next-generation vaccine platforms for COVID-19. *Nature Materials* **19**, 810–812 (2020).
3. Nur Altinörs, M. Future prospects of organ transplantation. *Organ Donation and Transplantation*, IntechOpen (2020). doi:10.5772/intechopen.94367.
4. Murabayashi, S. & Nosé, Y. Biocompatibility: Bioengineering Aspects. *Artificial Organs* **10**, 114–121 (1986).

5. Pandit, A. & Zeugolis, D. I. Twenty-five years of nano-bio-materials: Have we revolutionized healthcare? *Nanomedicine* **11**, 985–987 (2016).

6. Ibrahim, M. S., Sani, N., Adamu, M. & Abubakar, M. K. Biodegradable polymers for sustainable environmental and economic development. MOJ Bioorganic & Organic Chemistry 2(4), 192–194 (2018). doi:10.15406/mojboc.2018.02.00080.

7. Prasteen, P., Thushyanthy, Y., Mikunthan, T. & Prabhaharan, M. Bio-plastics-an alternative to petroleum based plastics. *International Journal of Research Studies in Agricultural Science* **4**, 2454–6224 (2018).

8. Horvath, A. Construction materials and the environment. *Annual Review of Environment and Resources* **29**, 181–204 (2004).

9. Biocompatibility: An overview I Science Direct Topics. https://www.sciencedirect.com/topics/materials-science/biocompatibility.

10. Donati, A. R. et al. Long-term training with a brain-machine interface-based gait protocol induces partial neurological recovery in paraplegic patients neurorehabilitation laboratory open. *Scientific Reports* 6(1), 1–16. (2016). doi: 10.1038/srep30383.

11. Hartmann, K. et al. Embedding a panoramic representation of infrared light in the adult rat somatosensory cortex through a sensory neuroprosthesis. *Journal of Neuroscience* **36**, 2406–2424 (2016).

12. Townsend, T. Five common permanent cardiac pacemaker complications. *Nursing in Critical Care* **13**, 46–48 (2018).

13. ISO - ISO 10993-4. Biological evaluation of medical devices: Part 4: Selection of tests for interactions with blood (2017). https://www.iso.org/standard/63448.html.

14. ISO - ISO 10993-4. Biological evaluation of medical devices: Part 4: Selection of tests for interactions with blood (2017). https://www.iso.org/standard/63448.html.

15. Peterson, L. H. *The Dynamics of Pulsatile Blood Flow.* http://ahajournals.org.

16. Vafa Homann, M., Johansson, D., Wallen, H. & Sanchez, J. Improved ex vivo blood compatibility of central venous catheter with noble metal alloy coating. *Journal of Biomedical Materials Research Part B Applied Biomaterials* **104**, 1359–1365 (2016).

17. Cerda-Cristerna, B. I. et al. Hemocompatibility assessment of poly(2-dimethylamino ethylmethacrylate) (PDMAEMA)-based polymers. *Journal of Controlled Release* **153**, 269–277 (2011).

18. Stoll, H. et al. Generation of large-scale DNA hydrogels with excellent blood and cell compatibility. *Macromolecular Bioscience* 17(4): 1600252 (2017).

19. Sanak, M., Jakieła, B. & Węgrzyn, W. Assessment of hemocompatibility of materials with arterial blood flow by platelet functional tests. *Bulletin of the Polish Academy of Sciences: Technical Sciences* **58**, 317–322 (2010).

20. Reviakine, I. & Braune, S. Preface: In focus issue on blood–biomaterial interactions. *Biointerphases* **11**, 029501 (2016).

21. Organ blood flow: An overview I Science direct topics. https://www.sciencedirect.com/topics/biochemistry-genetics-and-molecular-biology/organ-blood-flow.

22. Mechanobiology, Series On. Forces in cell biology. *Nature Cell Biology* **19**(6), 579 (2017).

23. Ng, A. P. & Alexander, W. S. Haematopoietic stem cells: Past, present and future. *Cell Death Discovery* **3**, 1–4 (2017).

24. Schreiber, G. The synthesis and secretion of plasma proteins in the liver. *Pathology* **10**, 394 (1978).

25. Strober, W. & Waldmann, T. A. The role of the kidney in the metabolism of plasma proteins. *Nephron* **13**, 35–66 (1974).

26. Palta, S., Saroa, R. & Palta, A. Overview of the coagulation system. *Indian Journal of Anaesthesia* **58**, 515–523 (2014).

27. Theopold, U., Schmidt, O., Söderhäll, K. & Dushay, M. S. Coagulation in arthropods: Defence, wound closure and healing. *Trends in Immunology* **25**, 289–294 (2004).

28. Millar, J. E., Fanning, J. P., McDonald, C. I., McAuley, D. F. & Fraser, J. F. The inflammatory response to extracorporeal membrane oxygenation (ECMO): A review of the pathophysiology. *Critical Care* **20**, 387 (2016).

29. Mamenko, M., Zaika, O., Boukelmoune, N., Madden, E. & Pochynyuk, O. Control of ENaC-mediated sodium reabsorption in the distal nephron by Bradykinin. *Vitamins and Hormones* **98**, 137–154 (Academic Press Inc., 2015).

30. Doolittle, R. F. The evolution of vertebrate blood coagulation: A case of yin and yang. *Thrombosis and Haemostasis* **70**, 24–28 (1993).

31. Doolittle, R. F. & Feng, D. F. Reconstructing the evolution of vertebrate blood coagulation from a consideration of the amino acid sequences of clotting proteins. *Cold Spring Harbor Symposia on Quantitative Biology* **52**, 869–874 (1987).

32. Kallikrein Kinin System: An overview | Science direct topics. https://www.sciencedirect.com/topics/medicine-and-dentistry/kallikrein-kinin-system.

33. The evolution of vertebrate blood clotting. http://www.millerandlevine.com/km/evol/DI/clot/Clotting.html.

34. Hirsh, S. L. et al. The vroman effect: Competitive protein exchange with dynamic multilayer protein aggregates. *Colloids Surfaces B Biointerfaces* **103**, 395–404 (2013).

35. Kappelmayer, J., Bernabei, A., Edmunds, L. H., Edgington, T. S. & Colman, R. W. Tissue factor is expressed on monocytes during simulated extracorporeal circulation. *Circulation Research* **72**, 1075–1081 (1993).

36. Sperling, C., Maitz, M. F., Grasso, S., Werner, C. & Kanse, S. M. A positively charged surface triggers coagulation activation through factor VII Activating Protease (FSAP). *ACS Applied Materials & Interfaces* **9**, 40107–40116 (2017).

37. Gorbet, M. B. & Sefton, M. V. Biomaterial-associated thrombosis: Roles of coagulation factors, complement, platelets and leukocytes. *Biomaterials* **25**, 5681–5703 (2004).

38. McGuigan, A. P. & Sefton, M. V. The influence of biomaterials on endothelial cell thrombogenicity. *Biomaterials* **28**, 2547–2571 (2007).

39. Peckham, S. M., Turitto, V. T., Glantz, J., Puryear, H. & Slack, S. M. Hemocompatibility studies of surface-treated polyurethane-based chronic indwelling catheters. *Journal of Biomaterials Science, Polymer Edition* **8**, 847–858 (1997).

40. Adams, R. L. C. & Bird, R. J. Review article: Coagulation cascade and therapeutics update: Relevance to nephrology. Part 1: Overview of coagulation, thrombophilias and history of anticoagulants. *Nephrology* **14**, 462–470 (2009).

41. Brotman, D. J., Deitcher, S. R., Lip, G. Y. H. & Matzdorff, A. C. Virchow's triad revisited. *Southern Medical Journal* **97**, 213–214 (2004).

42. Cervantes, J. & Rojas, G. Virchow's legacy: Deep vein thrombosis and pulmonary embolism. *World Journal of Surgery* **29**, S30–S34 (2005).

43. Boos, C. J. & Lip, G. Y. H. Blood clotting, inflammation, and thrombosis in cardiovascular events: Perspectives. *Frontiers in Bioscience* **11**, 328–336 (2006).

44. Watson, T., Shantsila, E. & Lip, G. Y. Mechanisms of thrombogenesis in atrial fibrillation: Virchow's triad revisited. *The Lancet* **373**, 155–166 (2009).

45. Castellano, J. M., Chinitz, J., Willner, J. & Fuster, V. Mechanisms of stroke in atrial fibrillation. *Cardiac Electrophysiology Clinics* **6**, 5–15 (2014).

46. Rao, A. K., Koike, K., Day, H. J., Smith, J. B. & Holmsen, H. Bleeding disorder associated with albumin-dependent partial deficiency in platelet thromboxane production: Effect of albumin on arachidonate metabolism in platelets. *American Journal of Clinical Pathology* **83**, 687–96 (1985).

47. Jørgensen, K. A. & Stoffersen, E. On the inhibitory effect of albumin on platelet aggregation. *Thrombosis Research* **17**, 13–18 (1980).

48. Morel, O., Jesel, L., Freyssinet, J. M. & Toti, F. Cellular mechanisms underlying the formation of circulating microparticles. *Arteriosclerosis, Thrombosis, and Vascular Biology* **31**, 15–26 (2011).

49. Hua, V. M. Targetin the procoagulant platelet.
50. Heemskerk, J. W. M., Matheij, N. J. A. & Cosemans, J. M. E. M. Platelet-based coagulation: Different populations, different functions. *Journal of Thrombosis and Haemostasis* **11**, 2–16 (2013).
51. Pham, T. T. et al. Hemodynamic aspects of reduced platelet adhesion on bioinspired microstructured surfaces. *Colloids Surfaces B Biointerfaces* **145**, 502–509 (2016).
52. Kulik, A., Saltzman, M. B. & Morris, J. J. Dabigatran after cardiac surgery: Caution advised. *Journal of Thoracic and Cardiovascular Surgery* **142**, 1288 (2011).
53. Meng, J. et al. Adhesion and interfacial fracture in drug-eluting stents. *Journal of Materials Research* **25**, 641–647 (2010).
54. Bridges, D. J. et al. Rapid activation of endothelial cells enables Plasmodium falciparum adhesion to platelet-decorated von Willebrand factor strings. *Blood* **115**, 1472–1474 (2010).
55. Mignot, C. et al. Perinatal-lethal Gaucher disease. *American Journal of Medical Genetics Part A* **120A**, 338–344 (2003).
56. Movafaghi, S. et al. Hemocompatibility of super-repellent surfaces: Current and future. *Materials Horizons* **6**, 1596–1610 (2019).
57. Golebiewska, E. M. & Poole, A. W. Platelet secretion: From haemostasis to wound healing and beyond. *Blood Reviews* **29**, 153–162 (2015).
58. Fröhlich, E. Action of nanoparticles on platelet activation and plasmatic coagulation. *Current Medicinal Chemistry* **23**, 408–430 (2016).
59. Meyers, K. M., Holmsen, H. & Seachord, C. L. Comparative study of platelet dense granule constituents. *American Journal of Physiology - Regulatory Integrative and Comparative Physiology* **243**, R454–R461 (1982).
60. Oshinowo, O. et al. Significant differences in single-platelet biophysics exist across species but attenuate during clot formation. *Blood Advances* **5**, 432–437 (2021).
61. Meyers, K. M., Holmsen, H., Seachord, C. L., Hopkins, G. & Gorham, J. Characterization of platelets from normal mink and mink with the Chediak-Higashi syndrome. *American Journal of Hematology* **7**, 137–146 (1979).
62. Fitch-Tewfik, J. L. & Flaumenhaft, R. Platelet granule exocytosis: A comparison with chromaffin cells. *Frontiers in Endocrinology* **4**, 77 (2013).
63. Brandt, E. et al. The β-thromboglobulins and platelet factor 4: Blood platelet-derived CXC chemokines with divergent roles in early neutrophil regulation. *Journal of Leukocyte Biology* **67**, 471–478 (2000).
64. Saleh, M., Stacker, S. A. & Wilks, A. F. Inhibition of growth of C6 glioma cells *in vivo* by expression of antisense vascular endothelial growth factor sequence. *Cancer Research* **56**, 393–401 (1996).
65. Walz, A., Dewald, B., Von Tscharner, V. & Baggiolini, M. Effects of the neutrophil-activating peptide NAP-2, platelet basic protein, connective tissue-activating peptide III, and platelet factor 4 on human neutrophils. *Journal of Experimental Medicine* **170**, 1745–1750 (1989).
66. Jung, F., Braune, S. & Lendlein, A. Haemocompatibility testing of biomaterials using human platelets. *Clinical Hemorheology and Microcirculation* **53**, 97–115 (2013).
67. Kuhbier, J. W. et al. Influence of direct or indirect contact for the cytotoxicity and blood compatibility of spider silk. *Journal of Materials Science: Materials in Medicine* **28**, 1–9 (2017).
68. Qian, Q., Nath, K. A., Wu, Y., Daoud, T. M. & Sethi, S. Hemolysis and acute kidney failure. *American Journal of Kidney Diseases* **56**, 780–784 (2010).
69. Vinchi, F. & Tolosano, E. Therapeutic approaches to limit hemolysis-driven endothelial dysfunction: Scavenging free heme to preserve vasculature homeostasis. *Oxidative Medicine and Cellular Longevity* (2013). doi: 10.1155/2013/396527.
70. Pittman, R. N. Oxygen Transport (2011).

71. Anderson, H. L., Brodsky, I. E. & Mangalmurti, N. S. The evolving erythrocyte: Red blood cells as modulators of innate immunity. *Journal of Immunology* **201**, 1343–1351 (2018).

72. Weber, M. et al. Blood-contacting biomaterials: In vitro evaluation of the hemocompatibility. *Frontiers in Bioengineering and Biotechnology* **6**, 99 (2018).

73. Arnaud, F., Higgins, A., McCarron, R. & Moon-Massat, P. F. Determination of methemoglobin and hemoglobin levels in small volume samples. *Artificial Cells, Nanomedicine, and Biotechnology* **45**, 58–62 (2017).

74. Bernhardt, I., C. Wesseling, M., Nguyen, D. B. & Kaestner, L. Red blood cells actively contribute to blood coagulation and thrombus formation. *Erythrocyte* (IntechOpen, 2019). doi: 10.5772/intechopen.86152.

75. Totea, G., Ionita, D., Demetrescu, I. & Mitache, M. M. In vitro hemocompatibility and corrosion behavior of new Zr-binary alloys in whole human blood. *Central European Journal of Chemistry* **12**, 796–803 (Versita, 2014).

76. Charles, A., Janeway, J., Travers, P., Walport, M. & Shlomchik, M. J. Principles of innate and adaptive immunity (2001).

77. Dunkelberger, J. R. & Song, W. C. Complement and its role in innate and adaptive immune responses. *Cell Research* **20**, 34–50 (2010).

78. Wetterö, J., Bengtsson, T. & Tengvall, P. Complement activation on immunoglobulin G-coated hydrophobic surfaces enhances the release of oxygen radicals from neutrophils through an actin- dependent mechanism. *Journal of Biomedical Materials Research* **51**, 742–751 (2000).

79. Wetterö, J., Askendal, A., Tengvall, P. & Bengtsson, T. Interactions between surface-bound actin and complement, platelets, and neutrophils. *Journal of Biomedical Materials Research - Part A* **66**, 162–175 (2003).

80. Andersson, J., Ekdahl, K. N., Lambris, J. D. & Nilsson, B. Binding of C3 fragments on top of adsorbed plasma proteins during complement activation on a model biomaterial surface. *Biomaterials* **26**, 1477–1485 (2005).

81. Nilsson, B., Ekdahl, K. N., Mollnes, T. E. & Lambris, J. D. The role of complement in biomaterial-induced inflammation. *Molecular Immunology* **44**, 82–94 (2007).

82. Newton, K. & Dixit, V. M. Signaling in innate immunity and inflammation. *Cold Spring Harbor Perspectives in Biologyold Spring* **4**, a006049 (2012).

83. Frenette, P. S. et al. P-selectin glycoprotein ligand 1 (PSGL-1) is expressed on platelets and can mediate platelet-endothelial interactions in vivo. *Journal of Experimental Medicine* **191**, 1413–1422 (2000).

84. Ghasemzadeh, M. et al. The CXCR1/2 ligand NAP-2 promotes directed intravascular leukocyte migration through platelet thrombi. *Blood* **121**, 4555–4566 (2013).

85. Yipp, B. G. & Kubes, P. NETosis: How vital is it? *Blood* **122**, 2784–2794 (2013).

86. Ghasemzadeh, M. & Hosseini, E. Intravascular leukocyte migration through platelet thrombi: Directing leukocytes to sites of vascular injury. *Thrombosis and Haemostasis* **113**, 1224–1235 (2015).

87. Respiratory burst: An overview | Science direct topics. https://www.sciencedirect.com/topics/agricultural-and-biological-sciences/respiratory-burst.

88. Roesslein, M., Hirsch, C., Kaiser, J. P., Krug, H. F. & Wick, P. Comparability of in vitro tests for bioactive nanoparticles: A common assay to detect reactive oxygen species as an example. *International Journal of Molecular Sciences* **14**, 24320–24337 (2013).

89. Delgado-Rizo, V. et al. Neutrophil extracellular traps and its implications in inflammation: An overview. *Frontiers in Immunology* **8**, 81 (2017).

90. Martinod, K. & Wagner, D. D. Thrombosis: Tangled up in NETs. *Blood* **123**, 2768–2776 (2014).

91. Sperling, C., Fischer, M., Maitz, M. F. & Werner, C. Blood coagulation on biomaterials requires the combination of distinct activation processes. *Biomaterials* **30**, 4447–4456 (2009).

92. Anderson, J. M. Chapter 4: Mechanisms of inflammation and infection with implanted devices. *Cardiovascular Pathology* **2**, 33–41 (1993).

93. Aflaki, E. et al. Macrophage models of gaucher disease for evaluating disease pathogenesis and candidate drugs. *Science Translational Medicine* **6**, 240ra73 (2014).

94. Moore, K. J. & Tabas, I. Macrophages in the pathogenesis of atherosclerosis. *Cell* **145** 341–355 (2011).

95. Bobryshev, Y. V., Ivanova, E. A., Chistiakov, D. A., Nikiforov, N. G. & Orekhov, A. N. Macrophages and their role in atherosclerosis: Pathophysiology and transcriptome analysis. *BioMed Research International* **2016**, 9582430 (2016).

96. Fajgenbaum, D. C. & June, C. H. Cytokine storm. *The New England Journal of Medicine* **383**, 2255–2273 (2020).

97. Sinn, S., Scheuermann, T., Deichelbohrer, S., Ziemer, G. & Wendel, H. P. A novel in vitro model for preclinical testing of the hemocompatibility of intravascular stents according to ISO 10993-4. *Journal of Materials Science: Materials in Medicine* **22**, 1521–1528 (2011).

98. Stang, K. et al. Hemocompatibility testing according to ISO 10993-4: Discrimination between pyrogen- and device-induced hemostatic activation. *Materials Science and Engineering C* **42**, 422–428 (2014).

99. Li, Z. & Kawashita, M. Current progress in inorganic artificial biomaterials. *Journal of Artificial Organs* **14**, 163–170 (2011).

100. Nomura, N. Artificial organs: Recent progress in metals and ceramics. *Journal of Artificial Organs* **13**, 10–12 (2010).

101. Erbulut, D. U. & Lazoglu, I. Biomaterials for improving the blood and tissue compatibility of total artificial hearts (TAH) and ventricular assist devices (VAD). *Biomaterials for Artificial Organs*, 207–235 (Elsevier Inc., 2010). doi: 10.1533/9780857090843.2.207.

102. Fischer, M., Maitz, M. F. & Werner, C. Coatings for biomaterials to improve hemocompatibility. *Hemocompatibility of Biomaterials for Clinical Applications: Blood-Biomaterials Interactions*, 163–190 (Elsevier Inc., 2018). doi: 10.1016/B978-0-08-100497-5.00007-0.

103. Kim, T. G., Shin, H. & Lim, D. W. Biomimetic scaffolds for tissue engineering. *Advanced Functional Materials* **22**, 2446–2468 (2012).

104. Li, J. et al. Investigation of enhanced hemocompatibility and tissue compatibility associated with multi-functional coating based on hyaluronic acid and Type IV collagen. *Regenerative Biomaterials* **3**, 149–157 (2016).

105. Luo, R. et al. In vitro investigation of enhanced hemocompatibility and endothelial cell proliferation associated with quinone-rich polydopamine coating. *ACS Applied Materials & Interfaces* **5**, 1704–1714 (2013).

106. Everett, W. et al. A material conferring hemocompatibility. *Scientific Reports* **6**, 1–12 (2016).

107. Cheng, Y. T., Rodak, D. E., Wong, C. A. & Hayden, C. A. Effects of micro- and nano-structures on the self-cleaning behaviour of lotus leaves. *Nanotechnology* **17**, 1359–1362 (2006).

108. Marmur, A. The lotus effect: Superhydrophobicity and metastability. *Langmuir* **20**, 3517–3519 (2004).

109. Feng, L. et al. Super-hydrophobic surfaces: From natural to artificial. *Advanced Materials* **14**, 1857–1860 (2002).

110. Raghavendra, G. M., Varaprasad, K. & Jayaramudu, T. Biomaterials: Design, development and biomedical applications. *Nanotechnology Applications for Tissue Engineering*, 21–44 (Elsevier Inc., 2015). doi:10.1016/B978-0-323-32889-0.00002-9.

111. Braune, S., Grunze, M., Straub, A. & Jung, F. Are there sufficient standards for the in vitro hemocompatibility testing of biomaterials? *Biointerphases* **8**, 1–9 (2013).

112. Zhang, L. et al. The influence of surface chemistry on adsorbed fibrinogen conformation, orientation, fiber formation and platelet adhesion. *Acta Biomaterialia* **54**, 164–174 (2017).

113. Aguilar, M. R., Rodríguez, G., Fernández, M., Gallardo, A. & San Román, J. Polymeric active coatings with functionality in vascular applications. *Journal of Materials Science: Materials in Medicine* **13**, 1099–1104 (2002).

114. Balasubramanian, V. & Slack, S. M. Effects of fibrinogen residence time and shear rate on the morphology and procoagulant activity of human platelets adherent to polymeric biomaterials. *ASAIO Journal.* **47**, 354–360 (2001).

115. Hemolysis assay: An overview | Science direct topics. https://www.sciencedirect.com/topics/medicine-and-dentistry/hemolysis-assay.

116. Clauser, J. C. et al. Hemocompatibility evaluation of biomaterials: The crucial impact of analyzed area. *ACS Biomaterials Science & Engineering* (2021). doi: 10.1021/acsbiomaterials.0c01589.

117. Henkelman, S., Rakhorst, G., Blanton, J. & van Oeveren, W. Standardization of incubation conditions for hemolysis testing of biomaterials. *Materials Science and Engineering C* **29**, 1650–1654 (2009).

118. Sperling, C. et al. In vitro blood reactivity to hydroxylated and non-hydroxylated polymer surfaces. *Biomaterials* **28**, 3617–3625 (2007).

119. Gorbet, M. B., Yeo, E. L. & Sefton, M. V. Flow cytometric study of in vitro neutrophil activation by biomaterials. *Journal of Biomedical Materials Research* **44**, 289–297 (1999).

120. Fogelson, A. L. & Neeves, K. B. Fluid mechanics of blood clot formation. *Annual Review of Fluid Mechanics* **47**, 377–403 (2015).

121. Lima, B. et al. Controversies and challenges of ventricular assist device therapy. *American Journal of Cardiology* **121**, 1219–1224 (2018).

122. The pig as a model in blood coagulation and fibrinolysis research. https://www.researchgate.net/publication/286839969_The_pig_as_a_model_in_blood_coagulation_and_fibrinolysis_research.

123. Kosaka, R. et al. Improvement of hemocompatibility in centrifugal blood pump with hydrodynamic bearings and semi-open impeller: In vitro evaluation. *Artificial Organs* **33**, 798–804 (2009).

124. Jaffer, I. H. & Weitz, J. I. The blood compatibility challenge. Part 1: Blood-contacting medical devices: The scope of the problem. *Acta Biomaterialia* **94**, 2–10 (2019).

125. Anderson, J. M. Future challenges in the in vitro and in vivo evaluation of biomaterial biocompatibility. *Regenerative Biomaterials* **3**, 73–77 (2016).

126. De Jong, W. H., Carraway, J. W. & Geertsma, R. E. In vivo and in vitro testing for the biological safety evaluation of biomaterials and medical devices. *Biocompatibility and Performance of Medical Devices*, 120–158 (Elsevier Ltd., 2012). doi: 10.1016/B978-0-85709-070-6.50007-9.

127. Myers, D. K. et al. From in vivo to in vitro: The medical device testing paradigm shift. *ALTEX* **34**, 479–500 (2017).

8 Computational Hemodynamics

Guilherme B. Lopes Jr
Federal University of Pernambuco

Luben Cabezas-Gómez
University of Sao Paulo

Raquel J. Lobosco
Federal University of Rio de Janeiro

CONTENTS

DOI: 10.1201/9781003138358-10

8.1 INTRODUCTION

Computational hemodynamic is a field inside a field. Hemodynamic is the study of the dynamic of blood, since its agglomeration to flow, including turbulence in blood and rheology. Studying blood flows is an exceedingly difficult task, due to several different and complex phenomena, some of them not completely understood or explored yet.

Simulating hemodynamic by the general principles of computational fluid dynamics (CFD) is also more challenging. Particularly, issues and concepts must be evaluated since geometry to solver and results. As more phenomena involved as complex are the models, in order to simulate blood flows in large arteries could be completely different from small arteries due to other phenomena influencing such as the wall structure. The same occurs for VAD blood flow simulations which depend on several different phenomena such as turbulence, geometry, wall effects or recirculation zones.

Now, imagine another complication: flux machines! Water flux machines are difficult to simulate. Even nowadays, some 2-D and simplified methods from the 1960s are still being in use for reducing the complex dynamics of the flow inside a centrifugal pump, for example. But using blood and main fluid of a pump, all the complex issues are brought together.

It is not intended to afraid you, dear reader, about the subject of this chapter. But warn you that it is complex to indicate the extreme importance of this matter. Simulating blood pumps is difficult, but essential to develop and predict prototype behaviors.

This chapter was written for discussing the main topics of computational hemodynamic that bring doubts in beginners. Here, geometry and mesh are widely discussed, even though not conclusive. The most common equations are presented, and boundary conditions are treated. At the end, some CFD programs and their importance are cited.

Here, the most relevant subjects are explained, discussed, and treated. Obviously, there are many other subjects and information not treated here. Consider it as a lighter in the theme; this chapter opens the subject and brings some important discussions based on experience, which are priceless. This will guide you for understanding the derivative subjects and create your own path on this delightful field.

8.2 GEOMETRY AND DOMAINS

The first necessary understanding of the computational approach is related to setting the geometry and the domain applied. The domain and geometry of ventricular assist devices (VADs) are different and, somehow, complementary when treating about computational hemodynamic.

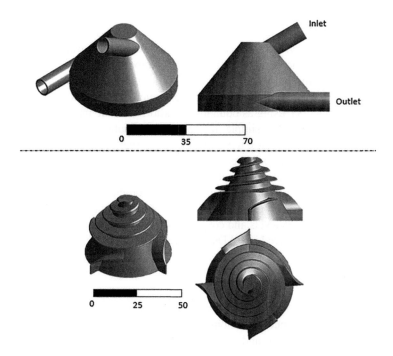

FIGURE 8.1   VAD geometry example from Ref. [1], described also in Ref. [2].

A VAD geometry is the solid, the physical prototype. Eventually, this geometry is a solid domain that might be or not used on the simulations. For example, there is a geometry tested by Ref. [1]. There are two overall geometry elements, and both are a solid domain (Figure 8.1).

A solid domain may be used on two different ways: on solid simulations or on fluid simulations as an interface with the fluid. For fluid simulation, the fluid domain is simulated, so it is essential to indicate to the software where there is fluid. So, by observing the geometry purposed in Ref. [1], the fluid domain is between the impeller and the body of the VAD.

The fluid domain may be unitary or multiple, depending on the computational approach for the moving impeller aiming to incorporate its rotation. In unitary domain, there is only one reference frame and a source of angular momentum is done to incorporate the rotation. It is also possible to use an interface between the fluid and solid domains and use adaptive mesh or the source on the interface region.

The multiple reference frame (MRF) consists of, on the other hand, using more than one domain to represent the total fluid domain. These domains will represent different phenomena condition to represent the region in question. The most common example is to create two domains: one rotating in the inner region, closer to the impeller, and other stationary in the outer region. So, the "source" of angular momentum is due to the nonstationary reference frame.

There are also some different approaches for basically (but not limited to) three general types of simulation.

8.2.1 STAGE APPROACH

On this approach, a fixed interface is separated by two different frames, representing the relative movement between two different solid impeller domains. For this reason, this is called stage simulations, because is useful for multiple-stage pumps.

It is created sequential domains in different reference frames and is simulated in order (inner to outer), using as boundary conditions on the interface the previous information. This method is simple and reduces computational costs on multiple-stage pumps but makes no sense to use out of these situations, due to very simplified effects, limited capacity to capture rotor-stator interactions, and to not considering transitional vortexes between the stages or transient effects. Usually, mean values are applied on the interface and no theta variations are computed as well.

In non-volumetric blood pumps, usually one-stage pumps are used since multiple stages increase hemolysis levels and coagulation inside the pump. So, this method is not common to be considered in VADs simulations.

8.2.2 FROZEN ROTOR-STATOR APPROACH

The frozen rotor-stator approach consists in making different reference frames and changing the cell reference conditions. The boundaries and interface remain the same during the simulation, and consider the adjacent cell zones. So, at least two reference frames are created: a non-inertial one closer to the impeller and an inertial one to the outer region.

The concept here is that, in the inner impeller region, the fluid flow in steady state is represented by a forced vortex approach, and the outer impeller region by a free vortex approach.

In pumps and mixers (generally speaking), both approaches are relevant and reach good results simulating and modeling rotating impellers, and mixed approach is also recommended when both phenomena (forced and free vortexes) are relevant.

This is very coherent in centrifugal and axial blood pumps if the interface is well positioned. An interface not physically coherent will produce nonphysical results. It is more reliable to position the interface as closer as possible to the impeller region.

For this approach, no transient behavior or phenomena are captured. Only steady-state phenomena are physically represented by this method, even if time marching methodology is applied, when a false-transient time marching is set for a steady-state simulation.

One possibility to reach a transient analysis for rotor position is to create several scenarios for each time and simulate it with this approach. But this only allows to analyze overall phenomena parameters.

8.2.3 SLIDING MESH

The sliding mesh is an approach applied to two different mesh groups, linked by one interface, where the quantities are transmitted from one to another. This method is applied when there are two adjacent regions in different moving frames where the entire mesh could have the relative position and the interface-wall conditions

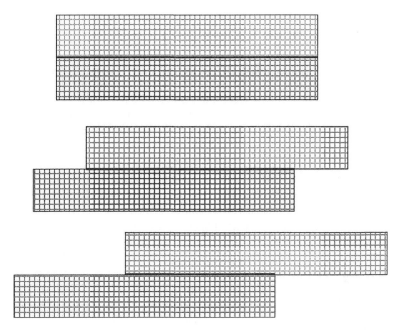

FIGURE 8.2   Translating sliding mesh approach example.

changed. In this kind of simulation, the mesh have a relative movement to a reference domain.

In Figure 8.2, an example of the sliding mesh is presented. In this example, the relative positions (between each other) are changed and so the interface and wall conditions applied to the problem.

This approach is very specific to problems in which the interface could be characterized by this relative movement between the domains and so its applications are specifics as well. Transforming interface to wall and changing the source-target elements of the interface are not simple when the boundaries are not limited.

Besides that, it is possible to compute transient-induced effects by changing this position according to time. Notice that it is also possible to create multiple adjacent groups of meshes, and not necessarily the distribution must be Cartesian, including rotational behaviors.

The sliding mesh is robust for transient or steady-state approach, but it is important to create correspondence to each mesh group very cohesive and the interpretation of the transient effects may be wrong if the mesh is not properly set and related to coherent boundary conditions.

This method has low costs compared to transient adaptive meshes and is useful in impeller-stator or multiple-stage types of pump, in which there is adjacent changes in regions with different reference frames are presented, and it is possible to create completely mesh zones where the boundaries can move and create a relative movement with the adjacent mesh zone.

Extra care must be done to not confuse MRF in frozen rotor and sliding mesh approaches: the first, the boundaries and interface are inertial and do not suffer alterations; the second interface changes the elements relation and connections, while the boundaries are moving with the mesh attached to them.

8.2.4 TRANSIENT ADAPTIVE MESHES OR TRANSIENT ROTOR STATOR APPROACH

When the rotor is considered changing its wall positions and the mesh needs to be remodeled, there is a completely mesh reorganization during each time step for capturing the new rotor blades position. In this case, there is a transient adaptive mesh approach.

This method is the most advanced and closer to the physical behavior, and so it has the highest computational costs applied. Also, it may be highly divergent for creating local and global flux divergences when the mesh is not well remodeled along time marching (considering explicit schemes).

On the other hand, some transient phenomena only can be completely captured by this method, for example, transient boundary layer detachment in sharp corners. The question is: are these specific phenomena relevant enough to justify the costs and possible accumulative errors?

Usually, the answer is no! It is much more desirable to invest on direct numerical simulations (DNS) than on this approach, including the guarantee of better mesh agreement, which is particularly difficult for transient adaptive meshes. Checking the mesh in each transient solution is impossible, so the quality of the mesh is not guaranteed.

However, when necessary, it is recommended to use a closer reference frame to the impeller, reducing the computational cost as much as possible. Notice that this method may be used with 1 reference frame as well, which is not recommended for high divergence chances.

8.3 MESH: RELEVANCE AND ITS INDEPENDENCY

In CFD, meshes have a relevant impact on the simulations. Convergence, accuracy, processing time, and phenomena capture are directly impacted for the mesh chosen.

A mesh (or grid) represents how the continuum domain is discretized, which means how this domain is subdivided (in elements) to represent and capture the phenomena. In fluid flow cases, the phenomena involved are complicated and require specific analyses based on a simple question with an exceedingly difficult answer: "How the flow are behaving on this scenario?"

The answer, as spoiled, is not simple, especially when relevant and significant turbulence and interface effects are presented. In these cases, the answer may be given by the simulation intended when the numerical modeling and approaches are physically coherent and real phenomena are represented by the simulation. So, a mesh must aid this representation.

In artificial hearts, such as VADs, the mesh gains even more relevance to the process. Turbulence and wall influence represent difficulties for mesh determination. Each phenomena type is relevant, and their influence could be undervalued if the other is overvalued. The balance and correct influence of each one starts with a representative mesh, and it is crucial for the simulation.

A mesh is composed by elements and group of elements. These elements will solve locally the phenomena using discretized equations and balances of conservative quantities. Each element solution feeds other element inlet information to be solved in this other element. After a certain number of elements, groups are formed, and the same discretized equations and balances might be applied to ensure that the conservation is maintained and reduces divergence on a global (not local) scale.

Even with great advances in commercial and free software for this purpose, to set a good mesh is still in the hands of the modeler (you!) to indicate it. But how to determine and create a good mesh?

The elements have important functions on CFD analysis. Usually, only the number of elements has been used for characterizing a mesh in studies along past 20 years. Maybe on a decade ago, it has been relevant enough, but nowadays it is crucial to observe other issues, as elements geometry; disposal and interface treatment; some quality parameters; and mesh density according to the simulation approach.

On the next subtopics, some particularly important discussions are presented to guide mesh determination and modeling choices, since a good mesh depends on each problem, approach, and boundary conditions, for example.

8.3.1 ELEMENT GEOMETRIES: TETRAHEDRAL VS HEXAHEDRAL

The elements geometry is the first to be considered. Some modeling conditions can interfere on the geometry choice of the elements in a mesh.

8.3.1.1 Overall Geometry

Difficult geometry demands difficulties for mesh determination. Sharp angles, small gaps, narrow passages, and divergent scales of dimensions are some of the most challenging overall geometry parts of a VAD. They cause ruptures and necessity of different mesh densities to comprehend these regions, which may cause nonadequacies on the mesh.

Besides these adequacy problems, the VAD geometry interferes directly with the choice of structured or unstructured meshes. Obviously, the prototype geometry is not the only factor in consideration but structured meshes are more limited to model these geometry difficulties.

8.3.1.2 Phenomena Expected

Diffusive and advective phenomena are quite different, so how to capture these phenomena as well. High-viscous and laminar fluid flows and their regions are easily captured by structured meshes. These phenomena are mostly diffusive, so the calculations element by element are performed and transmitted simply by adjacent elements by linear behavior and vectorial terms are just transmitted without local singularities. In other words, the properties flux directions are predictable.

In Figure 8.3, there is regularity in trespassing diffusive terms in this hypothetical situation. In these kinds of physical problems, structured meshes are truly relevant and can reach better results on a few interactions (explicit schemes) or better agreement with boundary conditions influence (implicit schemes).

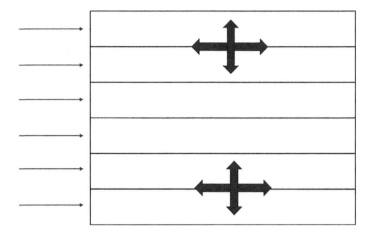

FIGURE 8.3   Diffusive properties flux transmission along structured mesh elements.

On the other hand, a turbulent flow is chaotic, so properties and vectors transitions are completely nonlinear and may cause instabilities, locally and globally. It means flux directions might be uncertain and singularities on elements (or group of them) will demand changing of the property's values there, which may cause instabilities in the simulation.

In turn, fluxes coming and going in different directions are well computed in unstructured meshes. In Figure 8.4, two different elements are hypothetically observed according to the fluxes in their boundaries.

Nondiffusive behaviors tend to creative difficulties on the balances of a structured element. The fluxes on them must be partitioned on the boundaries surfaces, which may cause nonphysical answers. The propagation of these pieces of information to surround cells, where the information is received, is done following the same "source" element, and must be corrected later.

Other problem is the dispersive errors that might be caused when there is an abrupt change of directions or incongruences on a small group of elements. This causes a

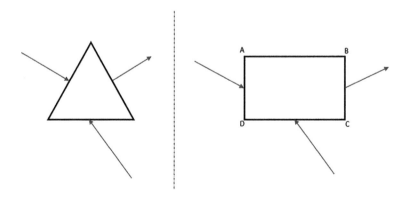

FIGURE 8.4   Property fluxes comparison between two kinds of elements in 2-D scenario.

dispersive error, which may be corrected by refinement, but it is problematic if high convective effects are presented, for example.

On explicit schemes, these analyses are essential to physical agreement, reducing interactions (and computational costs) and convergence. On implicit schemes, if the mesh is not correctly set, the simulation may diverge or incorporate directly the influence from the boundary conditions and produce nonphysical results to reach a numerical result.

8.3.1.3 Fluxes and Sources

On another point of view, theoretically the increasing number of faces produces results that are less influenced by element-by-element boundaries. For example, in a 2-D simulation, considering four faces should be more effective to capture fluxes than three faces. This is not true in general, except if both have similar shape, size, and distribution, so four-face elements in a unstructured mesh should be more appropriate than a three-face elements to capture convective effects and to consider the surroundings of the element and the propagation of its effects, if the same mesh density and distribution are respected.

A hypothetical influence of flux captures on the faces according to the increase in the number of faces is shown in Figure 8.5.

More the number of faces, more specific fluxes can be captured and their individual influences computed. This is different from the example of structured mesh

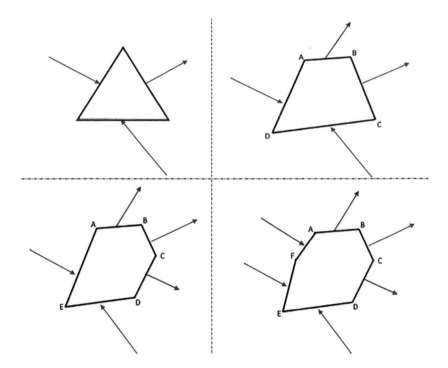

FIGURE 8.5   Hypothetical influence on flux captures when increasing the number of faces.

presented in Figure 8.4, since on unstructured meshes, this relevance and different directions can be computed.

Notice that even in unstructured meshes, these convective properties fluxes could not be well captured, but the chances are reduced. Although more faces on an element can contribute to accumulate errors as well. More faces indicate more diffusive errors and, if not necessary, dispersive errors.

Other difficulty is the adequacy and mesh generation. More faces create more nodes and mesh generation costs are considerable higher, sometime inviable. Besides, sharp-angled geometries difficult adequacy of the mesh, creating low quality form factors elements or even precluding to generate the mesh.

8.4 BEST PRACTICE

No conclusions may be done for choosing a best kind of mesh, because it will depend on these observations and other particularities. But there are some strong recommendations based on practice:

- Highly diffusive flows: structured and hexahedral meshes can capture diffusive effects.
- Turbulent flows: unstructured and tetrahedral meshes are considerably better than the other for the main flow.
- Sharp-angled geometries demand unstructured meshes to keep mesh quality, but the number of faces should be evaluated.
- Simpler the meshes, the simulation will perform. But remember that the mesh must capture the phenomena by representing the domain.

8.5 INTERFACE TREATMENT

First, an interface is a region between at least two different domains (fluids or solids). These different domains might have multiple uses and explanations, but the most common in VADs is to allow "sources" of quantities (as momentum) to indicate the influence of the impeller or propulsor system. Other possibilities are due to multiphase flows or boundary deformability and limitations.

In centrifugal or axial blood pumps, for example, the interfaces are necessary to insert the impeller influence on the flow, while in volumetric blood pumps, the interfaces are usually deformable to represent their movement and transfer momentum to the flow.

The interface works as a "source" of information for both domains on it. So information coming from one domain is transferred to the other along the interface surface, even if the elements are not confluents.

Confluent elements on the interface mean that on the interface, the elements of both sides have a single and coincident face, which is recommended for decreasing local instabilities and errors, but not essential.

Sometimes, different refinement meshes are intended for each domain, which may inviable confluent elements, usually for limit number of elements required by computational costs or Direct Numerical Simulation (DNS) approaches aimed on certain regions. In these cases, extra care is required for mesh quality parameters.

Interfaces are usually sensitive, but essential to simulate blood flows in VAD. The types of interface depend on the computational approach for simulating the internal flow and its relation to the impeller/propulsor system. Basically, two general types may be considered.

8.5.1 Stationary

Stationary interfaces are usually applied to centrifugal and axial blood pumps. The impeller rotation (even when small rotation speeds) demands a stationary interface to simplify this treatment. An approach of transient rotor/stator with adaptive meshes can also be applied, but computational costs and instabilities due to divergent fluxes could make the moving boundaries unviable.

8.5.2 Nonstationary

When the boundaries are not stationary, but it is not possible to determine separated and stationary domains or there is not symmetry axis for the moving parts, a nonstationary interface should be considered.

In nonstationary interfaces, adaptive or remodeled meshes are applied for each time instant or interval to consider this movement of the interface. There are several models for this task, but the principle is basic: recreate locally or totally the mesh on the new geometry scenario.

Clever, even though problematic. Imagine a geometry that demands millions of elements changing completely at each time step, or at least several thousands of elements at local.

There are also some approaches for considering both kinds of interface, named mixed interface treatments, aiming to reduce to local adaptive meshes only, so the program only considers part of the mesh, reducing computational costs.

8.6 QUALITY PARAMETERS

Several quality parameters could be used to quantify some qualitative approaches. Here, the most common and useful parameters are discussed.

8.6.1 Growth Rate

Growth rate is how the elements are increased or decreased along the domain. It is essential when considered how to focus the discretization and the transitions between elements from different regions.

High growth rates mean that the adjacent elements are increasing faster. This causes rapid transition and less mesh densities for a mesh. The first impact could represent higher local errors for divergence of fluxes on a surface in contact with more surfaces from adjacent elements. The second is not problem, when the flow phenomena are simple. When complex events are presented, low mesh densities might be not enough to represent them. Lopes [2] also brings a comparison of this parameter, as shown in Figure 8.6.

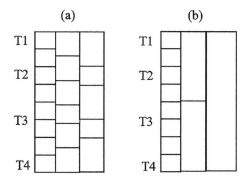

FIGURE 8.6 Different growth rate [Ref. 2].

TABLE 8.1

Skewness Parameter (Ansys Inc. Reference)

Skewness	Cell Quality
$S_k = 1.00$	Degenerate
$0.90 < S_k < 1.00$	Bad (sliver)
$0.75 < S_k < 0.90$	Poor
$0.50 < S_k < 0.75$	Fair
$0.25 < S_k < 0.50$	Good
$0 < S_k < 0.25$	Excellent
$S_k = 0.00$	Equilateral

8.6.2 SKEWNESS

Skewness is a parameter for reaching "ideal" element distribution: angles and dimensions. Ansys meshing, for example, represents skewness in a 0–1 coefficient according to Table 8.1.

Skewness is a truly relevant parameter for meshing quality determination, but it is not conclusive. Other shape parameters must be evaluated for regularity and shape for conclusions to analyze if the mesh is adequate for the problem.

8.6.3 ASPECT RATIO AND ASYMMETRY

Aspect ratio represents a relation between two different main dimensions from each element. These dimensions are the most relevant and representative from each element. So the aspect ratio represents how well distributed is the influence of the flow on that element.

Programs and their routines are directly influenced by this ratio. High aspect ratios can cause local divergence for considering more than one dimension directing than other, which may be intended casually, for example, in wall influence capture.

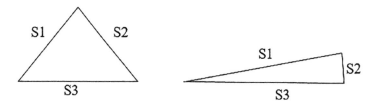

FIGURE 8.7   Comparison of elements with two different aspect ratios [Ref. 2].

Usually, low aspect ratios are more indicated for the flow simulation. They indicate regularity shape of the element when approximated to 1, and [2] represents a comparison between two 2-D triangular elements (Figure 8.7).

In (a), the low aspect ratio is clear, and in (b), the element has high aspect ratio. While is more recommended to focus on (a) kind elements, the (b) elements that are also relevant and could be deprecated. Ref. [2] indicates the relevance of high aspect ratio for capture wall effects of the subviscous boundary layer, while low aspect ratios are highly recommended for capture turbulent flows.

8.6.4   Mesh Independency Test

The independency test is a precision test. It tests how precise is your simulation when changing mesh density in the same overall conditions and types of mesh conception. When the simulations are precise, the mesh is independent, and from this point, refinement is not relevant to change the simulation results.

There are some practical procedures for realizing the mesh independency test.

- Create a Coarse Mesh: Using the conceptions of which regions to be more refined, kind of elements, interface approach, etc., it is recommended to generate a coarse mesh for your problem and to simulate it using a set of boundary conditions. A coarse mesh is usually more critical for representing the most extreme kinds of phenomena.
- Refine Your Mesh: Proceed with refinement and create new refined meshes based on the coarse mesh already done. The boundary conditions and conceptions must be the same of the first simulation.
- Graphical Analysis: Create a graphic with the results of your simulation according to a comparison parameter. This parameter must be representative of the simulation. For VAD, pressure difference between the inlet and outlet cannulas is classical. But when other analyses are intended, for example, friction on the impeller or stagnation points, other parameters might be considered: stress on the walls, recirculation total volume of fluid, or turbulent viscosity.
- Quantification: Relative deviation is common to be applied for comparing the results. As a precision test, the results are compared to each other, usually in sequence. Other parameters such as angular coefficient of three-point straight are also useful.

At least five different meshes must be tested for statistical relevance on mesh independency tests. The more meshes are tested, the more reliable is the result of the test and its conclusions. And it is always important to remember: it is a precision, not accuracy test!

8.7 FLUID DYNAMICS EQUATIONS

In this section, three of two-equation turbulence models are presented, considering that these are the models most used by the present authors in simulating VADs. However, in order to introduce this subject, first it is briefly commented about the Reynolds average procedure.

The Reynolds decomposition consists in separating variables into two parts: one that represents a mean value in time and the other related to the variable fluctuations. The mean time values refer to a time scale, which is large in relation to the turbulent fluctuations, but which is small regarding the macroscopic temporal scales. This decomposition procedure is written as:

$$\phi = \bar{\phi} + \phi' \tag{8.1}$$

where ϕ is the local temporal value of any scalar or vector variable, $\bar{\phi}$ represents the mean time value of this variable, and ϕ' represents its turbulent fluctuation value. Decomposing each variable in the mass conservation or continuity equation for an isothermal incompressible flow, it is obtained, in indicial notation, the next relation:

$$\frac{\partial V_i}{\partial x_i} = \frac{\partial \bar{V}_i}{\partial x_i} = \frac{\partial \bar{V}_i'}{\partial x_i} = 0 \tag{8.2}$$

In Equation (8.2), V_i represents the local instantaneous velocity vector, which is decomposed using Equation (8.1). Performing the same procedure for the Navier-Stokes equations results in:

$$\frac{\partial \left(\rho \bar{V}_i \right)}{\partial t} + \frac{\partial \left(\rho \bar{V}_i \bar{V}_j \right)}{\partial x_j} = -\frac{\partial \bar{p}}{\partial x_j} + \frac{\partial \bar{\tau}_{ji}}{\partial x_j} \tag{8.3}$$

In Equation (8.3) the body forces are not considered, ρ and p represent the fluid density and pressure, while x stands for the coordinate vector. After the Reynolds decomposition, the viscous stress tensor when it is considered a Newtonian fluid, $\bar{\tau}_{ji}$ is modeled by:

$$\bar{\tau}_{ji} = \mu \left(\frac{\partial \bar{V}_i}{\partial x_j} + \frac{\partial \bar{V}_j}{\partial x_i} \right) - \rho \overline{V_i' V_j'} \tag{8.4}$$

In Equation (8.4), the second term represents the denominated Reynolds stresses, which should be modeled to close the resulting system of conservative equations. This is performed by assuming a Newtonian fluid and considering the Boussinesq hypothesis for the turbulent viscosity, resulting in:

$$-\rho\overline{V_i'V_j'} = \mu_t\left(\frac{\partial\overline{V_i}}{\partial x_j} + \frac{\partial\overline{V_j}}{\partial x_i}\right) - \frac{2}{3}\rho k\delta_{ij} \tag{8.5}$$

Considering this equation, Equation (8.4) results in:

$$\overline{\tau}_{ji} = (\mu + \mu_t)\left(\frac{\partial\overline{V_i}}{\partial x_j} + \frac{\partial\overline{V_j}}{\partial x_i}\right) - \frac{2}{3}\rho k\delta_{ij} \tag{8.6}$$

In the above equations, μ and μ_t stand for the molecular and Boussinesq turbulent viscosities, respectively, k represent the turbulent kinetic energy, and δ_{ij} is the Kronecker delta operator. After the formulation of time-averaged mass and linear momentum conservative equations, relations to estimate the turbulent quantities (as μ_t and k should be obtained). This is presented in the following sections, repeating first the mass and linear momentum conservation, now considering the body forces and the equations commonly solved in CFD software, and presenting the most used two-equation models.

8.7.1 GENERAL CONSERVATIVE EQUATIONS

The general conservative equations commonly used to simulate the flow in a VAD are the continuity and momentum conservative equations. The energy conservation equation is commonly not used because the flow is assumed as isothermal. The equations are obtained considering the Reynolds decomposition and time-averaged procedure, previously presented.

A flow of a compressible fluid is modeled by the following general equations. Continuity equation:

$$\frac{\partial\rho}{\partial t} + \nabla(\rho U) = 0 \tag{8.7}$$

Momentum equation:

$$\frac{\partial(\rho U)}{\partial t} + \nabla(\rho U \otimes U) = -\nabla p' + \nabla\left(\mu_{\text{eff}}\left(\nabla U + \nabla U^T\right)\right) + B \tag{8.8}$$

where U is the local instantaneous velocity vector obtained after the Reynolds decomposition and time average, representing the mean time average value of the velocity vector (i.e., $U = \overline{V}$), B is the sum of body forces, μ_{eff} is the effective viscosity accounting for turbulence, and p' is the modified pressure. μ_{eff} and p' are given, respectively, by:

$$\mu_{\text{eff}} = \mu + \mu_t \tag{8.9}$$

$$p' = p + \frac{2}{3}\rho k \tag{8.10}$$

In the case of incompressible fluid and stationary flow, Equations (8.7) and (8.8) can be simplified as

$$\nabla(U) = 0 \tag{8.11}$$

$$\nabla(\rho U \otimes U) = -\nabla p' + \nabla\left(\mu_{\text{eff}}\left(\nabla U + \nabla U^T\right)\right) + B \tag{8.12}$$

In the VAD, the conservative equations need to be adapted for the MRF. Thus, the absolute velocity and the velocity of the reference system in relation to the inertial system are represented as:

$$U_r = U_{\text{abs}} - (\Omega \times r) \tag{8.13}$$

In the above relation, Ω stands for the angular velocity and r is the radius vector.

8.7.2 Most Common Turbulence Models

The most common turbulence models belong to the two-equation class of turbulence models, namely, the traditional k-ε model [3], the RNG k-ε model [4], and the SST (shear stress transport) model. The SST model was proposed by Ref. [5] from the k-ω turbulence model, initially formulated by Wilcox [6].

8.7.2.1 Standard k-ε Model

The standard k-ε model [3] introduces two new variables into the equation system. One is for the computation of the turbulent kinetic energy, k, m^2/s^2; and the other is for the calculation of the turbulence eddy dissipation, ε, m^2/s^3. The k-ε model uses the eddy viscosity concept, assuming that the turbulence viscosity is computed by:

$$\mu_t = C_\mu \rho \frac{k^2}{\varepsilon} \tag{8.14}$$

where C_μ is a model constant.

The quantities k and ε are computed directly from the resolution of the following differential transport equations:

$$\frac{\partial(\rho k)}{\partial t} + \nabla(\rho U k) = \nabla\left[\left(\mu + \frac{\mu_t}{\sigma_k}\right)\nabla k\right] + P_k - \rho\varepsilon \tag{8.15}$$

$$\frac{\partial(\rho\varepsilon)}{\partial t} + \nabla(\rho U\varepsilon) = \nabla\left[\left(\mu + \frac{\mu_t}{\sigma_\varepsilon}\right)\nabla\varepsilon\right] + \frac{\varepsilon}{k}\left(C_{\varepsilon_1}P_k - C_{\varepsilon_2}\rho\varepsilon\right) \tag{8.16}$$

Being C_{ε_1}, C_{ε_2}, σ_k, and σ_e model constants and P_k is the turbulence production tensor due to viscous forces. The buoyancy forces are not considered in the present work. This last term is modeled as:

$$P_k = \mu_t \nabla U\left(\nabla U + \nabla U^T\right) - \frac{2}{3}(\nabla \cdot U)\left(3\mu_t \nabla \cdot U + \rho k\right) \tag{8.17}$$

If the flow is incompressible, the mean velocity divergence is zero. In this case, the second term of Equation (8.17) does not contribute to the turbulence production. The standard k-ε model employs the values for the constants that were found by a comprehensive data fitting for a wide range of turbulent flows. The values of these constants are: $C_\mu = 0.09$; $C_{\varepsilon_1} = 1.44$; $C_{\varepsilon_2} = 1.92$; $C_k = 1.00$; and $\sigma_\varepsilon = 1.30$.

8.7.2.2 RNG k-ε Model

The *RNG k-ε* model is based on renormalization group analysis of the Navier-Stokes equations [4]. The transport equations for turbulence generation and dissipation are the same as those for the standard k-ε model, but the model constants differ. The equations for the momentum and continuity are also the same.

For the *RNG k-ε* model the transport equation for turbulence dissipation becomes:

$$\frac{\partial(\rho\varepsilon)}{\partial t} + \nabla(\rho U\varepsilon) = \nabla\left[\left(\mu + \frac{\mu_t}{\sigma_{\varepsilon\,\mathrm{RNG}}}\right)\nabla\varepsilon\right] + \frac{\varepsilon}{k}\left(C_{\varepsilon_1\,\mathrm{RNG}}P_k - C_{\varepsilon_2\,\mathrm{RNG}}\rho\varepsilon\right) \quad (8.18)$$

where

$$C_{\varepsilon_1\,\mathrm{RNG}} = 1.42 - f_\eta \quad (8.19)$$

and

$$f_\eta = \frac{\eta\left(1 - \dfrac{\eta}{4.38}\right)}{\left(1 + \beta_{\mathrm{RNG}}\eta^3\right)}; \quad \eta = \sqrt{\frac{P_k}{\rho C_{\mu\,\mathrm{RNG}}\varepsilon}} \quad (8.20)$$

The values of the constants are: $C_{\mu\,\mathrm{RNG}} = 0.085$; $C_{\varepsilon_2\,\mathrm{RNG}} = 1.68$; $\sigma_{k\,\mathrm{RNG}} = 0.7179$; and $\sigma_{\varepsilon\,\mathrm{RNG}} = 0.7179$.

8.7.2.3 Shear Stress Transport (SST) Model

The other two-equation turbulence model refers to the SST model taken from Ref. [24]. This model was proposed by Menter [5] and grew from the denominated baseline k-ω model in Ref. [24]. The baseline k-ω model makes use of the k-ε model in regions far away from the walls and the k-ω Wilcox model (cf. [6]) near the surface. The SST model is an improvement of the baseline k-ω model, considering the transport of the turbulent shear stress by a limitation of the eddy viscosity ν_t by the following equation:

$$\nu_t = \frac{a_1 k}{\max\left(a_1\omega,\ SF_2\right)} \quad (8.21)$$

where $\nu_t = \mu_t/\rho$ and S represents an invariant measure of the strain rate. F_2 is a blending function, which restricts the limiter to the wall layer computed by:

$$F_2 = \tanh\left(\mathrm{arg}_2^2\right) \quad (8.22)$$

with

$$\text{arg}_2 = \max\left(\frac{2\sqrt{k}}{\beta'\omega y'}; \frac{500v}{y^2\omega}\right) \qquad (8.23)$$

The turbulent kinetic energy k and turbulent frequency ω are computed by the following relations:

$$\frac{\partial(\rho k)}{\partial t} + \nabla(\rho Uk) = \nabla\left[\left(\mu + \frac{\mu_t}{\sigma_{k3}}\right)\nabla k\right] + P_k - \beta'\rho k\omega \qquad (8.24)$$

$$\frac{\partial(\rho\omega)}{\partial t} + \nabla(\rho U\omega) = \nabla\left[\left(\mu + \frac{\mu_t}{\sigma_{\omega 3}}\right)\nabla\omega\right] + (1-F_2)2\rho\frac{1}{\sigma_{\omega 2}\omega}\nabla k\nabla\omega + \alpha_3\frac{\omega}{k}P_k - \beta_3\rho\omega^2$$

$$(8.25)$$

The constants used in the SST model equations are: $\beta' = 0.09$; $\alpha_1 = 5/9$; $\beta_1 = 0.075$; $\sigma_{k_1} = 2$; $\sigma_{\omega_1} = 2$; $\alpha_2 = 0.44$; $\beta_2 = 0.0828$; $\sigma_{k_2} = 1$; and $\sigma_{\omega 2} = 1/0.856$.

The coefficients of the *SST* model are a linear combination of the corresponding coefficients of the underlying models:

$$\Phi_3 = F_2\Phi_1 + (1-F_2)\Phi_2 \qquad (8.26)$$

It should be noted that the stress tensor is computed from the eddy-viscosity concept. It is applied the Equation (8.7) for the conservation of mass.

8.8 BOUNDARY CONDITIONS AND WALL TREATMENT

At the end of the diastole, the heart's atria contract and pump the blood into the ventricles. In this heartbeat cycle, the shape and the volume of the heart periodically change. In this way, the process of defining the correct boundary condition for the numerical simulations can be really challenging depending on the complexity of the physical hypothesis.

Figure 8.8 illustrates six types of boundary conditions. A set of those conditions must be imposed on the geometry for achieving a solution of the differential momentum and mass equations [7].

1. For an *inlet*, the transported variables are specified on the boundary. If a fixed value is prescribed, the condition is classified as a Dirichlet boundary condition.
2. The *outlet* is usually a zero normal gradient, (Neuman condition) for all variables except for pressure that is defined as a fixed value.
3. The *symmetry* boundary condition represents the domain as a subregion by axes and planes of a segmented surface and can be applied to axisymmetric flows. Making use of that boundary condition can reduce the mesh size and decrease the computational cost.

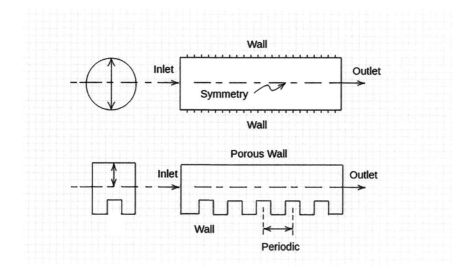

FIGURE 8.8   Boundary conditions main types.

4. A *periodic* condition represents a pair of identical boundaries that geometrically match. By the use of a periodic boundary condition, it is possible to solve a smaller geometry section of geometrical identical parts.
5. *Wall* boundary conditions must be defined as slip or non-slip. For the viscous flows, the non-slip conditions are applied.
6. A *porous wall* allows a mass flux through its length.

For an accurate modeling, it is important to notice that in the curved arteries, the centrifugal force causes a secondary flow, the perpendicular velocity of the flow produces a rotational flux in the outlet direction, and the flow becomes turbulent.

A schematic diagram of the combining possibilities for the boundary conditions is illustrated in Figure 8.9.

A rigid wall boundary is usually proposed as a simplified hypothesis. The flow modeling close to a solid edge requires by itself a special treatment.

In a near-wall region, the flow is dominated by the viscous force and a characteristic length. When the Reynolds number increases, the boundary layer thickness, δ, becomes much bigger than the characteristic length defined by the ratio between the kinematics viscosity and the speed fluctuation, in a general point of view, two scales govern the flow, and three layers are defined to deal with the physical process.

The viscous sublayer, the buffer layer, and the logarithmic region can be defined with the parameter known as y^+ (see Equation 8.27) that allows us to decide how small a mesh might be close to a wall [8]. Based on the y^+, the height value of the first cell mesh can be calculated; for a schematic illustration, see Figure 8.10.

$$y^+ = \frac{y u_\tau}{\upsilon} \tag{8.27}$$

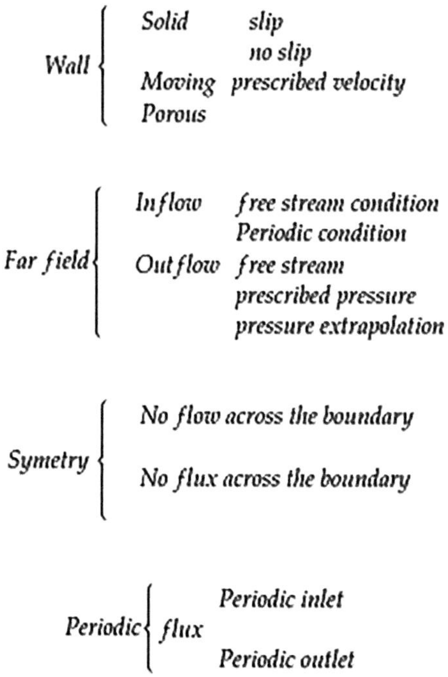

$$\text{Wall} \begin{cases} \textit{Solid} \quad \textit{slip} \\ \qquad\qquad \textit{no slip} \\ \textit{Moving} \quad \textit{prescribed velocity} \\ \textit{Porous} \end{cases}$$

$$\textit{Far field} \begin{cases} \textit{Inflow} \quad \textit{free stream condition} \\ \qquad\qquad \textit{Periodic condition} \\ \textit{Outflow} \quad \textit{free stream} \\ \qquad\qquad \textit{prescribed pressure} \\ \qquad\qquad \textit{pressure extrapolation} \end{cases}$$

$$\textit{Symetry} \begin{cases} \textit{No flow across the boundary} \\ \\ \textit{No flux across the boundary} \end{cases}$$

$$\textit{Periodic} \begin{cases} \qquad \textit{Periodic inlet} \\ \textit{flux} \\ \qquad \textit{Periodic outlet} \end{cases}$$

FIGURE 8.9   Schematic diagram of boundary conditions.

where y is the distance to the wall, y^+ is a nondimensional parameter, v is the viscosity, and ρ is the density.

The friction velocity can be defined as a function of the wall shear stress and the density, as shown by Equation (8.28).

$$u_\tau = \frac{\sqrt{\tau_w}}{\rho} \tag{8.28}$$

in which k is the von Kármán constant and E is the wall roughness.

1. The *viscous sublayer* ($y^+ < 5$) is the layer in which the flow is dominated by the viscous forces. In this region, the fluid shear stress is equal to the wall shear stress and the velocity profile is given by Equation (8.29).

$$y^+ = u^+ \tag{8.29}$$

2. In the *logarithmic layer* ($30 < y^+ < 500$), the flow is dominated by the turbulence (see Figure 8.3). The velocity profile obeyed a logarithmic function given by Equation (8.30).

$$u^+ = \frac{1}{k}\ln\left(Ey^+\right) \tag{8.30}$$

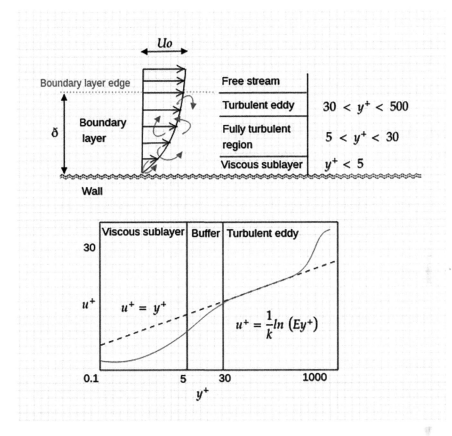

FIGURE 8.10 Sublayers in the region close to the wall.

3. Viscous and turbulent stresses are of similar magnitude in the **buffer layer**. In this near-wall region, the variables have large gradients and the velocity profile is not well defined.

In order to deal with the flow, close to a solid edge, two ways are usually proposed: either to integrate the turbulence to the wall or to use a specific function to the wall. The viscosity imposes the non-slip condition, which means that the fluid velocity on the wall is equal to the solid wall velocity.

The modified turbulence models deal with the viscous-affected region and resolve all the mesh down to the wall. The wall functions are empirical equations used to model the near-wall region; it connects the fully turbulent flow with the near-wall boundary for the momentum and the turbulence transport equations.

Using the wall function allows a reduction of the computational domain and the mesh size as the boundary layer does not have to be resolved. It substantially decreases the computational resources when the Reynolds number is high.

The wall function was first proposed in 1972 and suggests that the center of the first cell close to the wall is in a logarithmic layer [9]; when the cell center is positioned in the viscous sublayer, the approach is really accurate.

Some of the turbulence models that are heavily used in CFD, such as k-ε, do not perform properly in a region close to the wall; it is a good approach to the fully developed turbulence [10].

8.9   A VIEW ON CFD PROGRAMS

The so-called computational fluid dynamics (CFD) is a technique of computing and representing a fluid flow through numerical results of the fluid field properties. Traditionally divided into three independent main steps, it consists in preprocessing to generate the mesh and define the boundary conditions, a processing stage to run the solver and resolve the partial differential equations, and a post-processing step to graphically visualize the results, manipulate, and extract the data.

Due to the mathematical complexity of the momentum equation, the CFD software is still not such a trivial tool. Depending on the case of study to be simulated, it can demand a lot of computational effort. In this way, the processing performance of the software also plays a whole in the choice of the numerical tool.

The most famous CFD tools such as Ansys Fluent, Comsol, Star-CCM+, and OpenFoam allow users to solve a huge amount of high complexity problems in fluid dynamics especially when processing and paralleling the solver in supercomputers.

Therefore, there are still a lot of challenges to numerically represent a fluid dynamics phenomenon when the flow intricacy increases. Some of the numerical algorithms still have a lot to be improved on it. In this way, the biggest advantage of using a free open-source software, especially in the research area, consists specially in the fact that besides, it is free to use or distribute, the user can also modify the source code as needed.

The shared libraries for programming subroutines turn the use of open-source codes interesting also for programmers who want to develop new features for modeling fluid mechanics phenomenon and take the advantage of preimplemented functionalities such as the parallelization code or the implemented wall functions or so on. Due to that, many theses have been developed worldwide, which are intended to turn the implemented code into an OpenFoam solver. It also allows a single implemented routine to achieve a full disclosure while integrating a consolidated package [11].

In this way, OpenFoam software had a huge growth at its base in the last few years. The scientific CFD open source gained credibility at the universities through its convenience for new implementations and research validation of the implemented routines in comparison with the commercial packages.

Although it has benefits, the disadvantages also exist in using a noncommercial tool. The most critical limitation arises in the lack of an easy mesh manipulation functionality. The capabilities of Ansys icem CFD to generate a mesh are well known for its possibilities of meshing high-complexity geometries [12].

As mentioned in Section 8.3, the quality of a mesh interferes straight to the solutions of the differential equations through the computational domain. Depending on the mesh intricacy, using the commercial code is not just a matter of having a user-friendly interface, and it can even become a preclusion.

However, at the preprocessing stage, the mesh can be generated in any external utility and converted to a standard solver file extension. In this way, some limitations to generate a mesh can be mitigated [13]. For the specific purpose of post-processing, there is a visualization software. Some of the widespread commercial versions are Ensight, Fieldview, and tecplot.

The free software ParaView is integrated in the OpenFoam package as the post-processing module [14]. The internal version is called paraFoam, and it includes most of the basic capabilities for data visualization such as contour plots, vector plots, streamlines, and line plots besides some statistical and temporal functions. For more advanced post-processing, it can be useful for the user to use data science and python implementations to extract the results and manipulate the data. In this way, some probe or sampling functions can be set in the preprocessing stage to have specific data stored in a file.

Some external open-source toolboxes are available on the internet and can be coupled with OpenFoam. The rheoTool toolbox is, for instance, a programming pack capable of simulating generalized Newtonian fluids (GNF) and viscoelastic fluids under pressure-driven and electrically driven flows [15].

The rheoTool first version was developed in 2016 based on the viscoelasticFluid-Foam, an OpenFoam solver [16]. The library containing the viscoelastic fluid models is useful to represent non-Newtonian fluids with complex rheologies [17]. The tool can contribute to better represent the phenomena of blood flow in computational hemodynamic [18].

It is important to mention that some incompatibilities with software versions can sometimes be a limitation to manipulate coupled tools. That disadvantage occurs quite frequently while using a no commercial package, and it can be annoying for the user while updating from one version to another.

At the end, the user choice for a specific tool depends on a lot of criterions, including budget and cost benefits. First of all, it is necessary to be sure of choosing a tool capable of solving the problem to be solved. In a second step, all the criterions must be evaluated to estimate which tool better fits the demands.

8.10   FINAL REMARKS

In this chapter, a discussion is made of the main points of CFD applied to hemodynamics in blood pumps. Some experience is shared aiming to help beginners, to guide intermediates, and to encourage experts to philosophize [19–27]. The particularities are so many that it is impossible to reach the entire field in a chapter, but to think about and create your own path of study and guide, this chapter has fulfilled its goal.

As seen along the text, computational hemodynamics is a wide field with so many particularities. This remarkable scientific and technologic subject and its issues are somehow defying and bringing the possibility to advance in the development of blood pumps. The new marks of registration around the world, demanding certain specific information of blood pump functionalities, require computational hemodynamics.

In the future, more and more approaches are coming. The computational capability is being defeated year by year, which brings even more possibilities. New approaches come to add not necessarily to take a place and other come to complement. In this dynamic scenario, as many others, the knowledge is evolutionary and sequential.

We hope this chapter to be useful, and we are open to contribute anyhow in the future.

REFERENCES

1. Bock, E., P. Antunes, T. Leão, B. Uebelhart, J. Fonseca, J. Leme, B. Utiyama, C. da Silva, A. Cavalheiro, D. Santos Filho, J. Dinkhuysen, J. Biscegli, A. Andrade, C. Arruda. "Implantable centrifugal blood pump with dual impeller and double pivot bearing system: Electromechanical actuator, prototyping, and anatomical studies". *Artificial Organs*, 35(5), 437–442, 2011.
2. Lopes, G. B., Jr. Metodologia para Análise Computacional de Escoamento Sanguíneo em Dispositivos de Assistência Ventricular. Thesis. University of São Paulo, 2016.
3. Launder, B. E., D. B. Spalding. "The numerical computation of turbulent flows". *Computer Methods in Applied Mechanics and Engineering*, 3, 269–289, 1974.
4. Yakhot, V., S. A. Orszag, S. Thangam, T. B. Gatski, C. G. Speziale. "Development of turbulence models for shear flows by a double expansion technique". *Physics of Fluids A*, 4(7), 1510–1520, 1992.
5. Menter, R. F. "Two-equation Eddy-viscosity turbulence models for engineering applications". *AIAA Journal*, 32(8), 269–289, 1994.
6. Wilcox, D. C. *Turbulence Modeling for CFD*. DCW Industries: La Cañada, CA, 1993.
7. Versteeg, H. K., W. Malalasekera. *An Introduction to Computational Fluid Dynamics*. Bell & Bain: Glasgow, 2003.
8. Davidson, L. *An Introduction to Turbulence Models*. Chalmers University of Technology: Gothenburg, Sweden, 2003.
9. Spalding, D. B. "A single formula for the law of the wall". *Applied Mechanics*, 28(3), 455, 1961.
10. Kalitzin, G., G. Medic, G. Iaccarino, P. Durbin. "Near-wall behavior of rans turbulence models and implications for wall functions". *Computational Physics*, 204(205), 265–291, 2004.
11. OpenFOAM® Documentation. Online, Available at: https://www.openfoam.com/documentation/. Accessed on: 03-February-2021.
12. Ansys Inc. ICEM-CFD. Accessible in: https://www.ansys.com/-/media/Ansys/corporate/resourcelibrary/brochure/ansys-icem-cfd-brochure.pdf. Accessed on: 03-February-2021.
13. https://www.resolvedanalytics.com/theflux/comparing-cfd-software-part-2-open-source-cfd-software-packages. Accessed on: 03-February-2021.
14. ParaView Tutorial. Online. Available at https://www.paraview.org/tutorials/. Accessed on: 03-February-2021.
15. Pimenta, F., M. A. Alves. 2016, rheoTool, Available at https://github.com/fppimenta/rheoTool.Accessed on: 03-February-2021.
16. Favero, J., A. Secchi, N. Cardozo, H. Jasak. Viscoelastic fluid analysis in internal and in free surface flows using the software OpenFOAM. *Computers & Chemical Engineering*, 34(12), 1984–1993, 2010.
17. Pimenta, F., M. A. Alves. "Numerical simulation of electrically-driven flows using OpenFOAM." arXiv:1802.02843, 2018.

18. Valencia, A., M. G. Zarate, L. Badilla. "Non-newtonian blood flow dynamics in a right internal carotid artery with a saccular aneurysm". *International Journal for Numerical Methods in Fluids*, 50(6), 751–764, 2006.

19. Hochstuhl, J., M. Kassi, S. Elias, A. Ruhparwar, C. Karmonik, S. Chang. "Computational Fluid Dynamics (CFD): A reliable basis for therapy and surgical VAD strategy?" *The Journal of Heart and Lung Transplantation* 37 (4), S268–S269, 2018.

20. Zhang, Q., B. Gao, K. Gu, Y. Chang, J. Xu. "The study on hemodynamic effect of varied support models of BJUT-II VAD on coronary artery: A primary CFD study." *ASAIO Journal* 60 (6), 643–51, 2014.

21. Chiu, W.-C., M. J. Slepian, D. Bluestein. "Thrombus formation patterns in the HeartMate II VAD-clinical observations can be predicted by numerical simulations." *ASAIO Journal*, 60 (2), 237, 2014.

22. Chen, Z., S. K. Jena, G. A. Giridharan, S. C. Koenig, M. S. Slaughter, B. P. Griffith, Z. J. Wu. 2018. "Flow features and device-induced blood trauma in CF-VADs under a pulsatile blood flow condition: A CFD comparative study." *International Journal for Numerical Methods in Biomedical Engineering* 34 (2): e2924.

23. Song, X., H. G. Wood, D. Olsen. "Computational fluid dynamics (CFD) study of the 4th generation prototype of a continuous flow ventricular assist device (VAD)." *The Journal of Biomechanical Engineering*, 126 (2), 180–187, 2004.

24. Neidlin, M., C. Corsini, S. J. Sonntag, S. Schulte-Eistrup, T. Schmitz-Rode, U. Steinseifer, G. Pennati, T. A. S. Kaufmann. 2016. "Hemodynamic analysis of outflow grafting positions of a ventricular assist device using closed-loop multiscale CFD simulations: Preliminary results." *Journal of Biomechanics* 49 (13): 2718–2725.

25. Fan, H. M., F. W. Hong, G. P. Zhang, L. Ye, Z. M. Liu. "Applications of CFD technique in the design and flow analysis of implantable axial flow blood pump." *Journal of Hydrodynamics* 22 (4), 518–25, 2010.

26. Argueta-Morales, I. R., R. Tran, W. Clark, E. Divo, A. Kassab, W. M. DeCampli. "Use of computational fluid dynamics (CFD) to tailor the surgical implantation of a ventricular assist device (VAD): A patient-specific approach to reduce risk of stroke." *Journal of the American College of Surgeons* 211 (3), S26–S27, 2010.

27. Chen, Z., S. K. Jena, G. A. Giridharan, M. A. Sobieski, S. C. Koenig, M. S. Slaughter, B. P. Griffith, Z. J. Wu. "Shear stress and blood trauma under constant and pulse-modulated speed CF-VAD operations: CFD analysis of the HVAD." *Medical & Biological Engineering & Computing* 57 (4), 807–18, 2019.

9 Biofunctional Materials

Rosa Corrêa Leoncio de Sá
INPE National Institute for Space Research

CONTENTS

9.1 INTRODUCTION

Organic, inorganic, and existing cells come from phenomena resulting from chemical and physical interactions between the constituent surfaces of the surrounding and interfacial environment, usually by electrochemical affinity, connection sites, among other transport phenomena involved. This rule governs the impacting events that occur in matter as a function of time and determine its properties and characteristics (Buttiglieri et al., 2003; Etsion, 2005; Lopes et al., 2016; Masuzawa et al., 2003; Meyers et al., 2007; Murabayashi and Nose, 2013; Nakazawa et al., 1996; Neto et al.; 2020; Pfleging et al., 2015; Solheid et al., 2020; Takami et al., 2008; Xie et al., 2015).

The natural life cycle of each being can be interrupted by interferences or mutations, depending on its properties and the environment that remains over time; in this way, the characteristics of the material can be altered, in a natural or purposeful manipulated way, to promote improvements to a specific application.

Today, advances in science and technology in numerous areas have made it possible to manipulate these events for targeted use, as seen in the controlled release of drugs by nanodevices as a complementary alternative in chemotherapy processes to combat cancer, for example. In this case, nanoscale materials highly resistant to corrosion are used to transport certain drugs in different concentrations to the place where the diseased cells are located; most of the time, biomaterials are adopted to be eliminated by the living organism through excretion routes, such as urine and sweat, to carry out this *biofunction*.

A material is classified as *biofunctional* because it is biocompatible and capable of performing a certain function and/or activity on a living cell, tissue, system, and/ or organism; the surface of a material can also have biofunctional properties in isolation from its volume, just as an entire device can be biofunctional even if not all of its components are.

The biofunctionality of an implant is defined according to its ability to act with an appropriate response in a specific condition, which is influenced by the set of properties that enable it to perform a function similar to the one being replaced. The biomaterial can present biofunctional activity in a spontaneous, natural way, without the

DOI: 10.1201/9781003138358-11

205

need to be manipulated, altered; or through its modification and/or use, in a planned way for a certain purpose.

Normally, the performance of the material biofunction occurs in a specific location, either in cells of the internal and/or external biological tissue; the implantation method, on the other hand, can be invasive or not, occur in an isolated or systemic way, that is, its introduction can be done directly at the site of interest or through a systemic, circulatory route, for example.

After its introduction into the body, the biofunctional material can remain for hours, days, weeks, or even months and years; in this respect, the dynamic and synthetic toxic study must be considered and the particle release rate controlled.

Biomaterials capable of accelerating the mechanisms of tissue regeneration for patients' victims of high-grade burns perform several biofunctions simultaneously; after its introduction in the injured region, the release of drugs and substances with high anesthetic, anti-inflammatory, and antibacterial properties is activated, which accelerate the process of regeneration of the endothelial tissue up to the epidermis. This corrective mechanism prevents the introduction of bacteria in the site so that the tissue layers recover in a healthy and accelerated manner, in order to minimize scarring and the need for graft placement.

The chitosan polymer, derived from the shrimp shell, has already been applied for this purpose and also in the manufacture of reabsorbable suture threads with the release of healing particles, Table 9.1 and Figure 9.1.

The introduction of biofunctional surfaces in different types of materials stands out in terms of gaining high performance at a low cost. There are times when the volume material of the implant cannot be replaced due to its physical properties being ideal for the application, but the modification of its surface by the introduction of a thin film and/or particles of different scales and promotion of nano- and microscale textures allow the implant material to have a biofunctional action on the site of interest.

The ability of a biomaterial to promote metabolic changes in living cells and other systems is influenced, not only by its chemical composition but also by the topography of the material and the conditions of the implanted site. Usually, the phenomena resulting from the interaction in biomaterial interface and biological tissue are directly proportional to the surface profile, such as chemical composition and geometric aspect at all levels, mainly micro- and nanometric.

When a liquid droplet comes into contact with a solid, smooth surface, it displays the Young contact angle (θ). The wettability character, hydrophilic or hydrophobic ($\theta > 90°$), can be determined quantitatively from the measurement of this θ and qualitatively through the practical observation of the spread of the drop on the solid. The hydrophilic profile (from the Greek hydro = water + filico = attraction) indicates the affinity of a material with water, $\theta < 90°$ and superhydrophilic $\theta < 45°$; hydrophobic (from Greek phobic = repulsion) non-affinity $\theta > 90°$ and superhydrophobic $\theta > 150°$ (Figure 9.2).

According to the implant site and its biofunction, the most appropriate interaction profile is defined. Since the largest proportion of an organism consists of water, an average of 70%, rheological laws can be considered to predict the interaction

TABLE 9.1

Illustration, Main Characteristic of Nanomaterials Applied to Obtain Nanostructured Drugs

Nanomaterial	Illustration	Feature	Indication (Drugs)
Liposomes	80–300 nm	Spherical shell-like closed structures, formed from lipids, amphipathic, which spontaneously organize	Assist in the treatment of cancer (doxorubicin) treatment of cancer/ (Myocet® and DaunoXome®) treatment of mycoses visceral leishmaniasis (amphotericin B)
Magnetic nanoparticles	10–300 nm	Spherical particles can be coated with dendrimers, silane, gold, or hydrophilic polymers. The drug can be encapsulated in the shell or inside. Examples of metals: Co, Mn, Fe, and Ni and their oxides	Immunodiagnostics/(clinical cell separation) antibiotics/ (ciprofloxacin) chemotherapy/gemcitabine)
Solid lipid nanoparticles; nanoemulsions	80–300 nm	They are complex mixtures, where the nucleus is dense, due to the mixture of glycerides or triglycerides stabilized by surfactants	Osteoporosis/(indaflex)
Polymeric nanoparticles	10–100 nm	Nanospheres (the drug is solubilized inside, the nucleus being the polymeric matrix) or nanocapsules (the drug is surrounded by the polymeric matrix). Examples of polymers used in the synthesis of NP: polyacrylamide and polyacrylate; albumin, chitosan, DNA, and gelatin	Antineoplastic, lung cancer/ (carboplatin) colon cancer treatment/((5-fluorouracil, 5-FU) chemotherapy/ (nanoxel) chemotherapy/ (abraxane)
Dendrimers	1–10 nm	Dendrimers are macromolecules (branched polymers) with a well-defined size and structure. They may have the surface functionalized by different active groups, which generates specific links with drugs of interest	Mycoses and visceral cancer treatment/anti-inflammatory/ (ibuprofen and piroxicam)

Sources: Araki et al. (2017), Bock et al. (2008, 2011a,b, 2016), Hernandes et al. (2017), Nishida et al. (2009, 2017), Rodrigues et al. (2019), Uebelhart et al. (2013).

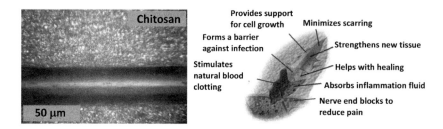

FIGURE 9.1 Optical microscopy of chitosan wire 4% glucosamine, 350× increase, and its benefits.

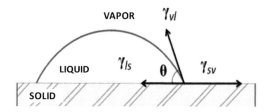

FIGURE 9.2 Scheme of a water drop on a solid surface and the representation of the surface tensions involved.

phenomena arising at the implanting circulating blood interface, for example; the solid portion, cellular activity, must also be taken into account.

9.2 BIOFUNCTIONAL MATERIALS FOR IMPLANTABLE MEDICAL DEVICES

The National Health Surveillance Agency (ANVISA) is the Brazilian organization responsible for standardizing, certifying, and supervising the entire life cycle of surgical instruments, equipment, and/or implantable medical devices. The requirements to be met must be proven through preliminary results obtained during the project development stages. The degree of risk is subdivided into classes, from I to IV, according to the properties and characteristics of the surrounding biological environment and the time of use of the item in question.

Medical devices that remain in direct contact with blood for an indefinite period, which are destined for intravenous implants, are classified as Class IV. Therefore, the biological environment must not compromise the implant's biofunctionality, by means of corrosive action, for example; as well as, the biomaterial cannot generate negative biological stimulus through hematological and/or immunological response to any system of the organism.

The biofunctional characteristic proves to be efficient and important in the optimization of Class IV implantable medical devices, which must consist of components capable of remaining stable for a minimum period of 5 years.

When an individual presents with severe heart failure (HF) due to low cardiac output, chronic ventricular failure, or "ventricular remodeling," the implantation of a ventricular assist device (VAD) specific to the clinical case is indicated (da Silva et al., 2011). This implant for mechanical circulatory assistance can be Class IV if kept in the body for more than 30 days, and its biofunction helps to "reverse" structural changes in the cardiac muscle, resulting in the functional improvement of the organ and the entire cardiovascular system.

From the geometric configuration of a VAD, it can be pulsatile, axial, or centrifugal; when axial or centrifugal, it basically consists of a rotor that remains suspended by a pivoting bearing system inside a vat with a geometry conducive to not generating hemolysis and irreversible deformation of blood components. According to the anatomical model of implantability, the VAD can have access cannulas to be connected to the ventricle outlet to the aorta; see Figures 9.3 and 9.4.

Regardless of the type of drive, electromechanical or pneumatic, and flow profile, pulsatile, axial, or centrifugal, the system of a biofunctional VAD must include a non-hemolytic blood pump, which proves good hemodynamic performance, in biocompatible material (non-cytotoxic, which do not degrade or deform during

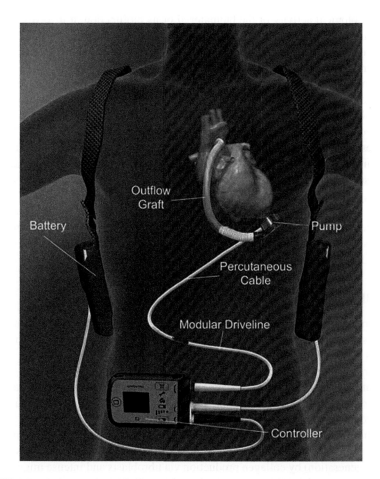

FIGURE 9.3   Anatomical positioning of the implantation of a VAD HeartMate.

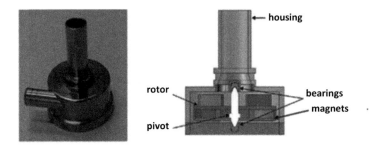

FIGURE 9.4 Aortic centrifugal VAD from the Institute Dante Pazzanese of Cardiology—University of São Paulo—and its components (see da Silva et al., 2011).

application time), an advanced electrical power device, and an intelligent control system with failure prevention (da Silva et al., 2011).

The biofunctional character of a total device is not restricted only to the chemical and biological activity of the biomaterial or its biofunction, it involves the entire design and manufacturing process of each component; the performance is shown according to the mobility, the assistance time, the toxicity and biodegradation of the biomaterial, and the clinical conditions of the patient.

The manufacturing processes and the choice of biomaterials applicable for each component must be planned to economically dispose of a final biofunctional product with high durability and reliability.

Of the most widely used biofunctional materials, 99.99% pure titanium (Ti) grade II is present in greater proportion due to its excellent chemical stability, promoting high durability and its hydrophilic profile, low wettability to the implant. Atoms on the surface react instantly with oxygen, so a titanium oxide nanolayer, titania ceramic, is chemically stable over the entire surface area.

Even though it is the main biomaterial used in the manufacture of long-lasting intravenous implantable components, blood triggers a thrombogenic response when it comes into contact with any non-endothelized surface; therefore, this interface must be improved.

9.3   BIOFUNCTIONALIZATION OF VAD COMPONENTS

The components of a VAD made of titanium are the blood chamber and its access cannulas and the rotor; whose surfaces remain in contact with circulating blood, constant shear stress by viscous and highly corrosive flow, the blood.

Several studies claim that an endothelized surface as an interface can attribute excellent biofunctionality as it presents a thromboresistant characteristic capable of minimizing the dose of anticoagulant and the hemolysis index (da Silva et al., 2011).

Hydrophilic surfaces with a microstructured scaffold characteristic can promote the formation of a neointimal layer in vivo in circulatory assist devices, if implanted for a long period; this process occurs after 20 weeks through neoangiogenesis (endothelial regeneration) by collagen production via fibroblasts and intense migration and cell adsorption. It is in this stage that the cells need anchoring points, scaffolds, of proportional dimension to the characteristics of the local biological tissue, which guarantee the biofixation and cell proliferation with no chance of detachment (Elias et al., 2001; de Sá et al., 2017a).

The process described above clearly describes the biofunctional performance attributed to an implant surface that is part of a medical device, which also performs an isolated biofunction.

The surfaces of permanent blood contact of the HeartMate III® centrifugal VAD, designed by Thoratec Corporation in Pleasanton, United States, are textured. The surface modification was performed to provide, in vivo, a thin layer of living cells, highly resistant to thrombus formation, on the implant surface. Figure 9.5 shows the texturing performed inside the cannulas, represented by sintered titanium microspheres, and at the base of the membrane by extruded polyurethane filaments.

After 17 years, this characteristic in the American VAD had efficiency proven through clinical evaluations for providing the formation of a biological neointima derived from the circulating blood under the modified surfaces; due to the characteristics of the biofilm formed (continuous thin film, well adhered and rich in collagen), patients received only infusion of aspirin and dipyridamole as anticoagulants.

Among the most suitable techniques and processes for modifying metal surfaces, those involving temperature control, the introduction of particles, and reagents as a function of time stand out, even more when the intention is to obtain a biofunctional material.

The application of precision tools using cutting, plasma phenomena and ultrafast lasers has gained prominence and preference when it is desired to obtain micro- or nanotexturing in a homogeneous and reproducible way.

In the plasma electrolytic oxidation (PEO) process, the material must be introduced in an electrolytic medium under high voltage; the oxidation of the substrate begins with the action of localized electrical discharges, the micro-arcs, as a function of time; which determine the growth rate of the oxide layer, its structure and chemical composition.

In 2017, titanium grade II sample surfaces were microtextured by PEO "step by step," through system improvements, according to comparative analysis of surfaces.

The results of physical-chemical characterization revealed a microtextured surface, homogeneous and characteristic of scaffolds, with the presence of pores and

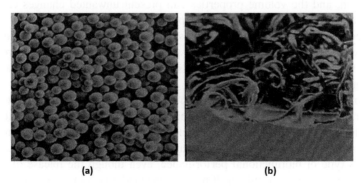

(a)   (b)

FIGURE 9.5 Textured surfaces of the VAD HeartMate®; microsphere in sintered titanium (40×) on the left and polyurethane filaments (80×) on the right.

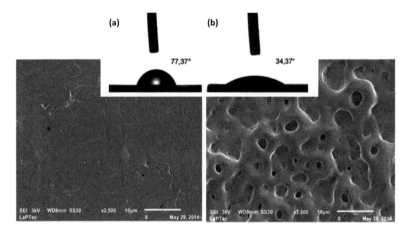

FIGURE 9.6 Micrograph of titanium surfaces: (a) polished, hydrophilic and (b) textured, superhydrophilic.

scaffolds Ø from 5 to 20 μm proportional dimension to the erythrocytes and endothelial cells (±7.5 μm), in Figure 9.6.

Consisting of titanium oxide (titania), this surface presented a more hydrophilic profile (B) compared to the profile seen in polished Ti (A). In vitro experiments with biological material were performed, hemodynamic and endothelial, and evidence of cellular anchoring could be perceived only on the modified surfaces.

This process is capable of modifying the surface of some metals without compromising the volume properties of the material; however, it must be automated in order to reproduce the results in materials of different geometries.

Other methods of surface modification, such as electrospinning, fiber bonding, phase inversion, solvent evaporation, and additive manufacturing, are also used in the manufacture of biofunctional materials and surfaces. Now, the process conditions, the morphological aspect, and the chemical composition of the resulting surface do not always meet the specific characteristics of the biological medium of interest, the biofunction, and the volume properties can present unwanted changes capable of compromising the performance of the implant.

For components that remain in a constant process of friction wear and also in contact with circulating blood, as with pivoting bearings used to keep the rotor suspended, temperature-resistant biomaterials, tension absorbers, and self-lubricants are highlighted.

Polymeric biomaterials usually do not release particles, they are better stress absorbers, but they cannot resist high temperatures; then, the energy resulting from the friction at the point of contact between the pivot and the support bearing generates deformation and compromises the performance of the VAD in general.

In this type of biofunctional performance, even though the release of particles as a function of time is minimal, it must be avoided and controlled, as well as the vibrational waves commonly resulting from pivoting sets in ceramic and glass, for example, alumina and zirconia.

One way to improve the biofunction of this important component is through the addition of diamond-like carbon molecules, diamond-like carbon (DLC), under its surface, whatever the material may be.

The plasma-enhanced chemical vapor deposition (PECVD) technique is capable of depositing a certain thin film on different materials, metals, and polymers of low and high temperatures through thermochemical reactions and plasma phenomenon between the substrate and reagents in vapor phase and vacuum condition.

DLC is a type of nanostructured amorphous carbon capable of providing excellent tribological properties, such as greater wear and corrosion resistance and low friction coefficient, in addition to being biocompatible and self-lubricating, that is, super biofunctional (de Sá et al., 2017b).

The 316 L stainless steel pivots, which make up the pivoting support system of a centrifugal VAD, had their surfaces coated in DLC by PECVD at the National Institute for Space Research (INPE), Brazil. As predicted, this coating attributed greater durability due to less frictional wear, noise, and vibration as confirmed by an in vitro durability test. Figure 9.7 shows this pivot before and after application the of the DLC and the corresponding microstructures.

This biofunctional attribution is highlighted when it comes to parts with complex geometry; the technique allows DLC steam to reach all areas of the surface, even at a negative angle. The rotor of the Spiral Pump® Extracorporeal Circulation Pump, Nipro, Brazil, made of polycarbonate can be uniformly coated, Figure 9.8. Even if used for a few hours during a surgical procedure, the lower viscous friction attributed by the DLC film collaborates a lot in the preservation of constituents of blood and reducing the dose of anticoagulants.

Of the different ways to *biofunctionalize* surfaces, those that apply in the cardio-vascular medical field deserve great attention and investment since the attributions are highly relevant in contributing to the better quality and life expectancy of countless patients who depend on the Unified Brazilian Health System.

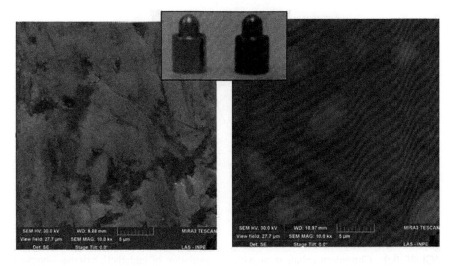

FIGURE 9.7   Pivot of the support system in stainless steel and DLC and its microstructures.

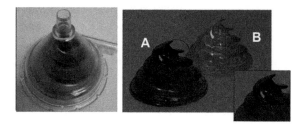

FIGURE 9.8   Spiral Pump® Extracorporeal Circulation Pump rotors, Nipro, Brazil.

The stent valve is a cardiovascular prosthesis of great demand that remains implanted in direct contact with blood and endothelial tissue for an indefinite period; its function is to unblock blood vessels that are victims of aneurysm and replace subsequent valves, which are consequently injured as an adaptive response to cardiovascular disease.

Well, the metallic stent is usually made of chromium-cobalt, an excellent biomaterial for such mechanical biofunction, but which allows the formation of pannus and growth of endothelial tissue around the stent; see Figure 9.9. This encapsulation leads to a new obstruction of the serious blood pathway, so the biofunction of the implant material should be improved.

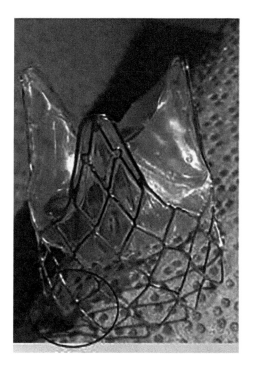

FIGURE 9.9   Chromium-cobalt stent with encapsulation of endothelial tissue—synthetic heart technology.

For this, the stent was subjected to chemical vapor deposition technique and a thin film in DLC highly resists fatigue and biocompatible material can be obtained; since then, new in vivo experiments have been carried out and it is possible to verify the absence of formation of "pannus." Here is yet another example of *biofunctionalizing* the surface of materials.

REFERENCES

Araki, S.Y., R.L. Stoeterau, P.C.F. Da Silva, M.A. Saito, J.R.C. De Sousa Sobrinho, A.L. Marques, D.F. De Sousa, E.G.P. Bock, and A.C.F. De Arruda. "Microstructure and tribology regarding precision studies of micro-sintered ceramic bearings for ventricular assist devices." In *Proceedings of the 17th International Conference of the European Society for Precision Engineering and Nanotechnology,* Hannover, *EUSPEN 2017,* 2017.

Bock, E., A. Ribeiro, M. Silva, P. Antunes, J. Fonseca, D. Legendre, J. Leme, et al. "New centrifugal blood pump with dual impeller and double pivot bearing system: Wear evaluation in bearing system, performance tests, and preliminary hemolysis tests." *Artificial Organs* 32, no. 4 (2008): 329–33.

Bock, E., A. Andrade, J. Dinkhuysen, C. Arruda, J. Fonseca, J. Leme, B. Utiyama, et al. "Introductory tests to in vivo evaluation: Magnetic coupling influence in motor controller." *ASAIO Journal* 57, no. 5 (2011a): 462–65.

Bock, E., P. Antunes, T. Leao, B. Uebelhart, J. Fonseca, J. Leme, B. Utiyama, et al. "Implantable centrifugal blood pump with dual impeller and double pivot bearing system: Electromechanical actuator, prototyping, and anatomical studies." *Artificial Organs* 35, no. 5 (2011b): 437–42.

Bock, E., G.P. Bock, T. Leão, J. Fonseca, and A. Andrade. "Left ventricle failure and blood flow estimation for centrifugal blood pumps." *DAVid Publishing* 6, no. 3 (2016): 162–66.

Buttiglieri, S., D. Pasqui, M. Migliori, H. Johnstone, S. Affrossman, L. Sereni, M.L. Wratten, R. Barbucci, C. Tetta, and G. Camussi. "Endothelization and adherence of leucocytes to nanostructured surfaces." *Biomaterials* 24, no. 16 (2003): 2731–38.

da Silva, I., O. Horikawa, J.R. Cardoso, F.A. Camargo, A.J.P. Andrade, and E.G.P. Bock. "Single axis controlled hybrid magnetic bearing for left ventricular assist device: Hybrid core and closed magnetic circuit." *Artificial Organs* 35, no. 5 (2011): 448–53.

de Sá, R.C.L., N.C. da Cruz, J.R. Moro, T. Leão, A.J.P. de Andrade, and E.G.P. Bock. "Modification surface in medicine: Techniques with plasma in a centrifugal blood pump implantable." *Sinergia* 18, no. 2 (2017a): 91–94.

de Sá, R.C.L., R.L. Stoeterau, E. Drigo, B. Utiyama, J. Fonseca, E. Leal, T. Leão, M. Hermandes, A. Andrade, and E.G.P. Bock. "Textured layer of titanium oxide in titanium pure to endotheliale ventricular assist devices." In *Proceedings of the 17th International Conference of the European Society for Precision Engineering and Nanotechnology,* Hannover, *EUSPEN 2017,* 2017b.

Etsion, I. "State of the art in laser surface texturing." *Journal of Tribology* 127, no. 1 (2005): 248.

Hernandes, M.M.A.P., J.A.F. Da Rocha, M.A. Saito, S.Y. Araki, P. Silva, R.L. Stoeterau, and E.G.P. Bock. "Dimensional control in pre-sintered zirconia machining for double pivot micro bearings of blood pumps." In *Proceedings of the 17th International Conference of the European Society for Precision Engineering and Nanotechnology,* Hannover, *EUSPEN 2017,* 2017.

Lopes, G.B. Jr, L.C.C. Gómez, G.B., and E.G.P. Bock. "Mesh independency analyses and grid density estimation for ventricular assist devices in multiple reference frames simulations." *Technische Mechanik* 36, no. 3 (2016): 190–98.

Masuzawa, T., S. Ezoe, T. Kato, and Y. Okada. "Magnetically suspended centrifugal blood pump with an axially levitated motor" 27, no. 7 (2003): 631–38.

Meyers, S.R., P.T. Hamilton, E.B. Walsh, D.J. Kenan, and M.W. Grinstaff. "Endothelialization of titanium surfaces." *Advanced Materials* 19, no. 18 (2007): 2492–98.

Murabayashi, S., and Y. Nose. "Biocompatibility: Bioengineering aspects." *Bio-Medical Materials and Engineering* 23, no. 1–2 (2013): 1–7.

Nakazawa, T., K. Makinouchi, Y. Takami, J. Glueck, S. Takatani, and Y. Nosé. "Modification of a pivot bearing system on a compact centrifugal pump." *Artificial Organs,* 20, no. 3 (1996): 258–63.

Neto, S., J.R.C. Sousa Sobrinho, C. da Costa, T.F. Leão, S.A.M.M. Senra, E.G.P. Bock, G.A. Santos, et al. "Investigation of MEMS as accelerometer sensor in an implantable centrifugal blood pump prototype." *Journal of the Brazilian Society of Mechanical Sciences and Engineering* 42, no. 9, 1–10 (2020).

Nishida, M., O. Maruyama, R. Kosaka, T. Yamane, H. Kogure, H. Kawamura, Y. Yamamoto, K. Kuwana, Y. Sankai, and T. Tsutsui. "Hemocompatibility evaluation with experimental and computational fluid dynamic analyses for a monopivot circulatory assist pump" *Artificial Organs* 33, no. 4 (2009): 378–86.

Nishida, B.Y.T., G.A. Pereira, E. Drigo, M. Fonseca, R.B.B. Santos, M.A.G. Silveira, and E.G.P. Bock. "Prototype for optical applications that microscopically affect the cancer cell diagnosis in biological sciences." In *Proceedings of the 17th International Conference of the European Society for Precision Engineering and Nanotechnology,* Hannover, *EUSPEN 2017,* 2017.

Pfleging, W., R. Kumari, H. Besser, T. Scharnweber, and J.D. Majumdar. "Laser surface textured titanium alloy (Ti-6Al-4V): Part 1 - surface characterization." *Applied Surface Science* 355 (2015): 104–11.

Rodrigues, M., N.C. da Cruz, J.A.F. Rocha, R.C.L. Sá, and E.G.P. Bock. "Surface roughness of biomaterials and process parameters of titanium dioxide gritblasting for productivity enhancement." *The Academic Society Journal* 3, no. 2 (2019): 169–76.

Solheid, J.S., T. Wunsch, V. Trouillet, S. Weigel, T. Scharnweber, H.J. Seifert, and W. Pfleging. "Two-step laser post-processing for the surface functionalization of additively manufactured Ti-6Al-4V parts." *Materials* 13, no. 21 (2020): 1–18.

Takami, Y., T. Nakazawa, K. Makinouchi, R. Benkowski, J. Glueck, and Y. Nosé. "Material of the double pivot bearing system in the gyro C1E3 centrifugal pump." *Artificial Organs* 21, no. 2 (2008): 143–47.

Uebelhart, B., B.U. da Silva, J. Fonseca, E. Bock, J. Leme, C. da Silva, T. Leão, and A. Andrade. "Study of a centrifugal blood pump in a mock loop system." *Artificial Organs* 37, no. 11 (2013): 946–9.

Xie, D, Y.X. Leng, F.J. Jing, and N. Huang. "A brief review of bio-tribology in cardiovascular devices." *Biosurface and Biotribology* 1, no. 4 (2015): 249–62.

10 Bioceramics for VADs

Fernando dos Santos Ortega
Hospital Israelita Albert Einstein

CONTENTS

10.1 SHAFTS AND BEARINGS IN VADs: CHARACTERISTICS AND DEMANDS

Ventricular assist devices (VADs) are complex equipment, whose design and construction are a multidisciplinary challenge, as it involves knowledge of medicine, fluid mechanics, mechanical projects, programming, simulation, and control [1]. In addition, knowledge of the properties of the materials used to manufacture VADs is of paramount importance, as the use of inappropriate materials can cause problems ranging from equipment malfunction to premature failure or negative interactions with the patient's body, such as inflammation, rejection, hemolysis, among others [2].

While the first-generation VAD models tried to imitate the heartbeat, the second-generation models demonstrated that continuous flow pumps could act on the human body for long periods, with significant advantages, such as the elimination of valves and reduction of size, weight, consumption of energy, vibration, and noise. This finding paved the way for third-generation model designs, based on the concept of centrifugal pumps with hydrodynamically supported axles [3]. More recently, fourth-generation models have adopted rotors supported by magnetic levitation [4].

One of the central elements of a centrifugal pump is the pivot bearing system, as they support the mechanical load and operate at high speeds. Under these conditions, they can wear out, which releases fragments into the bloodstream and reduces the life span of these components. Moreover, in contact with blood cells, protein deposits

DOI: 10.1201/9781003138358-12

can accumulate on their surfaces [5]. Therefore, in addition to high strength, it is necessary to minimize the friction of the system, either by hydrodynamic support or by magnetic levitation. Although magnetic levitation virtually eliminates friction between moving parts, it is likely that both solutions will continue to be used in the design and manufacture of VADs.

10.2   WHERE DO MATERIAL PROPERTIES COME FROM?

The selection of materials used to manufacture each component of a given project is made primarily based on its properties, although other factors may be important, such as cost and manufacturing method, which is directly associated with the design of the part.

The properties of materials basically result from three factors: (i) the chemical composition, which determines the type of bond that will be established between the atoms that compose the material and the energy associated with them; (ii) the crystalline structure, which stems from the way as the atoms are spatially connected, forming well-defined geometric arrangements (it is important to note that the same composition may have its atoms spatially organized in different ways, resulting in different crystalline structures); and (iii) the microstructure of the material, which, on a larger scale, involves the spatial distribution of grains (extension of crystalline regions with the same composition and spatial orientation), grain boundaries, pores, and heterogeneities. These levels of matter organization are briefly described below, seeking to highlight some relationships with the properties of materials.

10.4.1   CHEMICAL BONDS

When two atoms become chemically bonded, the free energy associated with them is smaller than in the same two isolated atoms. To separate them, it is necessary to supply the same amount of energy that was dissipated when they were bonded. This energy can be applied in different ways: The fracture of a material occurs under the action of mechanical energy; the melting of a solid occurs by applying thermal energy; corrosive processes are nothing but the action of chemical energy; sufficiently energetic electromagnetic radiation promotes the photodegradation of some materials. In all cases, if the bonding energy is high, there will be greater difficulty for each of those processes to occur, resulting in materials that are stronger, have higher melting point, and are resistant to corrosion and photodegradation [6].

Ceramic materials have chemical bonds that vary between ionic and covalent. The energy associated with these types of bonds varies over a wide range, but in general, it is higher than the energy of metallic bonds and much higher than that of secondary bonds, which are determinants in the properties of polymers. Table 10.1 presents some typical bond energy for the different types of bonds.

Because of the bond type, ceramics have some well-defined characteristics: They have comparatively high melting points (ceramics are widely used as refractories that are essential for melting metals) and are chemically inert. Additionally, ceramics have high theoretical strength, although such values cannot be achieved because they

TABLE10.1
Typical Bond Strengths [7]

Type of Bond	Bond Energy (kJ/Mol)
Ionic	50–1,000
Covalent	200–1,000
Metallic	50–1,000
van der Waals	0.1–10
Hydrogen	10–40

are highly sensitive to defects like pores and surface scratches, which act as stress concentrators and drastically reduce their practical strength. Nevertheless, ceramic fibers are widely used to produce extremely strong composites, since their tiny diameters can contain only very small defects, with a reduced ability to degrade their strength.

10.4.2 CRYSTAL STRUCTURE

The crystal structure refers to the spatial arrangement of atoms in solids, forming a well-defined three-dimensional network where each atom has its position and neighboring atoms following a pattern that extends over long distances. The crystalline structure can be associated with several properties of the materials [6,7]. Perhaps, the clearest example of this is carbon, as illustrated in Figure 10.1. Graphite, diamond, nanotubes, and graphene are some of the various carbon allotropes and have very different properties. However, the only difference between them (except for the presence of tiny amounts of impurities) is the spatial arrangement of the carbon atoms. In the diamond, all carbons bond covalently, forming a very strong three-dimensional crystalline lattice that provides extreme hardness. In graphite, covalent bonds occur only in two directions, forming a plane structure of hexagonal rings. The connection between these planes is made by van der Waals forces, which are much weaker than covalent connections and allow one plane to slide over the other. Consequently, graphite is soft and is used as a solid lubricant, while diamond is extremely hard and is used as a cutting tool in the most extreme situations.

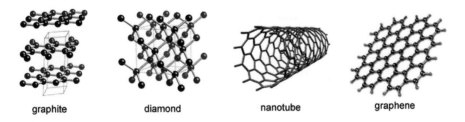

graphite   diamond   nanotube   graphene

FIGURE 10.1 Some of the carbon allotropes, illustrating how atoms can connect according to different patterns, resulting in very different properties.

Changes in crystal structure may be induced by small concentrations of impurities and by temperature. Zirconia (ZrO_2) is an example of ceramic material having excellent mechanical properties thanks to the possibility of inducing changes in its crystal structure in a controlled manner [8]. Zirconia has three crystal structures at atmospheric pressure: monoclinic at room temperature, tetragonal at temperatures between 1,170°C and 2,370°C, and cubic above 2,370°C. Its melting temperature is around 2,715°C. Figure 10.2a shows the phase equilibrium diagram of zirconia–yttria system. The density of monoclinic zirconia is 5.83 g/cm³, while the density of tetragonal zirconia is 6.10 g/cm³. When cooled from temperatures above 1,170°C, zirconia undergoes a volumetric expansion of 3%–5%. This phenomenon, known as stress-induced transformation toughening, has been used ingeniously to increase the toughness, that is, the resistance to crack propagation, of some ceramic materials [9]. In summary, when tiny zirconia particles are dispersed in a sufficiently rigid matrix, the strong compression it exerts can prevent the transformation of zirconia particles to the monoclinic phase, since they cannot expand. Thus, they are retained in a tetragonal form, in a metastable condition, at room temperature. However, as a crack starts to propagate in the material, there is a decrease in the compressive stress on the zirconia particles, allowing them to transform to the monoclinic form. The resulting expansion causes a strong compressive tension on the crack, which tends to close it and avoid it to grow. This toughening mechanism is schematically shown in Figure 10.2b. This strategy can be adopted to increase the toughness of other ceramics, such as alumina, but it has been used in zirconia itself, since small additions of ions such as Y^{3+}, Ca^{2+}, and Mg^{2+} make it partially stable at room temperature, in the tetragonal form.

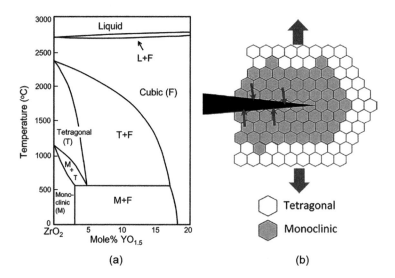

(a)   (b)

FIGURE 10.2   (a) Phase equilibrium diagram for ZrO_2-Y_2O_3 system up to 20 Mol% of yttria [10]; (b) sketch of the stress-induced transformation toughening mechanism for zirconia, showing the compressive stress on the crack [Ref. 11].

10.4.3 MICROSTRUCTURE OF MATERIALS

The microstructure of materials refers to morphological characteristics on a much larger scale than the atomic one, reaching tens of nanometers up to a few hundred microns. It consists of elements such as size, shape, and grain orientation; concentration, sizes, and location of pores; structure and thickness of grain boundaries. In the case of materials containing two or more phases, it also involves their proportion and spatial distribution. Figure 10.3 presents a SEM image of the microstructure of a polycrystalline alumina, showing some of these microstructural features.

The microstructure of ceramic materials plays a central role in defining their properties. Porosity, for example, directly affects properties such as density, translucency, thermal conductivity, hardness, strength, among others.

Although the type of atomic bond and crystal structure are crucial in determining the properties of materials, there is little freedom to modify the structure of matter at these levels, since it derives essentially from chemical composition and external factors such as temperature and pressure. These variables can often not be changed.

On the other hand, microstructural characteristics and their effects on the properties of materials acquire great importance, as they strongly depend on processing. Therefore, they can be modified by adjusting the various stages of the manufacturing process of materials in general, and particularly in ceramics [12].

The following topics will present an overview of the manufacturing process of ceramic materials, seeking to correlate the effects of some processing variables on the microstructure and consequently on the properties of these materials.

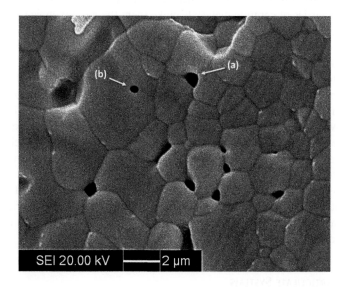

FIGURE 10.3 Example of a polycrystalline alumina microstructure, highlighting (a) an intergranular pore and (b) an intragranular pore. Grain boundaries are clearly shown, contouring grains with different sizes.

10.3   TRANSFORMING CERAMIC MATERIALS INTO CERAMIC PRODUCTS

Most manufacturing processes involve operations that deform the materials to the approximate final shape. When necessary, they are thinned to reach the dimensions defined in the project. This is how plastic granules, for example, soften when heated and can be injected into molds where they become stiff after cooling, acquiring the geometry defined by the mold cavity. In the softened state, they can also be pressed through a hole, forming tubes and different profiles. Aluminum, steel, and other metallic alloys are melted and cast into molds that contain cavities with the negative of the desired shape. Furthermore, metal ingots can be heated to temperatures below their melting point, but high enough to achieve the ability to undergo large plastic deformations and can then be laminated, forged, stamped, etc. Machining operations can be employed, either to remove small amounts of material for dimensional adjustment, or to produce complex geometries by removing larger amounts of material from an ingot or bar.

Ceramic materials, however, for reasons already discussed, have a very high melting point. Even if they are melted, the microstructures formed after cooling are difficult to control and, generally, unfavorable for many properties of technological interest. In addition, ceramics are not ductile, but rather brittle, even when heated. Therefore, they cannot undergo the plastic deformation necessary to be molded [13]. Finally, ceramics are widely used as cutting tools, due to their excellent hardness and wear resistance, which makes any attempt to machine ceramic materials demand long times and high costs. Such operations are usually limited to removing minimal amounts of material, just to improve the surface finish.

It is found that, due to the type of chemical bond and aspects of the crystal structure, the properties of ceramic materials make them the natural choice when refractoriness, rigidity, hardness, and wear resistance are desired. But at the same time, such properties make impossible the direct use of conventional forming techniques applied to metals and polymers.

Fortunately, this seemingly challenging issue has been settled for thousands of years. By experiencing with raw materials extracted from the vicinity of riverbeds, the first human groups soon realized it was possible to obtain a material with excellent plasticity, which could be shaped to produce anything from simple bricks to objects with fine details. Moreover, after being heated enough, these objects developed some strength and, if some components were added, they could become impervious to fluids like water. Indeed, ceramic materials are among the first artifacts manufactured by countless civilizations and constitute important archaeological records [14].

The following sections describe how the use of powdered raw materials enables a large number of manufacturing processes, from simple and traditional to the most recent technologies.

10.3.1   PARTICULATE SYSTEMS

Most processes used to manufacture ceramic products use powdered raw materials. This is mainly due to two factors [12]:

i. Particulate systems can develop different consistencies as a liquid is added, allowing the use of forming techniques traditionally used in the manufacture of other materials;

ii. The particle surface is a region where excess energy is stored due to the abrupt interruption of chemical bonds in the crystalline lattice. This surface energy favors the sintering process, in which ceramic parts acquire strength and changes from a simple powder compact to a ceramic material, under the action of temperature.

These two aspects are briefly described below.

10.3.2 CONSISTENCY

Consistency may be understood as the way a powder–water system responds to a shear stress. It can be classified as granular solid, plastic mass, or liquid suspensions, as the ratio of water to powder increases. The main reason why the water content changes the mechanical response of the material is outlined in Figure 10.4.

When a small amount of water is added to a ceramic powder (typically below 10%), small menisci are formed at the points of contact between particles that result in cohesive capillary forces. At the same time, such menisci reduce the friction between the particles, favoring the relative slipping between them. As a result, particles clump together to form small granules that can deform under the action of a shear stress. This consistency is used to form parts by dry pressing, since a lubricating film covering the particles favors their movement during compaction, while cohesive capillary pressure increases the green strength [15].

If the amount of water is increased enough to cover all the particles and fill in the empty spaces between them, the system develops plasticity. This property refers to the ability of deforming continuously under the action of shear stress and sustaining

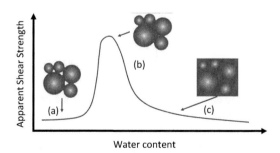

FIGURE 10.4   The apparent shear strength changes with increasing the water/powder ratio: (a) For low water content, the powder behaves as a granular solid, as the water is placed at contact points between particles; (b) As the amount of water increases, it eventually fills all the empty spaces between particles and forms a lubricating film between them that enables the sliding of particles under shear; (c) As the amount of water increases, the thickness of the liquid film between particles increases and the consistency gradually changes to a soft paste and eventually it becomes a liquid suspension.

its shape after the removal of this stress. The apparent shear strength is maximum, and the material requires great effort to be deformed, which allows it to keep its shape, even in the case of bulky and heavy parts. This is the consistency required for extrusion, plastic pressing, turning, among others involving plastic deformation of the material [16].

Finally, as the water-to-powder ratio increases, the particles become separated by an increasingly thick liquid layer and can move more easily. As a result, the flow resistance is gradually reduced, and the plastic mass becomes a soft paste and eventually reaches the liquid consistency of a suspension, or slip. Several manufacturing processes take advantage of liquid consistency, from slip casting to self-flowing refractory castables. In these processes, a liquid suspension fills a mold and, through the action of a wide variety of mechanisms, hardens inside the mold, accurately reproducing the geometric details or textures present on its surface [17].

The above discussion was restricted to the water-to-powder ratio, which is the most basic variable that determines the consistency of a ceramic mass. Many other factors affect the consistency of particulate systems, such as particle size distribution, particle shape, powder dispersion, organic and inorganic additives, pH, and temperature. Clays, for example, generally have good plasticity due to the presence of natural organic compounds in their composition, in addition to particles with the shape of tiny hexagonal flakes. On the other hand, technical ceramics produced with synthetic powders may develop plastic behavior only with the use of additives known as plasticizers. The role of each of these factors is beyond the scope of this chapter but is extensively described in the ceramics engineering literature [12].

10.3.3 DENSIFICATION

When a solid breaks, two new surfaces are formed. Atoms that were inside the solid are now located on new surfaces and have somewhat unsatisfied chemical bonds. This situation leads to increased energy in this region, associated with Gibbs free energy through the following relationship:

$$\gamma = \left(\frac{\partial G}{\partial A} \right)_{P,T,n} \tag{10.1}$$

where G is the Gibbs free energy (J), A is the solid surface (m^2), and γ is the specific surface energy (J/m^2), which corresponds to the rate of change of Gibbs free energy in relation to the surface area of the solid at constant pressure, temperature and quantity of matter γ depends on the crystalline direction and is affected by impurities on the surface [6].

As a solid is fragmented into millions of tiny particles, a certain amount of energy is stored on the newly created surfaces, which originally did not exist. Therefore, the finer a ceramic powder, the more energy is stored on its surfaces. Since changes in matter always occur in the direction of reducing Gibbs free energy, it is natural that a very fine powder tends to have its surface area reduced. Thermodynamically, this is the driving force for sintering to occur. However, when analyzing such a transformation considering the kinetic aspect, it appears that nothing occurs at room temperature due to the very low atomic mobility. It is necessary to increase the kinetic energy of atoms by providing thermal energy, which allows atomic diffusion in the solid state to occur. Thus, when heating a very fine compacted powder, the atoms have their mobility greatly increased and move, seeking to reduce the surface area. Particles that were initially only in contact bind chemically and the empty spaces between them gradually shrink, so that the solid–gas interfaces are gradually replaced by new solid–solid interfaces, forming grain boundaries [6,7,12]. These changes are outlined in Figure 10.5.

However, the idea that pores always shrink during sintering is wrong. In fact, in some situations, they can remain stable or even increase in size. For the purposes of this chapter, it is unnecessary to understand the reasons for this behavior, which are well described in the literature [6]. However, it is necessary to understand a key aspect: One of the factors that determine if a pore will increase or decrease in size is the number of particles that surround it, also known as coordination number, which essentially results from the combination between the pore size and the particle size. A small pore in relation to the average particle size will be surrounded by few of them, while a larger pore will have more particles around it. It happens that there is an equilibrium angle at the triple junction between the grain contour that was formed and the solid–gas surface, called dihedral angle.

As mass transport begins by diffusion in the solid state, the combination between dihedral angle and coordination number creates a curvature of the surface surrounding the pore. Figure 10.6 presents an example simplified by a flat representation, in which it is observed that: (i) For a pore with only three neighbors, the curvature will be concave in relation to the pore; (ii) in the hypothetical case of a 120° dihedral angle, the interface between the grains and the pore will be flat; and (iii) for a pore with eight neighbors, the surface will be convex.

It is important to note that the chemical potential of an atom at the surface of a solid is affected by its curvature, being greater on convex surfaces and less on concave surfaces. As a result, the solid gas interface always moves toward its center of curvature, whereas flat interfaces tend to be stable [6,7].

Based on this reasoning, to achieve maximum pore elimination during sintering, it is necessary that the ceramic powder has the best compaction possible. That is, the particles must fit in such a way that the empty spaces between them are minimal, generating small pores with few neighbors. As the compaction departs from this ideal condition, the compacted powder will have greater porosity and the pores will be larger, preventing them from being eliminated.

Another very important phenomenon occurs during sintering and microstructure formation, which is grain growth. Remember that Equation (10.1) refers to the solid–gas surface (γ_{SG}), indicating that the process occurs in the direction of densification. However, it can be modified to be applied at the solid–solid interface, referring to the new grain boundaries formed (γ_{GB}). For this reason, as the solid–gas interface decreases due to pore shrinkage, grain growth begins, driven by the tendency to reduce Gibbs free energy, now seeking to reduce the area of grain boundaries. Thus, thermodynamics teaches that the grain size cannot be reduced during sintering, which would imply an increase in the solid–solid interface [12].

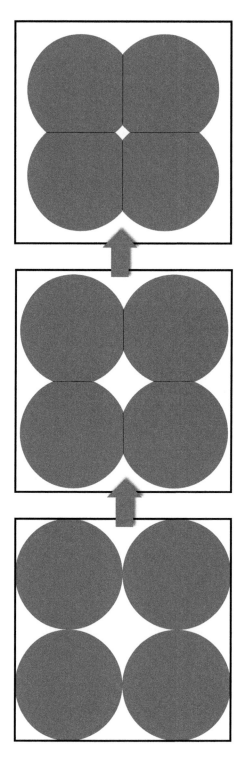

FIGURE 10.5 In a compacted powder, the particles just touch each other. As the sintering process begins, chemical bonds are formed at the points of contact between them and, gradually, this region extends, forming the grain boundaries. At the same time, the pore volume decreases, leading to a volumetric contraction of the piece, which in advanced ceramics normally exceeds 20%.

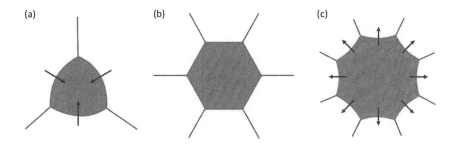

FIGURE 10.6   The curvature of the surface surrounding the pore determines how it moves, always toward the center of curvature. In this flat representation, the pore (gray) is surrounded by (a) three neighbors, shrinking; (b) three neighbors, being stable; (c) three neighbors, expanding.

Sintering is an extensive and complex issue, and there are still many aspects that are not yet fully understood. We did not address sintering with liquid phase formation, in which a small fraction of the material melts, wetting the particles and favoring densification. In addition, impurities present in the composition are often segregated to the particle surface, or to the grain boundary, which changes the interfacial energy and the dynamics of the process. Although these topics are strongly related to microstructure formation, consequently, to the properties of a ceramic body, they are not the focus of this chapter. For the reader interested in delving into these topics, there is extensive material in the literature [6,12,18].

10.4   CERAMIC FABRICATION PROCESSES

Given the above, it is observed that, although ceramic materials have properties that prevent the direct use of techniques widely used to manufacture plastic or metallic parts, the use of particulate raw materials makes such processes perfectly possible [13]. Thus, products as diverse as dishes, spark plugs, tiles, ceramic capacitors, refractories, sanitary ware, dental ceramics, and ceramic bearings for VADs are manufactured following essentially the same approach: The powdered raw material is compacted to the desired geometry and sintered to chemically bond particles, which reduce porosity and develop strength. However, for each product, there is an adequate shaping process (sometimes more than one), which depends on the type of raw material, the dimensions and shape of the final piece, and the ability to form a microstructure that favors the desired properties.

Bearings used in VAD must have high mechanical and wear resistance, in addition to being biocompatible. Biocompatibility is a property that depends more on the composition and crystalline structure than on the microstructure, being practically unaffected by the manufacturing process. Nevertheless, strength and wear resistance are typical properties of technical ceramics and can be strongly influenced by the microstructure.

Perhaps the most complete analysis of bearing wear in VADs, the work by Sundareswaran et al. analyzed the wear of 183 bearings used in left ventricular assist devices, after being explanted from patients with an average use time of 363 ± 349 days [19]. The results showed a very low wear rate (median bearing wear rate for patients supported for at least 1 year was $0.30\,\mu m$/year), sufficient to estimate a service life several times greater than the average survival time of patients. The material used to produce the VAD bearings studied was monocrystalline alumina, sometimes called jewel corundum, sapphire, or ruby, depending on the type of impurity present. Single crystals can be considered the ideal microstructure in this case, since they have no porosity and no grain boundaries, which are microstructural features usually related to mechanical properties degradation. However, the manufacture of single crystals cannot be carried out using the traditional powder compaction and sintering approach, but only through slow crystal growth processes, followed by tedious grinding and polishing with diamond tools, which greatly increases costs [20,21]. On the other hand, the very low wear rate verified in that work indicates that the use of polycrystalline ceramic bearings might be adequate and should be studied as an alternative to a more economical and faster manufacturing process. In fact, attempts to measure the wear of polycrystalline ceramic bearings have shown that it is very low [22]. In this case, the key is to obtain a microstructure that favors high strength and wear resistance.

Porosity is a microstructural characteristic that impairs both properties. In addition, the decrease in grain size benefits both properties [6,23]. Therefore, the microstructure of bearings used in VADs should ideally be free of porosity and have the minimum possible grain size. These characteristics lead us to two conclusions:

i. The raw material must consist of particles as small as possible, providing high specific surface area, which favors densification and can potentially result in a polycrystalline microstructure with small grain size.
ii. The particles must be compacted as efficiently as possible, so that the empty spaces between them are minimal, associated only with the small interstices located between the particles.

In this case, optimizing size distribution for improved particle packing is not an option to reduce porosity, although it is widely used in the manufacture of various ceramic products. This is because this approach involves the use of large particles, which accommodate smaller particles in their interstices and so on, significantly reducing the empty spaces in the compact (Figure 10.7a). Evidently, the resulting microstructure will present large grains, impairing the mechanical performance. Therefore, one must learn to work with very fine powders (typically, $D < 1.0\,\mu m$) with narrow particle size distribution.

As particle size decreases to the colloidal range, the specific surface area increases and favors densification during sintering. On the other hand, the larger surface area causes higher internal friction, hindering the movement of particles during the compaction process, which makes it difficult to achieve high relative density [24]. Furthermore, colloidal particles are mainly controlled by cohesive van der Waals forces, which favor agglomeration, as opposed to the good fluidity of granular particles, over which inertial forces (associated with their weight) predominate. Particle

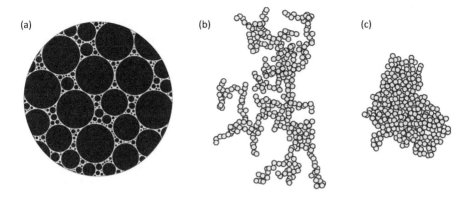

FIGURE 10.7   (a) Raw materials with wide particle size distribution can favor a high packing density, if designed so that smaller particles fill the interstices between the larger ones; (b) Monodispersed colloidal particles in which van der Waals forces predominate tend to form agglomerates with low packing density and large voids within the structure; (c) Monodispersed colloidal particles in which a strategy of opposing the van der Waals cohesive forces has been adopted can be well compacted, leaving only tiny (but numerous) interparticle pores with a low coordination number and good sinterability.

agglomerates are disordered, poorly compacted structures (Figure 10.7b) containing pores with high coordination number and they are generally not eliminated during sintering.

Therefore, to obtain a microstructure with minimal porosity and small grain size, it is necessary to use a manufacturing process capable of compacting colloidal ceramic particles (<1 μm), avoiding their natural tendency to agglomeration and providing green parts with as low a porosity as possible. For monodispersed spherical particles, the maximum compaction is around 0.63–0.65 of the particle density [25], which corresponds to a volumetric shrinkage of 35%–37% of a ceramic compact during sintering to full density. Even if the material is compacted as well as possible, some porosity usually persists after sintering, unless special sintering techniques are employed, such as hot isostatic pressing (HIP) or spark plasma sintering [26–28]. Such strategies are used for ceramic compounds that do not densify with conventional sintering (generally, ceramics with a predominance of covalent bonds, e.g., SiC, Si_3N_4, AlN), or when it is necessary to completely eliminate the porosity, which makes the ceramic transparent [29]. In the case of ceramic bearings for VAD, a dense microstructure (normally a porosity below 0.5% is well accepted in advanced ceramics) with a small grain size is the goal, not transparency. In fact, ceramic oxides whose properties could fulfill the requirements for VAD bearings, such as polycrystalline alumina and zirconia, can achieve very good mechanical properties under careful conventional processing conditions.

Ceramic manufacturing processes can be classified according to the mass consistency into dry compaction, plastic forming, and liquid forming, as discussed in Section 3.1.1 (Figure 10.4). Advanced ceramics have been produced by extrusion [16,30], but this technique has been used mainly when the part geometry has a regular cross section along one direction, such as honeycomb filters for catalysis [31], and when one dimension is much larger than the others, such as tubular parts [30,32]. Dry pressing has been widely used to produce advanced ceramics, although it requires careful preparation of ceramic powder, which involves granulation in a spray dryer, where organic additives are added to increase the plasticity of granules, guaranteeing their deformability during compaction. However, an intrinsic characteristic of this process is the formation of a compaction gradient in the green parts, which should be avoided in applications that require great reliability, as previously discussed [12,13].

Compaction gradients are more intense in pieces produced by uniaxial pressing. Cold isostatic pressing using flexible elastomeric molds immersed in oil can greatly reduce the compaction gradient but does not eliminate it. Considering that VAD bearings have small dimensions, this problem is not as serious as in larger parts, because the difference in porosity between the regions with maximum and minimum compaction is generally not large enough to put the process at risk. However, the porosity achieved by liquid forming processes tends to be less than that obtained by dry compaction, even in isostatic pressing. It may seem strange to the reader who is not familiar with ceramic processing that a powder compacted by isostatic pressing at 200 MPa has greater porosity than a compact obtained with the same powder by casting an aqueous suspension in a plaster mold, without any external pressure. But this is what is observed in practice, especially for ceramic powders with a high fraction of colloidal particles [33].

10.4.1 COLLOIDAL APPROACH

As part of 110th anniversary celebration, the American Ceramic Society elected the 11 best papers published in the *Journal of the American Ceramic Society* since 1898 [34]. Among these papers, only one was devoted to ceramic processing, whose title is *Powder Processing Science and Technology for Increased Reliability* [35]. In this paper, F. F. Lange recognizes the limitations of conventional processing techniques and launches the fundamentals of colloidal processing of ceramics. He establishes that the low reliability of technical ceramics, especially in terms of mechanical behavior, results from microstructural heterogeneities due to the inability of manufacturing processes to provide highly homogeneous compacts from colloidal ceramic powders. Among the main strength-limiting heterogeneities, organic or inorganic inclusions, hard aggregates formed by particles joined by strong bonds, and soft agglomerates formed by the action of van der Waals forces are highlighted.

In summary, the colloidal approach consists of preparing suspensions with colloidal ceramic powders in which, by controlling forces of either electrostatic or steric nature, a repulsive field is created between particles that exceeds the attractive van der Waals forces, inducing them to remain separated and suspended in a liquid medium [36]. This is called a colloidal dispersion. The most common approach for controlling the interaction between particles consists of manipulating the density of surface electrical charges (especially in aqueous media), either by simply adjusting the pH or by using anionic or cationic surfactants and polyelectrolytes, commonly called dispersants or deflocculants. Otherwise, in non-aqueous media, another approach usually works better, which consists of employing short to medium chain surfactants with the capacity to strongly adsorb onto the particles, while having high solubility in the liquid. This creates a steric barrier that prevents the colloidal particles from approaching, keeping the system dispersed. There is a vast literature describing in detail the mechanisms of dispersion of powders in liquids, including those for non-aqueous media [37–40].

In the dispersed state, inclusions and large aggregates can be removed by filtration, while agglomerates can be destroyed by inputting some mechanical energy through milling, sonication, and high shear mixing. Once separated, the strong repulsion between particles prevents them from agglomerating again. In this condition, the sedimentation rate of particles is very low, since it is proportional to the square of the particle diameter [41]. As the size of isolated particles is much smaller than that of agglomerates, the suspension is considered stable. Drying of the suspension for later use in ceramic processing should not be done, as it would reintroduce previously eliminated defects. Thus, obtaining green parts must be done by liquid forming processes.

One of the most striking effects associated with the balance between attractive and repulsive interparticle forces in a suspension is observed when it changes from the flocculated to the dispersed state: There is a drastic reduction in its apparent viscosity. This is because a flocculated suspension traps a large fraction of the liquid phase in the voids within particle agglomerates. When a repulsive field is created between particles, the structure breaks up and releases this water into the suspension, facilitating the flow of the particles. The effect is the same as adding water to a thick paste. Well-dispersed suspensions can therefore be prepared with a high solid concentration, approaching a practical limit where the particles are very close, separated by a thin layer of liquid. This condition is sufficient for particles having the mobility necessary to achieve liquid consistency, since they remain under strong repulsive interaction. Consequently, particles self-organize in a very compact pattern, minimizing the empty spaces between them, which explains the high packaging efficiency in powder compacts obtained through liquid forming processes.

The practical limit of concentration of solids in a suspension appears in the classic Krieger–Dougherty model [42], given by:

$$\eta_r = \left(1 - \frac{\phi}{\phi_{max}}\right)^{-[\eta]\phi_{max}} \tag{10.2}$$

where η_r is relative viscosity (ratio between the suspension and the liquid viscosities), ϕ_{max} is the maximum volume fraction, and $[\eta]$ is the intrinsic viscosity, which is expected to be 2.5 for spheres. ϕ_{max} varies a lot, as it is affected by particle shape, size distribution, dispersion, and shear rate, but can be experimentally estimated. A simulation considering a ϕ_{max} value of 0.63, which is a reasonable approach for monodispersed spherical particles [25], is shown in Figure 10.8 to highlight how the relative viscosity varies with the concentration of solids ϕ.

Notice that an increase in the solid volume fraction from 0.3 to 0.5 raises the relative viscosity from 2.8 to 12, while an increase from 0.59 to 0.61 raises it from 80 to 229. In fact, as the fraction of solids approaches the maximum value, the relative

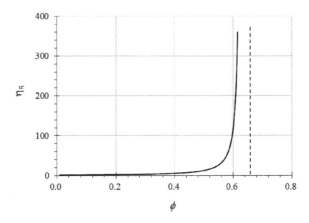

FIGURE 10.8 Effect of the volumetric fraction of solids in a suspension on the relative viscosity, according to the Krieger–Dougherty model, for maximum solid fraction of 0.63, as indicated by the dashed line [Ref. 42].

viscosity grows asymptotically to infinity, which can be associated with the loss of fluidity of the suspension. In the vicinity of ϕ_{max}, a small reduction in the water content due to evaporation, for example, may change the suspension to a stiff body. This behavior has been ingeniously applied in some liquid manufacturing processes, as discussed below.

Once stable suspensions of colloidal particles have been obtained, they can be used in a myriad of processes to manufacture ceramic parts [43,44], potentially generating polycrystalline microstructures containing small grains and very low porosity. In any case, the suspension must undergo some process capable of transforming it from a fluid to a solid stiff enough to be removed from the mold and subjected to drying and sintering. Such processes were classified by J. Lewis [40] into three categories: (i) fluid removal; (ii) particle flow, and (iii) gelation. The first two cases use exactly the approach discussed above, in which a small reduction in the amount of water in the suspension causes it to solidify, provided the solid concentration is close to its maximum value.

The first case includes slip casting, a process widely used to fabricate from sanitary ware to advanced ceramic pieces with complex shape [12,45]. This process consists of pouring the stable suspension into a plaster mold, whose porosity provides a capillary pressure that drains the water from the suspension, leading to the formation of a liquid saturated particle cake on the surface of the mold. In this case, the most fluid removal is accomplished by the capillary pressure. This process can be accelerated by applying pressure on the slip or vacuum under the mold surface, as the rate of cake formation is strongly reduced due to the low permeability of colloidal particle compacts [46]. Other processes based on fluid removal that have grown in industry include robocasting [40,47], which is a kind of 3-D printing of ceramics, and tape casting, which has been widely used to produce thin ceramic sheets [48]. In both cases, the ratio between the vaporization surface and the volume of the deposited layer is large, which favors a quick vaporization of the liquid phase, stiffening the material.

Consolidation through particle flow occurs in the presence of a field that induces particles in suspension to move in a given direction and be deposited on a surface. This field can be gravitational (sedimentation [49], centrifugation [50]) or electric (electrophoretic deposition), when the deposition of electrically charged particles occurs on an oppositely charged electrode [51,52]. Such processes can result in compacts with high packing density, but they still have not been adopted in industry, compared to other techniques.

The consolidation of colloidal dispersions has been achieved by another approach, generically called gelling, referring to the liquid to solid transition. However, the mechanisms involved can be completely different [40,44]. One of the first processes in this category was the gel casting [53], which is based on the polymerization of organic monomers dissolved in the liquid phase of the suspension. After careful preparation using the principles of colloidal processing, the suspension receives a small addition of a chemical initiator, before being transferred to a mold where the polymerization occurs. The monomers dissolved in the liquid phase must be of two types: one containing a single double bond and the other containing two double bonds. This leads to the in situ formation of a reticulated hydrogel in the liquid phase, which involves the dispersed particles and immobilizes them. The formation of the hydrogel drastically changes the consistency of the suspension, making it a rigid body within the mold, although all the water still remains in the system. Due to the cross-linking of the polymer chains, the material has good mechanical strength and, after drying, can even be machined before sintering [54].

An important advantage of the gel casting process is that it can be quickly implemented with minimal changes to conventional liquid ceramic manufacturing processes. Figure 10.9 presents a general flowchart with the main steps of colloidal

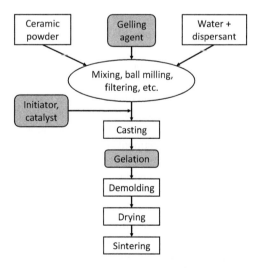

FIGURE 10.9 General flowchart of a conventional ceramic manufacturing process, showing the steps commonly used in colloidal processing (white boxes) and the addition of boxes highlighted in gray, showing the minor changes needed to adapt it to the gel casting process.

processing. The highlighted boxes show the components or modifications required to adapt the conventional route for the gel casting process.

Although there was initially some opposition to the wider use of this process due to the toxicity of the acrylamide-based monomers used, less toxic alternatives were quickly identified [55,56], breaking the initial resistance and enabling its use by industry. Other gelling systems have been investigated, such as agarose [57], alginate [58], gelatin [59], and egg white [60], all being generically called gel casting process, since they are based on the change in suspension consistency due to gelation.

10.4.2 MANUFACTURING PROCESSES FOR VAD BEARINGS

The geometry of bearings for VADs can be specific to each project, but, in general, they are simple parts and with small dimensions. Thus, the manufacture of such parts could be done by cold isostatic pressing, since there should be no problems associated with the compaction gradient, as discussed earlier. However, colloidal processing has the potential to generate results far superior to those obtained by dry compaction. Thus, processes such as slip casting and gel casting can be used to manufacture bearings for VAD with good results in terms of microstructure, provided that the precautions inherent to the colloidal processing previously discussed are used, in addition to raw materials with high purity, narrow size distribution, and high specific surface area.

In both cases, split molds facilitate the extraction of the compact, avoiding damage to the piece, especially for those obtained by slip casting, since they have much lower green strength than those obtained by gel casting.

Additionally, the surface finish of the mold should be the best possible, so that the green part is already produced with a good finish, minimizing the need for adjustments and facilitating polishing after sintering.

A fundamental characteristic for the good performance of the part is its surface finishing, which must be the best possible. Post-sintering operations can be done to adjust the dimensions of the part and improve the surface finish. However, machining operations on sintered parts are slow and expensive. Very hard ceramics, such as those used in VAD bearings, must be machined using diamond tools [12]. Ideally, the dimensional control in the manufacturing process should be good enough so that only fine abrasives are used in the final machining to obtain close tolerances and smooth surface finishes. Particularly in the case of the gel casting process, the good green strength allows small adjustments to be made easily by green machining, ensuring greater dimensional reproducibility of the parts [54]. Sometimes, a blank part is pre-sintered to develop some resistance and machined to the desired shape before final sintering [61]. This approach has been used in dentistry associated with CAD-CAM systems, and the shrinkage of the part in the final sintering must be considered when designing the part to be machined [62].

Post-machining procedures are applied to obtain further improvements in properties and to achieve the required surface finish for VAD bearings. The most common of these is lapping, which involves the use of very fine abrasive particles in a paste and is applied to the piece with felt or fabric. To obtain significant improvements, a polishing sequence must be adopted using abrasives with successively smaller grit sizes. For some structural applications, polishing to 1 μm grit diamond pastes may be sufficient. But for applications that involve wear resistance, such as, seals and VAD bearings, the use of finer grit, on a nanoscale, is necessary [12].

Tribological performance can be improved by depositing a high-strength film on the bearing surface. Diamond-like carbon (DLC) has been widely used for this purpose in several biomedical applications [63], as it provides a surface with low friction coefficient and high wear resistance and it is a biocompatible material [64], even when tested specifically in contact with blood, which is particularly important for VAD applications [65]. However, there are still few studies addressing long-term testing of DLC-coated bearings for VAD.

10.4.3 SUMMARY AND CONCLUDING REMARKS

Throughout its development, the VAD design evolved from pulsatile pumps to centrifugal pumps, which have the shaft and bearing as key parts for smooth operation and durability in an environment that involves direct contact with the patient's blood. Ceramic materials have a set of properties that make them the natural choice for the manufacture of these components, which require high reliability, mechanical performance, and biocompatibility. Polycrystalline ceramic bearings can meet the requirements for application in VAD bearings, provided they are produced with microstructures capable of enhancing the necessary properties, such as high hardness and low friction coefficient, which lead to high wear resistance, in addition to high mechanical resistance and biocompatibility. Some of these properties can be enhanced through careful control of the ceramic microstructure, mainly involving small grain size and minimal porosity. These characteristics are mainly developed during sintering, evolving from characteristics of the ceramic powder compact that are closely linked to the manufacturing process. The colloidal processing of ceramic materials proposes a set of care and procedures that allow obtaining ceramic compacts with high packing density and microstructural homogeneity using raw materials with submicrometric particle size and high specific surface area. Thereafter, it favors obtaining microstructures that result in superior properties, resulting in greater reliability. The principles involved in colloidal processing can be applied in various liquid forming processes for ceramic materials, such as slip casting and gel casting, which are widely used in the manufacture of several types of advanced ceramics. In addition to the microstructure, the surface finish is of fundamental importance for the performance of bearings for VAD and must be obtained through careful polishing. The coating of the surface with films that provide improved tribological performance and biocompatibility is a well-established procedure and is a promising alternative, but still lacks more testing to investigate possible local and systemic effects.

The advancement of ceramic bearing technology for VAD involves the application of a robust methodology of testing and the development of equipment and techniques so that polycrystalline parts with different compositions, such as Al_2O_3, ZrO_2, $MgAl_2O_4$, and SiC, obtained through different processing routes, applying the principles of colloidal processing, having a polished surface and/or coated with wear-resistant films, can be tested and evaluated, both *in vitro* and *in vivo*.

REFERENCES

1. M. Hosseinipour, R. Gupta, M. Bonnell, and M. Elahinia, "Rotary mechanical circulatory support systems," arXiv, September 24, 2017. doi: 10.1177/2055668317725994.
2. T. Michael. *Maul, Mechanical Blood Trauma in Circulatory-Assist Devices.* Momentum Press: New York, 2015.
3. N. Moazami et al., "Axial and centrifugal continuous-flow rotary pumps: A translation from pump mechanics to clinical practice," *Journal of Heart and Lung Transplantation*, vol. 32, no. 1, pp. 1–11, 2013. doi: 10.1016/j.healun.2012.10.001.
4. D. L. Joyce and L. D. Joyce, *Mechanical Circulatory Support.* Oxford University Press: Oxford, 2019.
5. J. M. Stulak et al., "Adverse events in contemporary continuous-flow left ventricular assist devices: A multi-institutional comparison shows significant differences," *Journal of Thoracic and Cardiovascular Surgery*, 151, no. 1, pp. 177–189, 2016. doi: 10.1016/j.jtcvs.2015.09.100.
6. M. W. Barsoum, *Fundamentals of Ceramics.* CRC Press: Boca Raton, FL, 2019.
7. C. B. Carter and M. G. Norton, *Ceramic Materials.* Springer: New York, 2013.
8. J. F. Shackelford and R. H. Doremus, *Ceramic and Glass Materials: Structure, Properties and Processing.* Springer: New York, 2008.
9. R. C. Garvie, R. H. Hannink, and R. T. Pascoe, "Ceramic steel?" *Nature*, vol. 258, no. 5537, 1975. doi: 10.1038/258703a0.
10. K.-J. Hwang, M. Shin, M.-H. Lee, H. Lee, M. Y. Oh, and T. H. Shin, "Investigation on the phase stability of Yttria-stabilized zirconia electrolytes for high-temperature electrochemical application," *Ceramics International*, vol. 45, no. 7, 2019. doi: 10.1016/j.ceramint.2018.09.026.
11. P. Palmero, L. Montanaro, H. Reveron, and J. Chevalier, "Surface coating of oxide powders: A new synthesis method to process biomedical grade nano-composites," *Materials*, vol. 7, no. 7, 5012–5037, 2014. doi: 10.3390/ma7075012.
12. D. W. Richerson and W. E. Lee, *Modern Ceramic Engineering.* CRC Press: Boca Raton, FL, 2018.
13. T. Chartier, "Ceramic forming processes," in P. Boch and J.-C. Niepce (eds), *Ceramic Materials.* ISTE: London, UK, pp. 123–197, 2007.
14. R. B. Heimann and M. Maggetti, *Ancient and Historical Ceramics: Materials, Technology, Art, and Culinary Traditions.* E. Schweizerbart'sche Verlagsbuchhandlung: Stuttgart, 2014.
15. W. Zheng, T. Cui, H. Li, and Y. Yang, "Novel dry-suspension granulation process for preparing pressed powders of ceramic tiles," *Powder Technology*, vol. 377, 2021. doi: 10.1016/j.powtec.2020.09.003.
16. F. A. Mesquita and M. R. Morelli, "Plastic forming of Al_2O_3 ceramic substrates," *Journal of Materials Processing Technology*, vol. 143–144, 2003. doi: 10.1016/S0924-0136(03)00293-0.
17. W. M. Sigmund, N. S. Bell, and L. Bergström, "Novel powder-processing methods for advanced ceramics," *Journal of the American Ceramic Society*, vol. 83, no. 7, 2004. doi: 10.1111/j.1151-2916.2000.tb01432.x.
18. M. N. Rahaman, *Ceramic Processing and Sintering.* CRC Press: Boca Raton, FL, 2017.
19. K. S. Sundareswaran, S. H. Reichenbach, K. B. Masterson, K. C. Butler, and D. J. Farrar, "Low bearing wear in explanted HeartMate II left ventricular assist devices after chronic clinical support," *ASAIO Journal*, vol. 59, no. 1, pp. 41–45, 2013. doi: 10.1097/MAT.0b013e3182768cfb.
20. V. Pishchik, L. A. Lytvynov, and E. R. Dobrovinskaya, *Sapphire.* Springer US: Boston, MA, 2009.

21. M. S. Akselrod and F. J. Bruni, "Modern trends in crystal growth and new applications of sapphire," *Journal of Crystal Growth*, vol. 360, 2012. doi: 10.1016/j.jcrysgro.2011.12.038.
22. E. Bock et al., "New centrifugal blood pump with dual impeller and double pivot bearing system: Wear evaluation in bearing system, performance tests, and preliminary hemolysis tests," *Artificial Organs*, vol. 32, no. 4, pp. 329–333, 2008. doi: 10.1111/j.1525-1594.2008.00550.x.
23. D. H. Buckley and K. Miyoshi, "Friction and wear of ceramics," 1984.
24. K. Kendall, "Influence of powder structure on processing and properties of advanced ceramics," *Powder Technology*, vol. 58, no. 3, 1989. doi: 10.1016/0032-5910(89)80109-3.
25. V. Baranau and U. Tallarek, "Random-close packing limits for monodisperse and polydisperse hard spheres," *Soft Matter*, vol. 10, no. 21, pp. 3826–3841, 2014. doi: 10.1039/c3sm52959b.
26. M. H. Bocanegra-Bernal, C. Domínguez-Rios, A. Garcia-Reyes, A. Aguilar-Elguezabal, J. Echeberria, and A. Nevarez-Rascon, "Hot isostatic pressing (HIP) of α-Al_2O_3 submicron ceramics pressureless sintered at different temperatures: Improvement in mechanical properties for use in total hip arthroplasty (THA)," *International Journal of Refractory Metals and Hard Materials*, vol. 27, no. 5, 2009. doi: 10.1016/j.ijrmhm.2009.05.004.
27. H. Mingsheng, L. Jianbao, L. Hong, G. Gangfeng, and L. Long, "Fabrication of transparent polycrystalline Yttria ceramics by combination of SPS and HIP," *Journal of Rare Earths*, vol. 24, no. 1, 2006. doi: 10.1016/S1002-0721(07)60365-2.
28. V. Nečina and W. Pabst, "Influence of the heating rate on grain size of alumina ceramics prepared via spark plasma sintering (SPS)," *Journal of the European Ceramic Society*, vol. 40, no. 10, 2020. doi: 10.1016/j.jeurceramsoc.2020.03.057.
29. Z. Xiao et al., "Materials development and potential applications of transparent ceramics: A review," *Materials Science and Engineering: R: Reports*, vol. 139, 2020. doi: 10.1016/j.mser.2019.100518.
30. F. Händle, Ed., *Extrusion in Ceramics*. Springer: Berlin, Heidelberg, 2007.
31. S. Hosseini, H. Moghaddas, S. Masoudi Soltani, and S. Kheawhom, "Technological applications of honeycomb monoliths in environmental processes: A review," *Process Safety and Environmental Protection*, vol. 133, 2020. doi: 10.1016/j.psep.2019.11.020.
32. D. Liang, J. Huang, H. Zhang, H. Fu, Y. Zhang, and H. Chen, "Influencing factors on the performance of tubular ceramic membrane supports prepared by extrusion," *Ceramics International*, 2020. doi: 10.1016/j.ceramint.2020.12.235.
33. F. S. Ortega, R. G. Pileggi, P. Sepulveda, and V. C. Pandolfelli, "Optimizing particle packing in powder consolidation," *American Ceramic Society Bulletin*, vol. 78, no. 8, pp. 106–111, 1999.
34. https://ceramics.org/publications-resources/journals/11-best-papers.
35. F. F. Lange, "Powder processing science and technology for increased reliability," *Journal of the American Ceramic Society*, vol. 72, no. 1, 1989. doi: 10.1111/j.1151-2916.1989.tb05945.x.
36. P. C. Hiemenz and R. Rajagopalan, Eds., *Principles of Colloid and Surface Chemistry*, Revised and Expanded. CRC Press: Boca Raton, FL, 2016.
37. T. F. Tadros, Ed., *Colloid Stability*. Wiley-VCH Verlag GmbH & Co. KGaA: Weinheim, Germany, 2010.
38. Ł. Zych, R. Lach, and A. Wajler, "The influence of the agglomeration state of nanometric $MgAl_2O_4$ powders on their consolidation and sintering," *Ceramics International*, vol. 40, no. 7, 2014. doi: 10.1016/j.ceramint.2014.02.066.
39. J. Cesarano, I. A. Aksay, and A. Bleier, "Stability of aqueous alpha-Al_2O_3 suspensions with poly(methacrylic acid) polyelectrolyte," *Journal of the American Ceramic Society*, vol. 71, no. 4, 1988. doi: 10.1111/j.1151-2916.1988.tb05855.x.

40. J. A. Lewis, "Colloidal processing of ceramics," *Journal of the American Ceramic Society*, vol. 83, no. 10, 2004. doi: 10.1111/j.1151-2916.2000.tb01560.x.

41. R. Buscall, "The sedimentation of concentrated colloidal suspensions," *Colloids and Surfaces*, vol. 43, no. 1, 1990. doi: 10.1016/0166-6622(90)80002-L.

42. I. M. Krieger and T. J. Dougherty, "A mechanism for non-newtonian flow in suspensions of rigid spheres," *Transactions of the Society of Rheology*, vol. 3, no. 1, 1959. doi: 10.1122/1.548848.

43. J. Yu, J. Yang, and Y. Huang, "The transformation mechanism from suspension to green body and the development of colloidal forming," *Ceramics International*, vol. 37, no. 5, 2011. doi: 10.1016/j.ceramint.2011.01.019.

44. W. M. Sigmund, N. S. Bell, and L. Bergström, "Novel powder-processing methods for advanced ceramics," *Journal of the American Ceramic Society*, vol. 83, no. 7, 2004. doi: 10.1111/j.1151-2916.2000.tb01432.x.

45. A. G. Dobrovolskiy, "Development of slip moulding methods," *Ceramurgia International*, vol. 3, no. 4, 1977. doi: 10.1016/0390-5519(77)90063-1.

46. D. S. Adcock and I. C. McDowall, "The mechanism of filter pressing and slip casting," *Journal of the American Ceramic Society*, vol. 40, no. 10, 1957. doi: 10.1111/j.1151-2916.1957.tb12552.x.

47. J. A. Lewis, "Direct ink writing of 3D functional materials," *Advanced Functional Materials*, vol. 16, no. 17, 2006. doi: 10.1002/adfm.200600434.

48. M. Jabbari, R. Bulatova, A. I. Y. Tok, C. R. H. Bahl, E. Mitsoulis, and J. H. Hattel, "Ceramic tape casting: A review of current methods and trends with emphasis on rheological behaviour and flow analysis," *Materials Science and Engineering: B*, vol. 212, 2016. doi: 10.1016/j.mseb.2016.07.011.

49. R. Buscall, "The sedimentation of concentrated colloidal suspensions," *Colloids and Surfaces*, vol. 43, no. 1, 1990. doi: 10.1016/0166-6622(90)80002-L.

50. X. Xu and H. Cölfen, "Ultracentrifugation techniques for the ordering of nanoparticles," *Nanomaterials*, vol. 11, no. 2, 2021. doi: 10.3390/nano11020333.

51. L. Besra and M. Liu, "A review on fundamentals and applications of electrophoretic deposition (EPD)," *Progress in Materials Science*, vol. 52, no. 1, 2007. doi: 10.1016/j.pmatsci.2006.07.001.

52. S. Yamaguchi and T. Yao, "Development of bioactive alumina-wollastonite composite by electrophoretic deposition," 2005.

53. A. C. Young, O. O. Omatete, M. A. Janney, and P. A. Menchhofer, "Gelcasting of alumina," *Journal of the American Ceramic Society*, vol. 74, no. 3, 1991. doi: 10.1111/j.1151-2916.1991.tb04068.x.

54. A. M. Riviello and F. dos S. Ortega, "Effect of gel chemistry on the machinability of green SiC parts produced by gelcasting," *Materials Science Forum*, vol. 727–728, 2012. doi: 10.4028/www.scientific.net/MSF.727-728.1596.

55. F. S. Ortega, P. Sepulveda, and V. C. Pandolfelli, "Monomer systems for the gelcasting of foams," *Journal of the European Ceramic Society*, vol. 22, no. 9–10, 2002. doi: 10.1016/S0955-2219(01)00486-1.

56. M. A. Janney, O. O. Omatete, C. A. Walls, S. D. Nunn, R. J. Ogle, and G. Westmoreland, "Development of low-toxicity gelcasting systems," *Journal of the American Ceramic Society*, vol. 81, no. 3, 2005. doi: 10.1111/j.1151-2916.1998.tb02377.x.

57. E. Adolfsson, "Gelcasting of zirconia using agarose," *Journal of the American Ceramic Society*, vol. 89, no. 6, 2006. doi: 10.1111/j.1551-2916.2006.01040.x.

58. H. Akhondi, E. Taheri-Nassaj, H. Sarpoolaky, and A. Taavoni-Gilan, "Gelcasting of alumina nanopowders based on gelation of sodium alginate," *Ceramics International*, vol. 35, no. 3, 2009. doi: 10.1016/j.ceramint.2008.04.023.

59. F. S. Ortega, F. A. O. Valenzuela, C. H. Scuracchio, and V. C. Pandolfelli, "Alternative gelling agents for the gelcasting of ceramic foams," *Journal of the European Ceramic Society*, vol. 23, no. 1, 2003. doi: 10.1016/S0955-2219(02)00075-4.

60. X. Liu, K. Li, C. Wu, Y. Zhou, and C. Pei, "Egg white-assisted preparation of inorganic functional materials: A sustainable, eco-friendly, low-cost and multifunctional method," *Ceramics International*, vol. 45, no. 18, 2019. doi: 10.1016/j.ceramint.2019.08.152.

61. J.-Z. Li, T. Wu, Z.-Y. Yu, L. Zhang, G.-Q. Chen, and D.-M. Guo, "Micro machining of pre-sintered ceramic green body," *Journal of Materials Processing Technology*, vol. 212, no. 3, 2012. doi: 10.1016/j.jmatprotec.2011.10.030.

62. N. F. Amat, A. Muchtar, H. Z. Yew, M. S. Amril, and R. L. Muhamud, "Machinability of a newly developed pre-sintered zirconia block for dental crown applications," *Materials Letters*, vol. 261, 2020. doi: 10.1016/j.matlet.2019.126996.

63. G. Dearnaley and J. H. Arps, "Biomedical applications of diamond-like carbon (DLC) coatings: A review," *Surface and Coatings Technology*, vol. 200, no. 7, 2005. doi: 10.1016/j.surfcoat.2005.07.077.

64. L. Mattei, F. di Puccio, B. Piccigallo, and E. Ciulli, "Lubrication and wear modelling of artificial hip joints: A review," *Tribology International*, vol. 44, no. 5, 2011. doi: 10.1016/j.triboint.2010.06.010.

65. M. Fedel, A. Motta, D. Maniglio, and C. Migliaresi, "Surface properties and blood compatibility of commercially available diamond-like carbon coatings for cardiovascular devices," *Journal of Biomedical Materials Research Part B: Applied Biomaterials*, vol. 90B, no. 1, 2008. doi: 10.1002/jbm.b.31291.

11 Tribology in Ceramic Biomaterials

Rodrigo Lima Stoeterau
Polytechnic School of the University of São Paulo

CONTENTS

Ceramic materials, as discussed in the previous chapter, show excellent results in mechanical applications that require high wear resistance. If they were not fragile to impact and prone to formation of fragile cracks, the ceramic materials would already be the majority of applications that involve contact of moving parts (Xiao et al. 2020).

An important property for its use as a biomaterial is its relative chemical inertia, which is, most of the time, associated with biocompatibility as they are normally used in hip prosthesis, to replace the femur and acetabulum (Araki et al. 2017; Florentino et al. 2019).

Its use in orthopedics is not only common, but also promising in cases of joints, since it can solve a problem of difficult solution, the replacement of living cartilaginous tissue. The moving parts can be replaced by ceramic implants with excellent performance, low wear, and relatively long life cycle (Laang et al. 2016).

Thus, the science that studies friction and develops materials and technologies that make it possible to improve the mechanical performance of these parts that are in constant contact is tribology. The first analysis that can be performed is the study of the dynamics involved in the system (Miranda and Faria 2014).

After massive use by the orthopedic medical community, the cardiology discovered the importance of tribology to develop better stents and vascular grafts, heart valves, and ventricular assist devices (VADs) (Bock et al. 2005; Neto et al. 2020). With ceramic pivot bearings, the miniaturization of blood pumps, the emergence of axial pumps and centrifugal pumps, and the important paradigm shift in assistance by non-pulsatile pumps were possible. Xie et al. (2015) presented a very interesting review of the entire history of bio-tribology in cardiovascular devices.

In this chapter, we will present design strategies and methodologies to develop pivot bearings for VADs, from the elementary concepts of contact mechanics to experimental setup and controlling of the process and materials evaluated (Yamane et al. 2008; Sundareswaran et al. 2013).

DOI: 10.1201/9781003138358-13

11.1   CONCERNS REGARDING CONTACT BEARING DESIGN FOR USE IN VADs

Among the various design requirements associated with a VADs design, many have a strong dependence on the types of pivot bearings that will be used to support the rotor, Figure 11.1.

Despite the existence of several bearing options for use in engineering, VAD design requirements limit the choices to three basic types: (a) rolling element bearings; (b) contact bearings; and (c) magnetic bearings, as shown in Figure 11.2.

11.2   THE CONTACT BEARING DESIGN

Contact bearings, also called jewelry bearings or pivoted bearings, exhibit a rare combination of unique design characteristics that make them attractive for several applications, and their main advantages and disadvantages are shown in Table 11.1 (Figure 11.3).

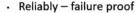

- Reliably – failure proof
- Biocompatibility
- Life (performance over time)
- Bearings low friction
- Vibration free
- Hemolysis proof
- Debris proof
- Dynamically controllable
- Low complexity

FIGURE 11.1   Main requirements associated with the VAD project.

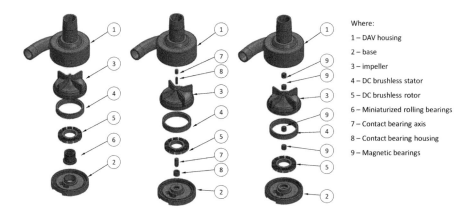

Where:
1 – DAV housing
2 – base
3 – impeller
4 – DC brushless stator
5 – DC brushless rotor
6 – Miniaturized rolling bearings
7 – Contact bearing axis
8 – Contact bearing housing
9 – Magnetic bearings

FIGURE 11.2   Sectional view showing the detail of a VAD rotor supported by contact bearings.

TABLE 11.1

Main Advantages and Disadvantages Associated with Contact Bearings

Main Advantages	Main Disadvantages
• Low friction	• Low load capacity
• Ability to operate in harsh environments	• Assembly clearance sensitivity
• Rigid	• Sensitivity to impacts
• Accurate	
• Miniaturized	
• Long life	
• Oscillating movements	

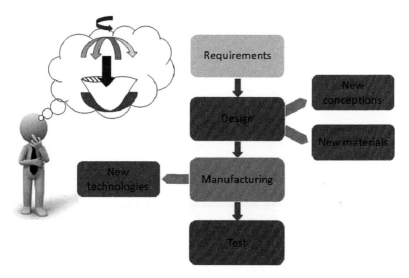

FIGURE 11.3 Process of developing contact bearings.

The operation principle of the soft contact is based on the nature of the Hertz contact. The Hertz contact theory is a classic theory of contact mechanics; although the derivation of the theory is relatively difficult, the final solution is a set of simple analytical equations that relate the geometry of bodies in contact with the loads, material properties of the bodies, and surface features in the contact region. The Hertz contact theory is derived from the analytical solution of the elasticity theory equations under the mid-space approach. According to this approach, the surfaces in contact are infinitely large half-spaces, and the pressure profile assumes that the shape of the bodies in contact can be approximated in the form of parabolas, spheres, ellipses, or cylinders. The simplifying hypotheses arising from the classical theory of elasticity apply; these consider small elastic or elastic-plastic deformation in the contact region, and homogeneous material (Popov 2010; Johnson 1987; Timoshenko and Goodier 1971) (Table 11.2).

TABLE 11.2

(a) Hertz Contact Ratio for Point Contacts and (b) Hertz Contact Ratio for Linear Contacts

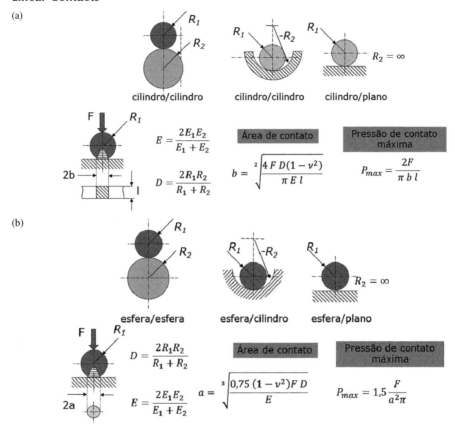

(a)

cilindro/cilindro   cilindro/cilindro   cilindro/plano

$$E = \frac{2E_1 E_2}{E_1 + E_2}$$

$$D = \frac{2R_1 R_2}{R_1 + R_2}$$

Área de contato

$$b = \sqrt[2]{\frac{4\,F\,D(1 - v^2)}{\pi\,E\,l}}$$

Pressão de contato máxima

$$P_{max} = \frac{2F}{\pi\,b\,l}$$

(b)

esfera/esfera   esfera/cilindro   esfera/plano

$$D = \frac{2R_1 R_2}{R_1 + R_2}$$

$$E = \frac{2E_1 E_2}{E_1 + E_2}$$

Área de contato

$$a = \sqrt[3]{\frac{0{,}75\,(1 - v^2)F\,D}{E}}$$

Pressão de contato máxima

$$P_{max} = 1{,}5\frac{F}{a^2 \pi}$$

Table 11.3 shows the finite element analysis for the Hertzian contact between the axis and the base of a contact bearing used in a VAD. The results in (a) are for a tribological pair with ANSI 1045 steel shaft and 6061 T6 aluminum alloy base, whereas the results in (b) show the contact for a 90% alumina shaft against a polymer base high density (peek); both simulations were performed for the same input conditions.

Confronting the results, it is possible to observe that the choice of the tribological pair is important for the proper performance of the bearing. The use of a pair of materials with a remarkably high hardness ratio, case (b), causes deformation to be concentrated on a single element, increasing the contact area, resulting in an increase in the resistive torque frictional forces.

The selection of a tribological pair with a hardness ratio closer to one improves the distribution of contact deformations, reducing the resistive torque. The need for a device that allows the adjustment of the contact pressure is recommended to guarantee the perfect functioning.

TABLE 11.3

Effect of the Choice of the Tribological Pair on Contact Deformations

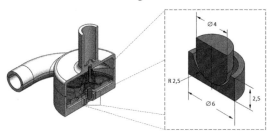

Axis - ANSI 1045		Axis - 90% Al2O3	
Tensile strength, ultimate:	585 MPa	Tensile strength, ultimate:	221 MPa
Modulus of elasticity:	206 GPa	Modulus of elasticity:	276 GPa
Hardness, Brinell:	170	Hardness, Brinell:	705
Hardness, Vickers:	174.76	Hardness, Vickers:	926.67
Base - Al 6061 T6		**Base - PEEK**	
Tensile strength, ultimate:	310 MPa	Tensile strength:	96,5 MPa
Modulus of elasticity:	68.9 GPa	Modulus of elasticity:	6.48 GPa
Hardness, Brinell:	95	Hardness, Vickers:	745
Hardness, Vickers:	106	Hardness, Shore D:	85

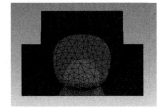 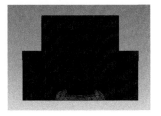

An important point regarding the use of contact bearings in VADs is associated with the manufacture of their constituent elements. Dimensional tolerances are not a critical point, associated with the design and manufacture of contact bearings for VADs; however, special care must be taken with respect to geometric tolerances and surface finishing. Precision manufacturing processes are recommended to achieve the tolerances and finish necessary for the good performance of this type of bearings. It is recommended that the finishing by fine removal processes, such as polishing, be employed to guarantee the surface finish and the removal of the geometric imperfections resulting from the other employed processes.

Table 11.4a and b shows the results of analyses of the upper and lower axes and their respective bases, showing the geometric profile and the characteristics of the surfaces (Johnson, 1987). All parts in this case were manufactured by conventional processes, without fine finishing processes.

The analysis of Table 11.4b clearly shows the geometric errors of manufacture; the presence of bumps in the center of the semi-spherical caps of the bases is a fact of instability for the operation of the resulting bearings. The hubcaps tend to collapse

TABLE 11.4

(a) Geometrical and Surface Analysis of Contact Bearing Shafts Used in VADs and (b) Geometrical and Surface Analysis of a Contact Bearing Base Used in VADs

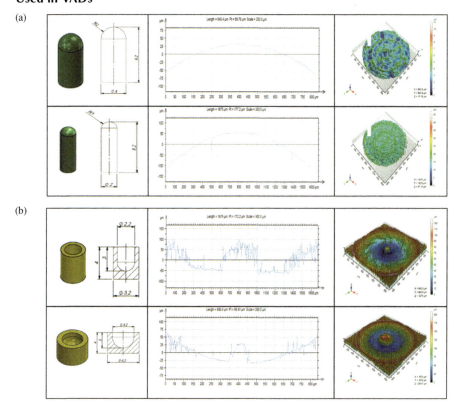

during use, generating debris that can be released into the bloodstream, or generate localized wear, which will result in a clearance in the rotor that can lead to loss of pumping efficiency, and even the collapse of the entire system. System by locking the rotor. The analysis of the optical profilometry of the central area of the spherical tip of the alumina shaft 90% of a counting bearing used in a VAD shows the periodic surface undulations from the manufacturing process, as well as imperfections in the central region. These observations reinforce the need to proceed with fine finishing operations to maximize the performance of the bearings, as this will be the contact region during the operation (Figure 11.4).

Imposing geometric errors at the base and axis and performing simulations using the finite element method are shown in Table 11.5. This allows us to observe that the presence of a projection in the center of the base (a) alters the contact condition and the intensity in the fields of deformation and stress when compared to the ideal contact condition presented in Table 11.4a. The presence of sphericity errors at the shaft

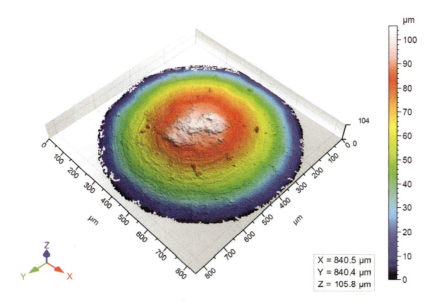

FIGURE 11.4 Optical profilometry of the central area of the spherical end of the bearing shaft.

TABLE 11.5

Simulation Imposing Geometric Errors on the Base and on the Axis of Contact Bearings

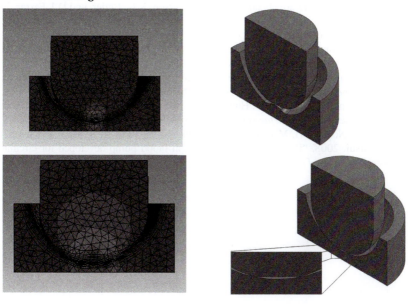

end changes the shape of the contact from point to linear, which results in an increase in resistive torque resulting from increased frictional forces, greater wear, and all the consequences associated with this.

Contact bearing is still one of the best and reliable options to support VAD rotors, but special attention must be concerned with material selection and manufacturing.

REFERENCES

Araki, S.Y., R.L. Stoeterau, P.C.F. Da Silva, M.A. Saito, J.R.C. De Sousa Sobrinho, A.L. Marques, D.F. De Sousa, E.G.P. Bock, and A.C.F. De Arruda. 2017. "Microstructure and tribology regarding precision studies of micro-sintered ceramic bearings for ventricular assist devices." *In Proceedings of the* 17th *EUSPEN 2017*, Hannover, Germany.

Bock, E.G.P., A.J.P. de Andrade, E.A.E. Wada, J.W.G. da Fonseca, J. Leme, D.E.C. Nicolosi, J.F. Biscegli. 2005. "A new concept of centrifugal blood pump using pivot bearing system: The conversion of the spiral pump inlet port." *Technology Meets Surgery International, São Paulo*, 4p, no. 1998: 2–5.

Florentino, P.C, S.Y. Araki, I.K. Fujita, A.A. Graciano, A.L. Marques Jr, and E.G.P. Bock. 2019. "Estudo da tribologia dos materiais bioinertes em aplicações ortopédicas e bombas de sangue." *The Academic Society Journal* 3(9): 261–268.

Johnson, K.L. 1987. *Contact Mechanics.* Cambridge University Press: Cambridge.

Laang, S.H., H.K. Tung, M.K. Lai, M. Husnain, and M. Ashraf. 2016. "Design of linear tribological wear tester." *Mechanical System Design* 1: 10.

Miranda, W.M., and M.T.C. Faria. 2014. "Finite element method applied to the eigenvalue analysis of flexible rotors supported by journal bearings." *Engineering* 6(3): 127–137.

Neto, S.S., J.R.C. Sousa Sobrinho, C. da Costa, T.F. Leão, S.A.M.M. Senra, E.G.P. Bock, G.A. Santos, et al. 2020. "Investigation of MEMS as accelerometer sensor in an implantable centrifugal blood pump prototype." *Journal of the Brazilian Society of Mechanical Sciences and Engineering* 42(9): 1–10.

Popov, V.L. 2010. *Contact Mechanics and Friction.* Springer: Berlin, Germany.

Sundareswaran, K.S., S.H. Reichenbach, K.B. Masterson, K.C. Butler, and D.J. Farrar. 2013. "Low bearing wear in explanted HeartMate II left ventricular assist devices after chronic clinical support." *ASAIO Journal* 59(1): 41–45.

Timoshenko, S.P., and J.N. Goodier. 1971. *Theory of Elasticity,* McGraw-Hill: New York.

Xiao, Z., S. Yu, S. Li, S. Ruan, L.B. Kong, Q. Huang, Z. Huang, et al. 2020. "Materials development and potential applications of transparent ceramics: A review." *Materials Science and Engineering R: Reports* 139: 100518.

Xie, D., Y.X. Leng, F.J. Jing, and N. Huang. 2015. "A brief review of bio-tribology in cardiovascular devices." *Biosurface and Biotribology* 1(4): 249–262.

Yamane, T., K. Nonaka, H. Miyoshi, O. Maruyama, M. Nishida, R. Kosaka, Y. Sankai, and T. Tsutsui. 2008. "Pivot wear of a centrifugal blood pump developed for circulatory assist." *Journal of Artificial Organs* 11(4): 232–237.

12 Surface Engineering of Biomaterials by Plasma Electrolytic Oxidation

César A. Antônio
FATEC – SO

Rosana F. Antônio
Centro Universitário FACENS

Elidiane C. Rangel and Nilson C. Cruz
São Paulo State University

CONTENTS

12.1 INTRODUCTION

In many situations, the performance of a given material in a biological environment is determined by the characteristics of its surface. In the human body, a material, along with being able to cause toxic effects and inflammatory reactions, may be subject to degradation by biological fluids. In particular, in the case of metallic biomaterials, corrosion products are generally salts of the metal, which, when in the extracellular environment, can be harmful to tissues, causing inflammation and subsequent tissue necrosis (Evans et al. 1974). Consequently, in addition to biocompatibility, chemical resistance is also a fundamental property for an artificial material to be well accepted by the organism. In this sense, biomaterials must have a set of physical, chemical, and biological properties in order to stimulate adequate responses from host tissues.

Depending on the nature of the interaction with living tissues, materials can be classified as bioinerts, when they do not induce any local response of the immune

DOI: 10.1201/9781003138358-14

249

system, biotolerables, when the response is minimum, and bioactives, which induce any specific biological response on the interface, enabling bonds between the tissue and the material (Davies and Hanawa 2016; Jasty 1992).

One may cite ceramics based on aluminum and titanium oxides, ultra-high-molecular-weight polyethylene, and some alloys containing chromium, vanadium, and titanium as the most used bioinert materials. Owing to their high strength, metals are important biotolerable biomaterials. A particularly important class are the bioactives materials such as bioglasses and calcium phosphate ceramics that, in spite of their relatively low mechanical strength, present exceptional biocompatibility.

Trying to get the best of two worlds, in recent years, a great amount of effort has been devoted to the development of materials combining the bioactivity and chemical resistance of ceramics with the mechanical strength of metals. In this sense, treatment techniques, such as those based on plasmas, which enable the adjustment of surface characteristics without affecting bulk properties, are very attractive. In this context, this paper presents some illustrative results obtained with plasma electrolytic oxidation (PEO), a versatile and experimentally simple technique for metallic biomaterial treatment.

12.2   SURFACE TREATMENT

Surface treatment techniques, such as plasma spray (Tejero-Martin et al. 2018), sol-gel (Owens et al. 2016), and biomimetic (Shin, Jo, and Mikos 2003) methods, and electrolytic process are very important options to improve the performance of a biomaterial. Among these techniques, plasma spray is the most used for commercial purposes. However, in addition to being a line-of-sight process, which makes difficult the treatment of complex-shaped pieces, the lacking of chemical interactions between the coating and the metal and high temperatures during the processing are noteworthy drawbacks (García-Sanz et al. 1997). On the other hand, the solgel technique has advantages such as low cost, low processing temperature, the possibility of covering large areas, and greater control over the characteristics of the deposited layer. However, poor mechanical properties are still a limitation to the widespread use of this technique.

Abe et al. (2001) have developed a biomimetic method to produce bioceramic films at room temperature, which enables the coating of temperature-sensitive materials, such as polymers. Such a method consists of soaking the substrate to be coated in a simulated body fluid (Kokubo and Takadama 2006) with ion composition similar to that of blood plasma. However, that is a time-consuming technique demanding, in some cases, more than a week of immersion to get a coating thick enough (Koju et al. 2017).

12.2.1   ELECTROLYSIS

The electrolytic processes are based on non-spontaneous oxidation–reduction reactions in systems composed of two metallic electrodes immersed in an electrolytic solution and connected to a power supply. The energized metallic surfaces react with ions in the solution, and coatings with a variety of chemical and physical properties can be grown on the electrodes. The formation process and the growth of these coatings depend on several parameters such as composition and concentration of electrolytes, current density, electrical conductivity, and temperature of the solution (Sul et al. 2001). In this way, surface characteristics such as chemical composition, morphology, roughness, wettability, wear and corrosion resistances, and thermal conductivity can be adjusted by modifying the treatment parameters (Araújo et al. 2019; Simchen et al. 2020; Nagay et al. 2019).

A particularly interesting version of the electrolytic process is the one frequently referred to as PEO (Yerokhin et al. 1999) or microarc oxidation (MAO). In the same way as in conventional electrolytic processes, this technique is also based on the application of a voltage between two electrodes immersed in an electrolytic solution and the sample to be treated is usually coupled to the anode (positive electrode) of the system similarly to what happens in anodizing treatments. However, the biggest difference between these two techniques is the voltage between the electrodes, which is significantly higher in PEO processes.

Essentially, at the beginning of the process, under low voltages, negative ions, mainly oxygen-containing species, are attracted to the sample surface, leading to the formation of an insulating oxide layer. At the same time, hydrolysis caused by the current flowing through the electrolyte results in intense gas evolution in the solution. As the voltage is increased, the molecules in the gas bubbles accumulated around the electrodes begin to be excited and ionized producing a tenuous glow discharge plasma surrounding the anode, as can be seen in Figure 12.1a, which shows photographs of an aluminum sample cut as LAPTEC during treatment with PEO in sodium silicate solution. The appearance of this plasma increases the density of ions in the vicinity of the electrodes, accelerating the coating growth. As this insulating layer becomes thicker, the potential drops and, consequently, the electric field through the coating becomes more intense, leading to the formation of small sparks that move quickly over the entire surface of the material, as can be seen in Figure 12.1b.

On those points where the electric field exceeds the dielectric strength of the coating and impact ionization is relevant, such sparks become more intense, transforming into electric microarcs, as can be seen in Figure 12.1c. Such microarcs are capable

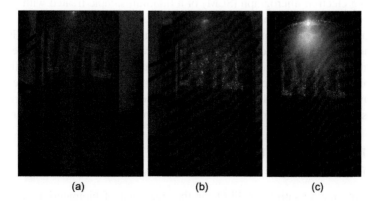

        (a)   (b)   (c)

FIGURE 12.1 Photographs of an aluminum sample at different stages during PEO treatment in sodium silicate solution with tenuous glow discharge plasma (a), formation of small sparks (b), and electric microarcs (c).

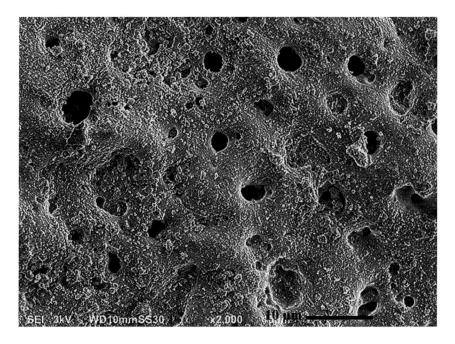

FIGURE 12.2   SEM illustrating the formation of pores on PEO-treated samples. The micrograph was acquired with a titanium sample treated for 5 minutes in a solution containing sodium glycerophosphate and calcium acetate.

of raising locally the temperature at values as high as 10^4 K (Yerokhin et al. 1999), which are high enough to melt locally the coating. The molten material reacts with the solution and is quickly cooled by the liquid and redeposited on the sample combined with electrolyte species. Likewise, the metallic substrate can also be melted when the microarcs are intense enough. With this, in addition to incorporating metal atoms into the coating, changes in surface morphology may also occur, with the formation of pores and other structures, as can be seen in Figure 12.2, which shows a scanning electron micrograph (SEM) of a titanium sample treated with PEO in a solution containing calcium and phosphorus.

Normally, the coatings produced by PEO are chemically and mechanically stable, are economically viable, and can be uniformly grown on objects with complex geometries without needing manipulating the sample. Furthermore, as it will be illustrated in the following section, the properties of the coatings can be tailored to best fit the requirements of a given application through the modification of treatment parameters, such as substrate and electrolyte compositions, applied voltage, and treatment time.

12.3   INFLUENCE OF PROCESS PARAMETERS ON THE PROPERTIES OF PEO-TREATED SAMPLES

To illustrate the versatility of PEO for the treatment of biomaterials, in the following sections, results obtained with titanium, tantalum, and aluminum samples treated by PEO are presented. The treatments have been performed in a water-cooled

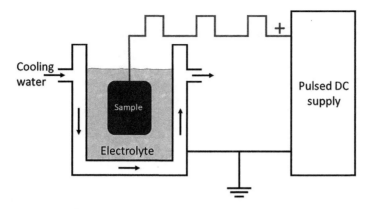

FIGURE 12.3 Schematic representation of experimental setup for the treatment of samples by PEO.

stainless-steel vessel, as depicted in Figure 12.3, applying DC pulses between the samples and the container walls, which also served as the cathode of the electrolytic cell. The composition of the electrolytic solutions has been chosen according to the nature of the substrates and the properties to be assigned to them. The influence of frequency, duty cycle and amplitude of the voltage pulses, and electrolyte composition on the properties of the coatings has been investigated.

12.3.1 INFLUENCE OF ELECTROLYTE COMPOSITION

In addition to supplying chemical species to be incorporated in the samples, the electrolyte composition has a great influence on important physical and chemical properties, such as roughness, porosity, crystalline phases, and wear and corrosion resistances of the coatings.

A SEM of a tantalum sample treated by PEO in an electrolytic solution containing calcium and phosphorus is shown in Figure 12.4. In this picture, some of the most common features resulting from the treatment can be noted. In addition to a large amount of different sized pores, one may note flat regions as those indicated by α. Such plateaus are formed on those regions where the microarcs are not intense enough to eject the molten material to the liquid solution forming the pores. Generally, those regions contain, predominantly, complex oxides of the substrate metal and some elements present in the electrolyte. In this particular case (Antonio et al. 2019), the coatings are formed mainly by Ta_2O_5 and $CaTa_2O_6$.

On those spots labeled as β, the breakdown of the dielectric strength of the coating produced microarcs intense enough to increase the local temperature and pressure and resulting in the ejection of material, such as a volcano does.

The molten metal is then quenched by the surrounding liquid and subsequently redeposited alloyed with species on the coating and in the electrolyte as one can clearly see in Figure 12.5, which shows SEM of a titanium sample treated by PEO in a solution containing sodium glycerophosphate, calcium acetate, and magnesium acetate. Owing to that, the coating chemical and structural compositions on those

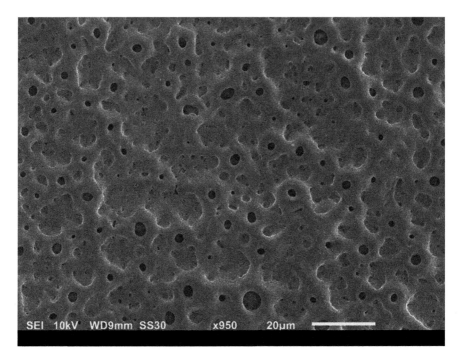

FIGURE 12.4 SEM of a tantalum sample treated for 300 seconds by PEO with pulses of 350 V, 100 Hz, in a solution containing sodium glycerophosphate and calcium acetate.

locations result from combinations of diverse forms containing species from the substrate, the coating, and the electrolyte, as revealed by results of chemical composition determination by X-ray electron energy-dispersive spectroscopy (EDS) indicated in the region labeled as β in Figure 12.5.

Where the temperature resulting from the microarcs is high enough, crystalline and complex structures can be formed as it can be observed in the region labeled as α in Figure 12.5. In this way, even complex structures such as hydroxyapatite can be deposited (Antônio et al. 2014).

As commented above, essentially, the characteristics of the coatings result from effects associated with the chemical species present in the solution and on the substrate and the intensity of the microarcs, as well. Therefore, the properties of the coatings can be tailored to best fit the requirements of a given application (Polo et al. 2020). As an illustration, Figure 12.6 shows the phase composition, determined by X-ray diffractometry, of PEO-treated titanium samples as a function of the proportion of magnesium acetate (*MgAcet*) added to electrolytes containing sodium glycerophosphate and calcium acetate. As it can be observed, while the crystalline structure of the coating grown in solutions without magnesium contains up to 80% of hydroxyapatite, the structure of sample treated with the addition of 0.08 M *MgAcet* is essentially titanium oxide in rutile and anatase forms. Furthermore, it is worthy to point out that the results reveal that the modification of the electrolyte composition even enables the modification of the relative proportion of the crystalline phases of a

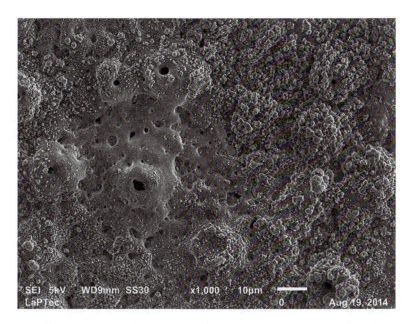

FIGURE 12.5   SEM of a titanium sample treated for 120 seconds by PEO with pulses of 480 V, 100 Hz, in a solution containing sodium glycerophosphate, calcium acetate, and magnesium acetate. The arrows indicate the chemical composition determined by EDS on the respective spots.

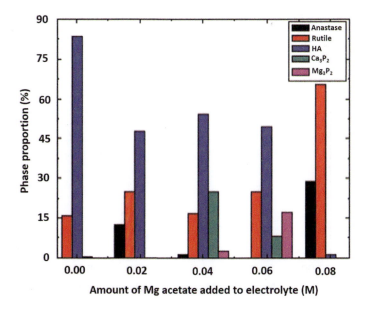

FIGURE 12.6   Phase composition of Ti samples treated by PEO with different proportions of magnesium acetate added to electrolytes of sodium glycerophosphate and calcium acetate. Treatments performed for 300 seconds at 500 V, 100 Hz.

given material. For instance, while TiO_2 is only present in rutile form in the sample produced with the addition of 0.06 M of magnesium acetate, the ratio of anatase to rutile proportions increases from 0.08 to 0.5 as the *MgAcet* concentration is reduced from 0.04 to 0.02 M. The larger proportion of rutile and its variation can be understood recalling that the anatase can be converted to rutile under heating to temperatures higher than typically 600°C. In addition, the enhancement of the concentration of ions in solution, as the amount of *MgAcet* is increased, leads to higher electric current and, consequently, higher power delivered to the samples and the higher the delivered power, the higher the sample temperature.

It is worthwhile remarking that the variation of the electrolyte composition also implies modifications of coating composition. This is evident in Figure 12.7, which presents the ratios of the concentrations of Ca to Mg and Ca to P, determined by Rutherford backscattering spectroscopy (RBS), on a 200-nm-thick layer on the surface of the coatings as a function of the proportion of *MgAcet* added to the electrolyte (Antônio et al. 2014). As one can note, the ratio Ca/Mg is roughly independent of the quantity of *MgAcet* when this is larger than 0.04 M. Furthermore, calcium is incorporated in larger proportions than phosphorus in all the studied situations, and, as the quantity of *MgAcet* is increased from 0.4 M, the ratio Ca/P abruptly increases. In conjunction, these results suggest that the incorporation of Mg in the coating occurs through the replacement of phosphorus atoms. Therefore, from the figure, it is possible to conclude that modifications of the solution composition affect differently the species in solution and the proportion they are incorporated in the coating. An important implication of fact is the possibility to select the species that will be

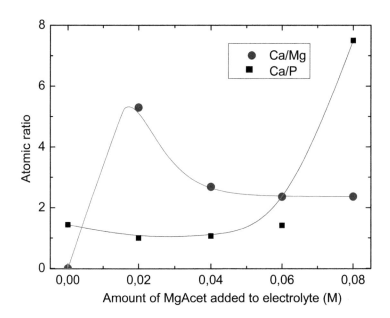

FIGURE 12.7   Ca/Mg and Ca/P concentration ratios in the surface of the coatings as a function of the proportion of magnesium acetate added to the electrolyte. Treatments performed for 300 seconds at 500 V, 100 Hz.

incorporated in larger (or smaller) proportions in the coating and, consequently, to tailor the surface properties.

12.3.2   Influence of Applied Voltage

The amplitude and the form (i.e., AC or DC, pulsed or continuous wave, duty cycle, etc.) of the applied voltage is another important parameter in PEO treatments. Essentially, whereas the amplitude determines the intensity of the microarcs, the voltage form determines their duration.

During DC treatments, the voltage is continuously applied to the substrate favoring the establishment of high thermal power arcs that may be deleterious for the quality of the coating, as it can be observed in Figure 12.8, which presents SEMs of aluminum samples treated by PEO in solution of sodium silicate at 350 V during treatment and the respective photographs taken by the end of the treatment. As it can be observed, the surface of sample grown under the condition with less intense microarcs (a) is smoother, and a very clustered and irregular surface is noted on the sample exposed to the stronger arcs (b).

The effect of intense microarcs on the quality of the coatings is yet more evident in Figure 12.9, where a SEM of a titanium sample treated by PEO under excessively high voltage (550 V) is shown. As it can be noticed, the arcs produced severe sputtering of material, resulting in flaws, large pores, and even cracks (indicated by the arrows) in the coating.

A possible way to circumvent such arcing problems is using voltage pulses, which means interrupting periodically the voltage, to avoid the conversion of microarcs into high power arcs. The effect of using such a technique can be observed in Figure 12.10, which presents SEMs of Ti samples treated by PEO in a solution containing sodium glycerophosphate, calcium acetate, and magnesium acetate with pulses of 480 V at various frequencies.

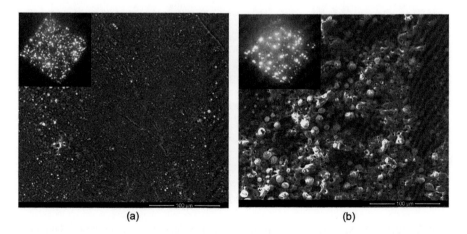

(a)   (b)

FIGURE 12.8   SEMs of aluminum samples treated by PEO in sodium silicate substrates under conditions that resulted in mild (a) and intense (b) microarcs.

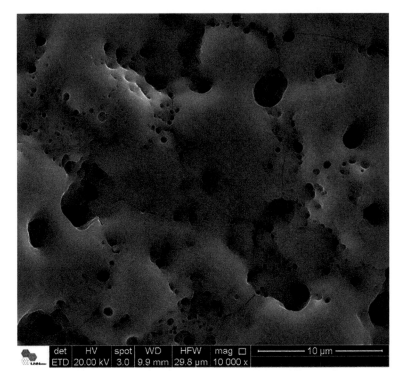

FIGURE 12.9 SEM of a Ti sample treated by PEO in electrolyte containing sodium glyc-erophosphate and calcium acetate. Treatments performed for 300 seconds applying 550 V DC. The arrows indicate cracks on the coating.

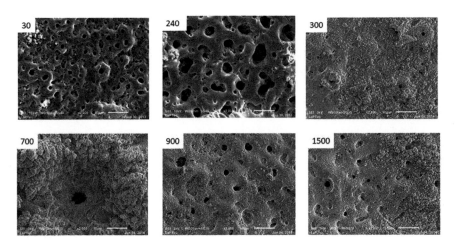

FIGURE 12.10 SEM of Ti samples treated by PEO in electrolytes containing sodium glyc-erophosphate, calcium acetate, and magnesium acetate with 480 V pulses with repetition rates of 30, 240, 300, 700, 900, and 1,500 Hz.

It is interesting to point out that any clear dependency of surface features on the variation of the frequency can be concluded from the results. For instance, when the frequency was increased from 30 to 240 Hz, an expressive increase in average pore diameter is observed. However, pores can barely be seen on the sample treated at 300 Hz. In addition, from this frequency, a granular structure begins to be formed on the treated samples, reaching its largest amount at 700 Hz and then decreasing for higher frequencies.

In order to understand the influence of the voltage frequency on the structure of the coatings, some aspects have to be taken into account. Firstly, according to the micrographs in Figure 12.10, the effect of increasing the frequency is, in a certain way, dependent on the frequency level itself. When the frequency is too low, the period during which the power is applied to the substrate is too short to significantly yield effects associated with the microarcs. Therefore, the main consequence of increasing the repetition rate in this low frequency range is the enhancement of the amount of energy delivered to the substrates. On the other hand, as the frequency is increased, the duration of the pulses decreases and, when frequency is excessively high, the pulses are too short to produce high power arcs and, consequently, smoother surfaces are produced. In this way, the morphology of the coatings is basically determined by the density of energy delivered to the surface by the microarcs.

It is evident from Figure 12.10 that the voltage frequency influences the composition of the coating, as well. Similarly, to what happens with morphology, the effect of the repetition rate is also dependent on the range of frequency. Under low frequencies, the coating growth is limited by the energy availability. As the frequency is increased, more energy is deposited on the sample, increasing the rates of reactions that result in the incorporation of species on the surface. However, beyond a certain frequency, the pulses become too short to significantly produce energetic microarcs and, consequently, high-temperature reactions. This supposition is corroborated by results such as those presented in Figure 12.11, which shows the proportion of crystalline phases detected in Ti samples treated by PEO in a solution of sodium glycerophosphate, calcium acetate, and magnesium acetate with pulses of 480 V at various frequencies. With this picture, it is possible to note that the higher the frequency, the lower the proportion of hydroxyapatite, the most complex crystalline phase detected in such samples.

The intensity of the microarcs can also be adjusted by inserting small negative components between the positive voltage pulses. In addition, the presence of negative pulses may have an important influence on the migration of charged particles in the solution and, consequently, on the coating composition and growth mechanism. As an illustration, Figure 12.12 presents the effect of different negative voltages on roughness and phase composition of coatings deposited on Ti samples. As it can be observed, setting the amplitude of the negative pulses enables one to produce rougher or smoother surfaces as well as to select the proportion of certain species or crystalline phases in the coating.

As shown in Figure 12.13, which presents a SEM of a PEO-treated Ti sample after fibroblast cell adhesion assay, the treatments are able to enhance surface biocompatibility, as the cells (indicated by the arrows) prefer to adhere to hydroxyapatite-rich regions instead of on those spots predominantly composed of titanium oxide.

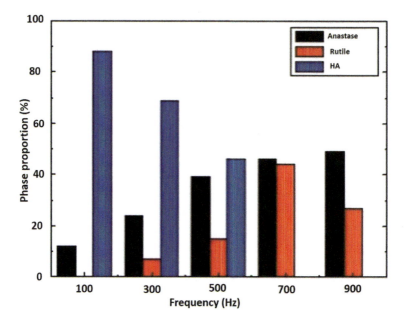

FIGURE 12.11 Proportion of crystalline phases detected on Ti samples treated by PEO in solution of sodium glycerophosphate, calcium acetate, and magnesium acetate with pulses of 480 V at various frequencies.

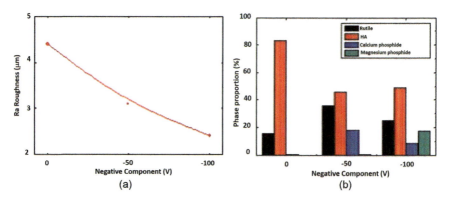

FIGURE 12.12 Roughness (a) and proportion (b) of crystalline phases of coatings produced by PEO under different amplitudes of negative pulses. Treatments performed in solutions of sodium glycerophosphate, calcium acetate, and magnesium acetate with pulses of 480 V, 100 Hz, and different negative components.

Finally, it is worthy to mention that the modifications produced by PEO treatments can even improve the bioactivity of biocompatible materials, such as titanium. As an exemplification, Figure 12.14 presents results of alkaline phosphatase (ALP) activity, which is an important indicator of cell differentiation, obtained with Ti samples as received and after coating with hydroxyapatite by PEO. As it can be observed,

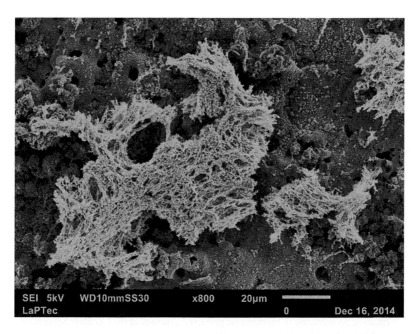

FIGURE 12.13 SEM of PEO-treated Ti sample after osteoblast cell adhesion assay. Treatment performed in sodium glycerophosphate, calcium acetate, and magnesium acetate solution with pulses of 480 V, 100 Hz.

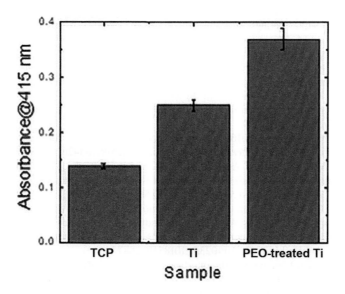

FIGURE 12.14 Results of alkaline phosphatase activity assay obtained with fibroblasts culture on titanium samples as received and coated with hydroxyapatite by PEO. Treatment performed in sodium glycerophosphate, calcium acetate, and magnesium acetate solution with pulses of 480 V, 100 Hz. TCP stands for the tissue culture plate, used as positive control.

the treatment increased in up to 50% the ALP (Bowers and McComb 1966) activity, suggesting a significant enhancement on the surface ability to induce the conversion of fibroblast cell into the bone on the material.

12.4 CONCLUSIONS

As illustrated above, PEO is a potentially useful technique for surface modification of metallic biomaterials. Experimentally simple, economically viable, and easily scaled up for industrial processes, PEO is a versatile tool that allows the production of surfaces with tailored morphology and chemical structure without changing the bulk properties of lightweight metals. Owing to that and the fact that the results of the treatment are strongly influenced by the processing parameters, PEO should always be considered as an important procedure to improve the performance of prosthesis and implants based on metals such as titanium, tantalum, niobium, magnesium, and their alloys.

REFERENCES

Abe, Y., M. Kawashita, T. Kokubo, and T. Nakamura. 2001. "Effects of solution on apatite formation on substrate in biomimetic process." *Journal of the Ceramic Society of Japan* 109 (1266). doi: 10.2109/jcersj.109.1266_106.

Antônio, C.A., N.C. Cruz, E.C. Rangel, R. de Cássia Cipriano Rangel, T. do Espirito Santo Araujo, S.F. Durrant, B.A. Más, and E.A.R. Duek. 2014. "Hydroxyapatite coating deposited on grade 4 Titanium by plasma electrolytic oxidation." *Materials Research* 17 (6). doi: 10.1590/1516-1439.286914.

Antonio, R.F., E.C. Rangel, B.A. Mas, E.A.R. Duek, and N.C. Cruz. 2019. "Growth of hydroxyapatite coatings on tantalum by plasma electrolytic oxidation in a single step." *Surface and Coatings Technology* 357. doi: 10.1016/j.surfcoat.2018.10.079.

Araújo, T.E.S., M. Macias Mier, A. Cruz Orea, E.C. Rangel, and N.C. Cruz. 2019. "Highly thermally conductive dielectric coatings produced by plasma electrolytic oxidation of aluminum." *Materials Letters* X3. doi: 10.1016/j.mlblux.2019.100016.

Bowers, G.N., and R.B. McComb. 1966. "A continuous spectrophotometric method for measuring the activity of serum alkaline phosphatase." *Clinical Chemistry* 12 (2). doi: 10.1093/clinchem/12.2.70.

Davies, J.E., and T. Hanawa. 2016. "4. Titanium and its oxide film: A substrate for formation of apatite." *Bone-Bio Material Interface.* doi: 10.3138/9781442671508-007.

Evans, E.M., M.A.R. Freeman, A.J. Miller, and B. Vernon Roberts. 1974. "Metal sensitivity as a cause of bone necrosis and loosening of the prosthesis in total joint replacement." *Journal of Bone and Joint Surgery: Series B* 56 (4). doi: 10.1302/0301-620x.56b4.626.

García-Sanz, F.J., M.B. Mayor, J.L. Arias, J. Pou, B. León, and M. Pérez-Amor. 1997. "Hydroxyapatite coatings: A comparative study between plasma-spray and pulsed laser deposition techniques." *Journal of Materials Science: Materials in Medicine*, 8, 861–65 Chapman & Hall Ltd. doi: 10.1023/A:1018549720873.

Jasty, M. 1992. "The bone-biomaterial interface." *The Journal of Bone & Joint Surgery* 74 (9). doi: 10.2106/00004623-199274090-00027.

Koju, N., P. Sikder, Y. Ren, H. Zhou, and S.B. Bhaduri. 2017. "Biomimetic coating technology for orthopedic implants." *Current Opinion in Chemical Engineering.* doi: 10.1016/j. coche.2016.11.005.

Kokubo, T., and H. Takadama. 2006. "How useful is SBF in predicting in vivo bone bioactivity?" *Biomaterials* 27 (15). doi: 10.1016/j.biomaterials.2006.01.017.

Nagay, B.E., C. Dini, J.M. Cordeiro, A.P. Ricomini-Filho, E.D. de Avila, E.C. Rangel, N.C. da Cruz, and V.A.R. Barão. 2019. "Visible-light-induced photocatalytic and antibacterial activity of TiO$_2$ codoped with nitrogen and bismuth: New perspectives to control implant-biofilm-related diseases." *ACS Applied Materials and Interfaces* 11 (20). doi: 10.1021/acsami.9b03311.

Owens, G.J., R.K. Singh, F. Foroutan, M. Alqaysi, C.M. Han, C. Mahapatra, H.W. Kim, and J.C. Knowles. 2016. "Sol-gel based materials for biomedical applications." *Progress in Materials Science.* doi: 10.1016/j.pmatsci.2015.12.001.

Polo, T.O.B., W.P. da Silva, G.A.C. Momesso, T.J. Lima-Neto, S. Barbosa, J.M. Cordeiro, J.S. Hassumi, et al. 2020. "Plasma electrolytic oxidation as a feasible surface treatment for biomedical applications: An in vivo study." *Scientific Reports* 10 (1). doi: 10.1038/s41598-020-65289-2.

Shin, H., S. Jo, and A.G. Mikos. 2003. "Biomimetic materials for tissue engineering." *Biomaterials.* doi: 10.1016/S0142-9612(03)00339-9.

Simchen, F., M. Sieber, A. Kopp, and T. Lampke. 2020. "Introduction to plasma electrolytic oxidation-an overview of the process and applications." *Coatings.* doi: 10.3390/coatings10070628.

Sul, Y.T., C.B. Johansson, Y. Jeong, and T. Albrektsson. 2001. "The electrochemical oxide growth behaviour on titanium in acid and alkaline electrolytes." *Medical Engineering and Physics* 23 (5). doi: 10.1016/S1350-4533(01)00050-9.

Tejero-Martin, D., M. Rezvani Rad, A. McDonald, and T. Hussain. 2018. "Beyond traditional coatings, a review on thermal sprayed functional and smart coatings." ArXiv.

Yerokhin, A.L., X. Nie, A. Leyland, A. Matthews, and S.J. Dowey. 1999. "Plasma electrolysis for surface engineering." *Surface and Coatings Technology.* doi: 10.1016/S0257-8972(99)00441-7.

13 Additive Manufacturing for VADs

Adriana Del Monaco De Maria and Evandro Drigo
Centro Universitário das Américas

CONTENTS

13.1 INTRODUCTION

Three-dimensional printing, technically known as rapid prototyping or additive manufacturing, corresponds to a set of techniques developed in the 1980s. Chuck Hull was an American physical engineer from the California state who contributed to the development of machines that use stereolithography in rapid prototyping. Since then, additive manufacturing has become popular and part of different areas of engineering, medicine, and even the food industry (Gross et al., 2014).

In medicine, computer assistive manufacturing (CAM) can contribute to a number of important areas, such as printing of complex clinical cases for biomodel surgical planning, using reconstruction of exam images, such as computed tomography and nuclear magnetic resonance, for example. It can also be used for making phantoms, calibration models for imaging equipment and, more recently, developed artificial organs and tissues using 3D bioprinting and tissue engineering techniques as the case of bone graft implants for the skull and even the development of a "mini heart" by the Tel Aviv University group in 2019 (Parthasarathy, 2014; Shapira et al., 2019).

In this chapter, we will discuss some of the contributions of additive manufacturing to the development of ventricular assist devices (VADs) and introduce some future perspectives of these devices.

13.2 VAD DEVELOPMENT STRATEGIES

In the development of circulatory assist devices, we are often faced with distinct strategic paths: from a blood-pumping geometry, the actuator (engine) is developed or starting with an actuator, the geometry of the nozzle itself is developed. A third way of development considered ideal for the perfect marriage of form/function is

DOI: 10.1201/9781003138358-15

the concomitant design of actuator + pump geometry, ensuring optimization of the project with this married couple; this is not a simple task, but in this sense, additive manufacturing technology presents itself as a tool of great value for the development of the project.

Additive manufacturing makes it possible to streamline the study of different geometries, previously indicated as promising in the stages of computer simulations, in a faster and cheaper way (Drigo et al. 2015; de Andrade 2019). With the possibility of making different physical prototypes that can be tested on hydrodynamic/cardiovascular simulation benches (Uebelhart et al. 2013; Leao et al. 2020; Fonseca et al. 2011), the chance of the project converging to a cost/benefit technology suitable for the application increases. Additive manufacturing not only allows the study of the geometries of rotors and casings of blood pumps but also the interaction with users; it can be through manufacture of anatomically reliable biomodels, which allow planning of the best surgical approach to implant and explant devices (Del Monaco et al. 2018; Sá et al. 2017).

13.3 MINIATURIZATION: TRANSVENTRICULAR AND TRANSCATHETER DEVICES

This miniaturization is also desirable in the conception of future VADs, making it possible to implant them using minimally invasive surgery techniques, such as transventricular devices as de Andrade (2019) discusses.

Another promising technique with a good future perspective is the transcatheter device. These VAD systems, when implanted by a minimally invasive route, such as catheterization, reduce the risks of infections and risks inherent to major surgical procedures. They can be used to support systemic or pulmonary circulation independently. For the development of a transcatheter device prototype, computer assistive design (CAD) and additive manufacturing technology were used for the project, as in Figures 13.1 and 13.2 as demonstrated by Del Monaco et al. (2019). The model consists of a small rotor and housing assembly, with a diameter of 7 mm and 2.5 cm in length (Figure 13.1) and an entry cannula.

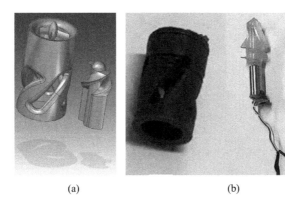

(a)   (b)

FIGURE 13.1 CAD rotor and housing assembly (a); additive manufactured rotor and housing assembly (b).

It has an anchoring system in the ventricle or in another position of interest, such as descending aorta, by a stent, avoiding suction of adjacent tissues through the entry cannula (Figure 13.2).

Its dimensions allow the implantation via minimally invasive catheterization (Figure 13.3).

Preliminary results of this project indicate that it is possible to have required partial circulatory support capacity, between 0.7 and 1.5 L/minute, with engine rotation in the range of 80–90,000 rpm, for this first prototype mentioned.

And furthermore, it is the opinion of the authors that the future of manufacture of VADs can be fully carried out by additive manufacturing, with the development of biocompatible materials (ceramics, metal alloys, and biopolymers) suitable for different processes (stereophotolithography, laser sintering, deposition cast material, etc.).

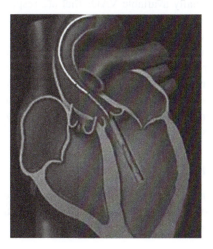

FIGURE 13.2 Transcatheter VAD anchoring system in the left ventricle example.

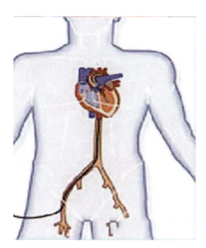

FIGURE 13.3 Minimally invasive possible route for implant, catheterization.

13.4   TET AND VADs—A POSSIBILITY FOR TOTAL IMPLANTABLE DEVICES

With the evolution and development of new materials and manufacturing techniques, it is possible to work on other aspects of the implant system in addition to VADs and their interaction with anatomical models. There are already commercially available 3D printing technologies for electronic circuits in complex geometries, which may be of great interest due to the nature of the application, paving the way for making the control and monitoring circuits inherent to the implant system. One of the possibilities is the application of these methods in the development of a transcutaneous energy transmission (TET) system for fully implantable VADs. TET is a wireless charger for batteries implanted in patients, eliminating the need for percutaneous cables used in commercially available VADs that are responsible for postoperative problems (infections) and the consequent increase in process costs (Silva 2018).

In this type of development, anatomical studies of the positioning of the coupling coils can be carried out—the external part and the implanted part (Figure 13.4); important not only for surgical planning but also for electromagnetic compatibility studies of the system (Drigo et al. 2017). In the future, perhaps the components themselves (conductors and insulators), such as electromagnetic coupling coils, can be directly manufactured in 3D printing, reducing their size and improving their implantability with flexible materials.

13.5   BIOPRINTING

Bioprinting is a recent technology of 3D printing in health used in tissue engineering and regenerative medicine for the production of 3D tissue structures, aiming at the construction of functional tissues and organs (Dernowsek, 2019).

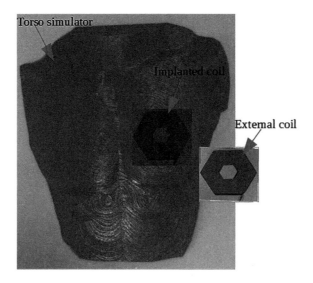

FIGURE 13.4   Anatomical torso simulator for testing the positioning of coupling coils.

The bioprinting process goes through practically the same steps of 3D printing, from image acquisition and treatment in CAD software, passing through the analysis of computer-aided engineering and CAM manufacturing, the difference being the biocompatible material (Barros, 2019).

Still within the possibilities of additive manufacturing, one can find the recent developments in the area of bioprinting techniques that aim at the impression of organs working with living cells.

Researchers developed the first prototype of heart with cells and vessels that became known worldwide; however, it did not have a capacity to conduct coordinated electrical impulses to guarantee the functioning of the heart as a contractile pump. In the case of cardiac muscles, the response to electrical stimuli and the targeted growth of muscle fibers are the biggest challenge when thinking about 3D bioprinting for the heart. In this sense, the development of bioabsorbable conductive biomaterials can be an important starting point for the success in the growth of oriented muscle fibers. A possibility for conductive polymeric biomaterial development is demonstrated in Venancio and Santos' (2010) work.

Perhaps, it is a long way in the case of an organ like the heart for bioprinting, it may take a few decades more of science development.

REFERENCES

Barros, W.F., "Proposed technical-economic feasibility for 3D assistive bioprinting by robotic manipulator". College of Pharmaceutical Sciences, Araraquara, 2019.

da Silva, E.D., "Nova abordagem na transmissão de energia transcutânea para dispositivos de assistência ventricular implantáveis." *Tese de Doutorado em Medicina/Tecnologia e Intervenção em Cardiologia*, Instituto Dante Pazzanese de Cardiologia, Universidade de São Paulo: São Paulo, 2018. doi: 10.11606/T.98.2018.tde-18092018-095803.

de Andrade, G.C., "Rotor for a transventricular blood pump rotor for a transventricular blood pump." 2019.

Del Monaco, A.D.M., E. Drigo, J.C.M. Lautert, S.S. Margarido, and T.Y. Miyashiro, "Case report: Auxiliary device for recreational use in a child with upper limb malformation, made by additive manufacture (3D printing)." *The Academic Society Journal* 2(4): 242–47, 2018.

Del Monaco, A.D.M., S.M. Margarido, J.C.M. Lautert, E.S. Drigo, and A.J.P. Andrade, "Dispositivo de assistência circulatória transcatéter – DACT". *Anais 6° OBI*, 2019.

Dernowsek, J., E. Pizzoni, *Do You Know What BIOMATERIAL*. BioEdTech: São Paulo, 2019.

Drigo, E., J. Leme, T. Leão, E. Bock, J. Fonseca, B. Utiyama, R. De, G. Andrade, and A.J.P. De Andrade. "Low cost assembly for flow visualization study on blood pumps" 4–6, 2015.

Drigo, E., J. Fonseca, T. Leão, E. Bock, C. Sartori, L. Lebensztajn, C. Silva, R. Nunes, and A. Andrade. "Transcutaneous energy transmission by capacitive coupling." *International Journal of Artificial Organs* 40 (8): 437, 2017.

Fonseca, J., A. Andrade, D.E.C. Nicolosi, J.F. Biscegli, J. Leme, D. Legendre, E. Bock, and J.C. Lucchi, "Cardiovascular simulator improvement: Pressure versus volume loop assessment" *Artificial Organs* 35(5): 454–58, 2011.

Gross, B.C. et al., "Evaluation of 3D printing and its potential impact on biotechnology and the chemical sciences". *Analytical Chemistry* 86(7): 3240–3253, 2014.

Leao, T., B. Utiyama, J. Fonseca, E. Bock, and A. Andrade, "In vitro evaluation of multi-objective physiological control of the centrifugal blood pump" *Artificial Organs* 44(8): 785–96, 2020.

Parthasarathy, J., "3D modeling, custom implants and its future perspectives in craniofacial surgery". *Ann Maxillofac Surg* 4: 9–18, 2014.

Sá, R., M. Hirata, E. Drigo, A. Del Monaco, T. Leão, J. Fonseca, B. Utiyama, A. Andrade, and E. Bock, "Preliminary results of in vitro endothelialization on plasma modified titanium surface." *International Journal of Artificial Organs* 40(8): 453, 2017.

Shapira, A., R. Edri, I. Gal, L. Wertheim, and T. Dvir. "3D printing of personalized thick and perfusable cardiac patches and hearts". *Advanced Science* 6(11): 1900344, 2019.

Uebelhart, B., B.U. da Silva, J. Fonseca, E. Bock, J. Leme, C. da Silva, T. Leão, and A. Andrade, "Study of a centrifugal blood pump in a mock loop system." *Artificial Organs* 37 (11): 946–949, 2013.

Venancio, E.C., and C.C.S. Santos, "Modificação de tecidos biocompatíveis através da síntese de polímeros condutores intrínsecos". *UFABC Anais III Simpósio de Iniciação Científica*, Santo André, 2010.

14 Laser Additive Manufacturing for the Realization of New Material Concepts

Wilhelm Pfleging and Juliana dos Santos Solheid
Karlsruhe Institute of Technology

CONTENTS

14.1 INTRODUCTION

In additive manufacturing (AM) processes, components are built up in layers from liquids, powders, wires, or foils using chemical or physical processes. Direct energy deposition (DED) or powder bed fusion (PBF) can be used as AM processes in which metal powder or wires are used to print dense metal layers on substrates or on free-form surfaces of existing components [1]. Metal powder (pure elements, element mixtures, or master alloys) or metal wires are melted at high speed and instantaneously deposited in layers on respective metallic substrates. In the case of the so-called laser cladding [2], this technology is generally used for applying coatings or for tool repairs. Compared to subtractive processes, additive processes save time and resources, as the material is only added where it is needed. Established steels, nickel-based alloys, or titanium alloys are typically used. However, it is also possible to

DOI: 10.1201/9781003138358-16

obtain completely new materials by in situ alloying of powder mixtures or to create material gradients by changing the powder mixture composition during the buildup [3]. High entropy alloys (HEAs) represent a new research field for future applications. These are formed from a large number of elements, all of which are present in similarly strong concentrations, e.g., alloys consisting of zirconium, niobium, hafnium, tantalum, or tungsten [4]. The alloys formed can generally be single-phase as well as multiphase mixed crystals. HEAs can often combine high strength and very good ductility. In situ alloying offers the unique possibility of fast material screening for the future production of new metallic components with outstanding mechanical properties at high temperatures. For a long time, the manufacture of refractory alloys was limited to vacuum arc remelting because of their high melting points. With laser-based methods, these metals are locally melted by the focused laser beam and deposited additively. In addition to material development, AM offers great design freedom in component design, which can be used, for example, for the development of load-optimized designs based on the bionic principle [5].

To add up to the versatility of AM, laser postprocesses can be used to modify the resulting surfaces of parts produced with such technologies [6–9]. The different types of laser sources commercially available assure their suitability in a wide range of applications, with continuous wave (cw) lasers being often used for the reduction of surface roughness, while pulsed lasers are being applied in the modification of surface functionalities and to enhance the geometry accuracy. Even with the prospect of being able to replace certain steps of AM process chain, adopting laser postprocesses as an additional step can also be proved beneficial when specific characteristics are required in the localized areas of final built components.

14.2 SHORT OVERVIEW OF AM PROCESSES AND RESPECTIVE APPLICATIONS

The technical term "additive manufacturing (AM)" describes a process of joining materials to create objects from three-dimensional (3D) model data, usually layer by layer, as opposed to subtractive manufacturing methods like milling or laser ablation. It is obvious that in the case of large-scale 3D objects, subtractive manufacturing will in general produce a larger amount of material waste than established AM methods. However, in the case of selective surface texturing or surface modification, subtractive methods become more advantageous. Especially the combination of AM and laser ablation provide new opportunities in the designing of 3D objects with local functionalities and biocompatibility as required for medical implants [9]. In Section 14.4, recent progress in this approach will be presented and discussed referring to biomedical surfaces and ventricular assist devices (VADs).

Synonyms for AM are additive manufacturing, additive processes, additive techniques, additive layer production, layer production, and free-form production. Before focusing on AM of metallic parts, let's go back to the beginning of AM technology. The first AM technology is based on an invention and patent of Chuck Hull in 1984, describing the application "for apparatus for production of three-dimensional objects by stereolithography," which is subsequently annotated as a stereolithography apparatus (SLA) [10]. In 1986, C. Hull founded 3D systems emerging the worldwide first commercialized rapid prototyping system, i.e., the first 3D printer, in 1987, the SLA-1. The related process is based on a laser-induced photopolymerization process, wherein a UV laser beam is scanned on a vat of a photopolymer resin. Three-dimensional prototypes are formed by curing the monomer resin layer by layer while in between each layer the build platform submerges deeper into the resin vat. Nowadays, the principle of this technology covers a broadscale range, from a submicron range up to several meters. Regarding submicron technology, the work of Kawata et al. [11] was a technical milestone, enabling subdiffraction-limited fabrication of micro-objects like the so-called micro-bull sculpture (Figure 14.1a). The new approach was to use femtosecond laser radiation and to initiate a 2-photon photopolymerization with subdiffraction-limited resolution as schematically described in Figure 14.1b by pushing the pulse energy close to the polymerization threshold. Already in 2015, the researchers from Oak Ridge National Laboratory were able to print cars (Figure 14.1c) or even buildings with up to a size of $11.5 \times 3.7 \times 4.0\,m^3$ [12]. The Shelby Cobra was printed using 20% carbon fiber–reinforced acrylonitrile butadiene styrene material. During large-scale polymer deposition, polymer pellets were heated to near molten temperatures and extruded layer by layer onto an out-of-the-oven build platform.

In addition to polymers, metallic alloys as material for AM technologies are of huge interest in research and development since more than a decade ago. Laser cladding/coating and laser metal deposition (LMD) for repairing damaged turbines and 3D metal printing for the rapid production of objects on a large scale became reliable technical approaches for small and medium batches.

In 2015, the Beijing University of Aeronautics and Astronautics demonstrated the 3D laser printing of a cockpit window frame assigned to a commercial aircraft (C919). The printing time for the frame took 55 days which is quite impressive considering that an aircraft manufacturer in Europe takes two whole years with a budget of about $2 million just to develop molds for making similar frames [13]. The Comac C919 is

"Micro Bull" (length 10 μm)

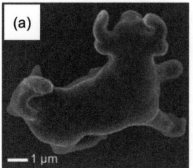

"Shelby Cobra" (2015)

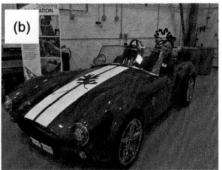

FIGURE 14.1 Scale range of AM technologies. (a) Microfabrication and nanofabrication at sub-diffraction-limit resolution by 2-photon–photopolymerization with laser-pulse energy above the polymerization threshold [Ref. 13]. (b) At Oak Ridge National Laboratory (ORNL) printed Shelby Cobra (est. 1965) by large-scale polymer deposition.

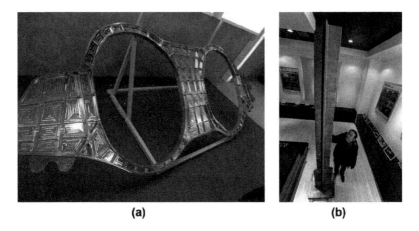

(a)   **(b)**

FIGURE 14.2 Selective laser sintering (SLS) for 3D printing of large scale objects made of titanium alloys for application in aircraft industry (a) C919 aircraft cockpit window frame [Ref. 17], (b) 5 m high wing carrier [Ref. 15].

China's first domestically built commercial aircraft. The Northwestern Polytechnical University (NPU) of China was producing within 25 days a 5 m-long titanium central wing spar for the C919 passenger plane (Figure 14.2) [14]. The LMD system at NPU was developed in 2013 for inert atmosphere printing of components with sizes up to $5 \times 2.5 \times 0.6\,m^3$, with an accuracy of about 1 mm [15].

The commercial aircraft manufacturer, Airbus, has been increasingly gaining the importance of laser sintering and melting of metal powders in aircraft manufacturing. The cabin bracket connector is used in the Airbus A350 XWB [14] (Figure 14.3).

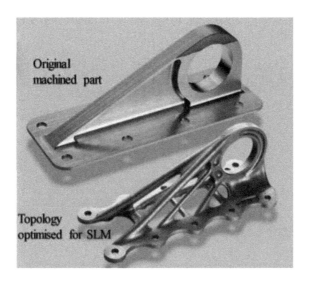

FIGURE 14.3 Titanium bracket connector for the Airbus A350 XWB optimized using additive manufacturing [Ref. 19].

The bracket was additively manufactured using the so-called LaserCUSING technology (Concept Laser GmbH), which is in principle working like the laser powder bed fusion (LPBF). In the past, the cabin bracket connector was milled and machined out of aluminum alloys. Now, it is a 3D-printed part, which is made out of titanium powder material with a more than 30% weight reduction. Mechanical milling of such aircraft parts leads to 95% of material waste, while with LPBF the percentage of the waste is only 5%. In AM, tools are not required to produce functional sample parts, thereby eliminating tool and mold costs. This also helps in identifying early-stage design errors and design optimization. In the past, Airbus projected 6 months to develop such components, which could be reduced to 1 month by establishing LPBF.

The exact knowledge and reliable prediction of the component behavior under the load conditions prevailing in the respective application are of essential importance for the establishment or broader application of AM technologies. The load-bearing capacity or the mechanical behavior of additively manufactured metallic structures is, as in the case of conventionally manufactured components, largely determined by the microstructure and thus by the thermomechanical conditions during processing. In a direct comparison of these conditions, however, there are significant differences between additive and conventional manufacturing processes. For example, the volume of material that is temporarily in the molten state during processing is much smaller in relation to the component to be manufactured with the AM process than with casting or welding, for example. In addition, due to the layered production method, there is a constantly repeated heat input. As a result, different solidification conditions as well as different thermal histories, i.e., different temperature–time paths, are to be expected. However, regarding component weight and optimized stability properties under a mechanical load, a topology optimization for achieving an optimal material distribution is strongly recommended. Topology optimization and selective laser melting were also applied during the manufacture of the above-mentioned lightweight aircraft bracket by achieving 30% weight reduction with an enhanced safety [18]. The use of construction principles from nature in technical applications, so-called bionic principles, is nowadays a common approach to enable lightweight constructions with optimized mechanical properties. In principle, material is mainly used where the greatest mechanical loads occur, while less material is distributed in places that have only a lower load, leading to the so-called cellular structures or materials [5].

The main types of AM of metallic objects with the most prospects of product marketing are based on electron beam (EB) processes or laser beam technologies. However, a more general approach in the classification of manufacturing technologies related to "additive manufacturing (metal)" is given in Ref. [1]. Based on this, a significantly more condensed overview is given in Figure 14.4.

Sheet lamination and especially laminated object manufacturing are derived from the principle of the first in 1991 commercialized AM techniques involving layer by layer lamination of paper material sheets, which in advance were cut using CO_2 laser [19]. Also, complex-shaped 3D metallic parts have been made starting from laser-cut metallic sheets and foils employing diffusion bonding, laser spot welding, brazing techniques, and Ultrasonic Additive Manufacturing (UAM).

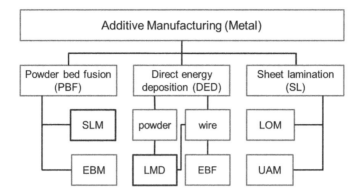

FIGURE 14.4 Overview of additive processes for metallic materials (EBM: electron beam melting, SLM: selective laser melting, LMD: laser metal deposition, EBF: electron freeform fabrication, LOM: laminated object manufacturing, UAM Ultrasonic additive manufacturing). The red-framed boxes are related to laser-based AM technologies.

More relevant in current research and development is the application of PBF) and DED technologies using electron or laser beam as possible heat sources.

Two EB-based AM technologies will be highlighted and shortly described due to their relevance in current AM applications:

- DED-electron beam free-form fabrication (EBF)
- PBF-electron beam melting (EBM)

DED-EBF is an AM technology using a mobile EB gun and a wire feeder within a vacuum chamber to fuse a deposited bead of metal, one bead at a time layer by layer. High deposition rates of about 6.8–18 kg/h can be realized for titanium or tantalum. However, the material selection is limited by the reliance on commercial sources of wire used by the process. One disadvantage is the slow cooling rate of the deposit within the vacuum environment and its potential effect on large grain growth and other metallurgical effects of the deposit. Advantages are that very large build volumes are possible and that the use of materials that are expensive, reactive, or with high melting points is possible due to the capability of high beam power and the high-purity vacuum environment [20].

PBF-EBM is an AM technology that selectively consolidates metal powders such as titanium, Inconel 718, and cobalt alloys to create 3D structures. Compared to conventional manufacturing processes, the EBM process is able to manufacture items with low volume and high value with reduced lead times. The method involves focusing an EB in a powder bed of metal particles to create a localized melt followed by resolidification that enables complex geometries to be fabricated layer by layer. The EBM system consists of an EB gun, vacuum chamber, building tank, and powder distribution mechanism. EBM systems are able to achieve scanning speeds of up to 8,000 m/s with an EB positioning accuracy of ± 0.025 mm and a single-layer thickness in the range of 0.05–0.2 mm [21] (Figure 14.5).

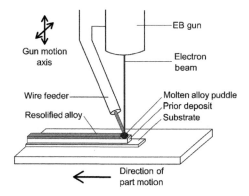

FIGURE 14.5 Schematic view of direct energy deposition process using e-beam and wire technology.

14.3 LASER ADDITIVE MANUFACTURING

In the following, laser-based AM technologies—selective laser melting (SLM) and direct/laser metal deposition (DMD/LMD)—will be introduced with regard to typical process parameters and characteristics.

SLM (or LPBF) is operating under inter-atmosphere (nitrogen and argon) in order to avoid oxidization of metallic powders such as aluminum and titanium and to avoid impurities in the respective 3D metallic object. The type of SLM operation is schematically shown in Figure 14.6.

As shown in Figure 14.6, powder material with typically mean diameter values up to 50 μm is spread onto a building plate driven by a blade or a wiper mechanism. The space between the surface of the building plate and the bottom edge of this spreading mechanism defines the single-layer thickness. This single-layer thickness is typically smaller than 100 μm. In PBF, the process parameters have to be carefully selected with regard to the single-layer thickness and the selected type of material. After deposition of a powder layer, a laser beam with an operation wavelength of about 1,064 nm is focused onto the powder bed and is scanned along the powder

- **Laser power:** 400-1000W

- **Growing rate:** 88 cm³/h

- **Building chamber:** 280x280x365mm³

- **Atmosphere:** (Ar, N₂)

- **Layer thickness:** 20μm – 90μm

- **Powder grain size:** 15-45μm

- **Roughness R_a** = 9-20μm (*as-built*)

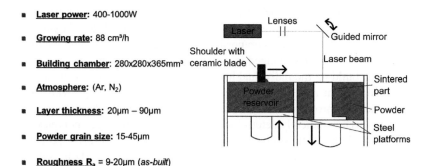

FIGURE 14.6 Process parameters and schematic view of principle selective laser melting operation.

surface in a sliced 3D CAD (computer-aided design)-defined pattern. The scanning strategy is also an important task due to the fact that it has a strong impact on the quality, microstructure, and defect formation. Once a single layer is completed, the building platform is stepwise moved down, and the procedure for a single-layer formation is repeated until the 3D build process is completed. It is worth mentioning that the laser beam exposure induces a melting depth into the previous layer to enable a full fusion of each layer into the previous (see also Figure 14.9). Consequently, the texture properties in the finished metallic part are less directional.

In Figure 14.6, the process parameters related to a commercial AM system (SLM 280, SLM Solutions Group AG [22]) are illustrated. The minimal achievable structure size is 150 µm with an as-built average surface roughness of 9–20 µm and a growing rate of up to 88 cm³/h. The material density of the final 3D object is in the range of 98.8% up to 99.9% of the pure alloy. It is also very common to apply a preheating platform depending on the process with adjustable temperature in the range of 20°C up to 200°C in order to reduce intrinsic mechanical stress formation.

The LMD process is also known as DED, DMD, or laser cladding. Previous applications of the process were limited to the processing of standard alloys (steel, titanium, or aluminum alloys), e.g., for the quick repair of damaged technical components or the application of protective layers. Technological and methodological progress is now opening up access to completely new fields of application such as "high throughput examinations" and "additive 3D production of samples and components" [23–26]. LMD can be used to create parts directly from a 3D CAD model by applying materials layer by layer. This technology offers a high degree of flexibility due to the possibility of modifying an existing design (substrate) and manufacturing macroscopically extended components. During LMD, metal powder (pure elements, element mixtures, and master alloys) is brought into the focus of a high-power laser beam (fiber laser; diode laser) at high speed, melted, and instantaneously deposited in layers on a substrate or component. The effect of the laser beam on the substrate or layer surfaces can also be used to generate a small weld pool in a controlled manner, in which, e.g., hard materials such as TiC are to be dispersed [27]. This makes alloys and metal–ceramic composites accessible (see Section 14.5). After rapid solidification, a material layer with a thickness of up to a few hundred micrometers is formed. The type of LMD operation is schematically shown in Figure 14.7. By repeatedly scanning the surface with the laser, multiple layers can be deposited on top of one another according to a given CAD/CAM model, and larger samples can be produced. The chemical compositions, the microstructures, and the resulting material properties can be changed in a controlled manner from layer to layer. The materials that build up the individual layers are very homogeneous with an adapted process management and can be characterized very precisely, e.g., with chemical analysis. The most promising alloys or composite materials for the respective applications can thus be efficiently determined and processed into larger, complex-shaped components with the LMD system through additive 3D manufacturing [26]. Typical process parameters are given in Figure 14.7. It is obvious that LMD in comparison to SLM is not as precise due to the higher layer thicknesses but enables a three times higher deposition rate. Furthermore, LMD offers outstanding prospects to develop new materials and components with designed properties.

- **Laser power:** 4kW

- **Growing rate:** 250 cm³/h

- **Building chamber:** 2000x1500x750mm³

- **Atmosphere:** (Ar, N_2, He)

- **Layer thickness:** >100μm – 500μm

- **Powder efficiency:** bis 90%

- **Powder grain size:** 45-150μm

- **Roughness R_a** = ~40μm (*as-build*)

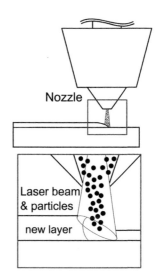

FIGURE 14.7 Process parameters and schematic view of principle "selective laser metal deposition" / "direct metal deposition."

14.3.1 FUNDAMENTAL ASPECTS OF LASER MATERIAL PROCESSING

Laser material processing is a technique based on irradiating a substrate surface with laser radiation at high intensities ($>10^5$ W/cm²). The optical energy is absorbed by the electronic system which subsequently transfers energy into the phonon system until thermal equilibrium is reached. For laser pulse lengths above 100 ps (10^{-12} s), thermalization of electrons and phonon occurs almost instantaneously, and the processes are denoted as thermal laser processing. Laser AM technologies for metals based on SLM and LMD are always thermally driven due to the required melting processes. Generally, a good understanding of heat transfer fundamentals is of great importance to comprehend the laser/material interaction and select the most appropriate system and parameters for a given application [8].

Initially, it is important to describe the characteristics of the laser beam as a heat source. Laser beams with Gaussian intensity profiles are widely adopted and can be expressed as a heat flux as shown in Equation 14.1:

$$Q'' = \frac{2AP_w}{\pi R_w^2} e^{\frac{-2\left(x^2+y^2\right)}{R_w^2}} \tag{14.1}$$

Where Q'' is the surface heat generation term, R_w is the distance from the center of the heat source, A is the laser absorption coefficient, and P_w is the laser power.

The generated heat interacts with the material in question. A simplified heat transfer equation to describe the heat dissipation within the part being processed is expressed in Equation 14.2:

$$\rho C_p \frac{\partial T}{\partial t} = k\nabla^2 T \tag{14.2}$$

where k is the effective thermal conductivity and C_p and ρ are the effective specific heat capacity and density of the material, respectively.

Although not all the optical laser energy is transformed into heat that will affect the process and properties of the final part, heat exchanges with the environment through convection and radiation (Stefan–Boltzmann law) are almost impossible to be avoided. Both heat losses can be described by Equations 14.3 for the former and 14.4 for the latter:

$$Q_{conv} = h(T_{amb} - T) \qquad (14.3)$$

$$Q_{rad} = \varepsilon\sigma(T_{amb}^4 - T^4) \qquad (14.4)$$

with h the convective heat transfer coefficient and ε and σ the surface emissivity and the Stefan–Boltzmann constant, respectively.

During several laser material processing, phase changes occur and the thermophysical properties of the material should be assessed accordingly.

It is worth mentioning that for ultrafast laser radiation the above-mentioned concept has to be modified by introducing a so-called two-temperature model [28]. The main advantage of using ultrafast laser processes is that melting or heat-affected zones can be almost avoided by minimizing thermal effects [29–31]. Therefore, ultrafast laser radiation is a preferred manufacturing tool for surface texturing and functionalization with structure details down to the nanometer range.

14.3.2 LMD Process Characteristics

The main objective is to refine metallic surfaces or to gain new functions through a coating. For this purpose, the metallic surface is melted in a locally limited manner with intense and focused laser radiation. Particles or powder mixtures are then sprayed into the molten bath. In this approach, the layers below are also melted again in order to achieve good adhesion and tight transition. The layered coating leads to an intrinsic heat treatment of the underlying areas. First of all, the melting temperature is reached on the top layer, and the layers below experience a repeated temperature control, which in some cases can reach the melting temperature. Thus, periodic heating of the individual layers takes place. This means that the microstructure and the internal stress of the lower layers will be adjusted depending on the process parameters and the number of layers. The main process characteristics of LMD are as follows:

- Transport of metal powder (pure elements, element mixtures, and master alloys) at high speed
- Melting in the focus of a high-power laser beam
- Locally thin melt pool on substrate or layer surfaces
- Layered structure on a 2D/3D substrate/component
- Alloying and dispersing (e.g., hard materials)

Hereby, the nozzle configurations for guiding the powder material play an important role regarding the requested application scenario. Conical ring nozzles provide a small powder focus diameter suitable to establish 0.5-mm width tracks. Another design is denoted as multijet nozzle with a large powder focus to enable melt tracks with a width in the range of 1–3 mm and typically applied laser powers above 1,000 W. This nozzle design is suitable for 3D positioning of the laser and powder injection relative to the building platform. Finally, the lateral nozzle arrangement that enables an efficient powder application is strongly depending on the building and laser scanning direction. The later nozzle design is not suitable for a flexible building up of 3D components.

14.3.3 DEFECTS, STRUCTURES, AND TEXTURES

During laser AM, a huge number of different types of defects can be observed. In the following list, the commonly observed defects are listed and shortly described:

- During solidification, gas bubbles can become trapped in the molten bath, which are caused by excessive stirring of the molten bath, porosity of the powder raw material, or evaporation of alloying elements and can lead to formation of gas pores.
- Rapid solidification of the weld pool can lead to trapped porosity as the gas does not have enough time to exit the weld pool.
- Contraction cavities, so-called balling, can form when isolated pockets of liquid solidify separately from the remaining melt. The contraction stresses during the solidification of the terminal liquid are sufficient to pull the semisolid material apart and create a contraction cavity (Figure 14.8).
- Incorrect surface preparation can lead to contamination of the weld pool, which affects the surface tension and adhesion of the coating to the substrate.
- Laser scan overlap mismatch can result in porosity in the overlap region if the deposit is excessively large as this reduces the contact angle and prevents complete merging of adjacent lines.

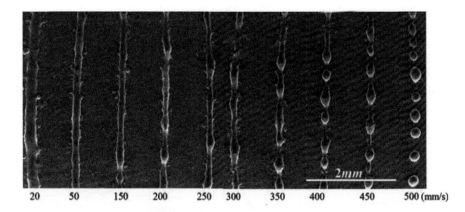

FIGURE 14.8   SEM images showing the balling characteristics of single scan tracks under different laser scan speeds (material: 316-L). Reprinted with permission from Nusser, C., Wehrmann, I., and Willenborg, E. *Physics Procedia*, 12, 462–471, 2011. Copyright 2017, IOP Publishing, Ltd.

- Residual stresses, heat and solidification cracks by volume change or shrinkage due to solidification
- Pore formation due to locally high laser absorption, e.g., at hatch turning points (Figure 14.9a)
- Layer delamination due to heat accumulation and residual stress release

Normally, due to orientation-dependent properties, such as the interface energy between the solid and liquid phase, the crystal growth parallel to heat dissipation would take place in the direction of <001> for metals with a cubic structure, i.e., in the direction of the temperature gradient. This is the direction of crystallization with the greatest growth rate. When the laser is slowly scanned over the surface, a crystalline and columnar-like growth is caused toward the substrate. With increasing laser advance speed, the alignment of the microstructure growth will then be increasingly inclined with respect to the substrate normal. The grain size, on the other hand, essentially depends on the cooling rate. The resulting texture can also be influenced by varying the laser scan filling direction from layer to layer (Figure 14.9a). The fact that the underlying layers can be melted again (Figure 14.9b) creates a new structure with a disruption of the preferred texture alignment.

Another important factor that influences the structure is the Marangoni convection (Figure 14.9b). The Marangoni convection is derived from the temperature dependence of the surface tension of the melt. The Gaussian intensity distribution of the laser causes a temperature profile on the melt. The surface tension depends on the temperature. If the surface tension decreases with increasing temperature, i.e., if it has its minimum in the center of the weld pool, then a movement of the melt toward the edges of the melt pool is caused on the surface. The Marangoni convection thus causes a melting bath turbulence, which in turn influences the texture in the later resolidified material.

Local adjustment of the microstructure and texture can be simply realized by controlling the laser power during the LMD process as shown in Figure 14.10. The average grain size is in the range of 80 μm while applying a low laser power of 400 W, but the grains are less columnar crystalline. The texture is less pronounced with regard to <101> parallel to the building direction (BD). Adjusting the process parameters to higher laser power (1,000 W), on the other hand, causes a significant increase in the grain size, resulting in an average diameter of 235 μm. At the same time, the intensity of the <001> texture in relation to the BD is increased from 1.9 to 3.7. However, the cubic form of the crystals is lost due to the rotation of the scanning direction from layer to

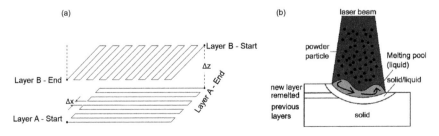

FIGURE 14.9 Process parameters disturbing a preferred texture grow in laser AM. (a) Laser scanning and hatch strategy. (b) Impact of Marangoni convection during laser processing.

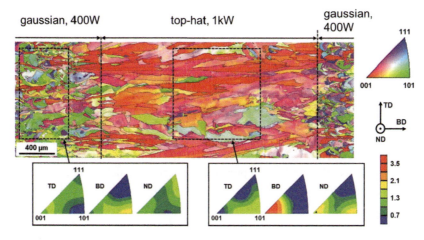

FIGURE 14.10 Microstructure analyses for a LMD produced X2CrNiMo17-12-2 steel sample by applying different laser power. The inverse pole figure mapping reveals that two different types of microstructures were formed. A fine-grained microstructure was obtained for low laser power (400W) while a columnar-grained coarse microstructure was achieved for high laser power (1000W). Also the respective textures in building direction (BD) differ significantly showing a strong <001> intensities for the columnar-grained material and much weaker intensities for the fine-grained regions [Ref. 36].

layer (see Figure 14.9a) in successive layers used in the case of this sample. In the transition areas regarding the change in laser power, no defects such as pores, delamination, or keyholes could be detected as possible indications of insufficient or excessive melting. The transition from the completely globular to the completely columnar crystalline microstructure in the lower area of the sample takes place over a distance of ~400μm and thus takes place over several layers. In contrast, the transition from columnar crystalline to globular microstructure appears to be significantly sharper, with the <001> texture being lost. Complementary hardness mappings confirm the basically very steep transitions between areas of high hardness (400 W) and low hardness (1 kW), whereby differences between the respective transition areas could not be resolved. The competing effects from the solidification parameters (thermal gradient and speed of the solidification front) and epitaxial growth as well as molten bath turbulence associated with Marangoni convection (see Figure 14.9b) certainly play an important role.

14.4 LASER POSTPROCESSING OF ADDITIVE MANUFACTURED PARTS

In this section, laser-based postprocess for improvement of surface quality by roughness reduction, termed laser polishing, and for modification of surface functionalities, named surface functionalization will be introduced with regard to typical process characteristics.

Laser polishing consists of irradiating the part's surface with a laser beam, thus generating a molten layer that is redistributed and resolidified to create a surface with lower roughness [34,35].

As shown in Figure 14.11, a cw laser with an operational wavelength of about 1064 nm scans the surface of the workpiece submitted to laser polishing. Typically, the mean laser spot diameter has a value of 100 μm, which can easily be increased by altering the laser focusing offset. Other process parameters that highly influence the processing outcome are the laser scanning speed, hatch distance, and laser power. Significant surface roughness reduction, from 6.9 to 0.8 μm, was obtained by repeating the laser polishing processing three times with a laser power of about 300 W, scanning speed of about 1,200 mm/s, and hatching distance of about 50 μm for a laser beam with a diameter of 100 μm. It is worth mentioning that the process is also characterized by deep-melted and heat-affected zones (HAZ) with consequent microstructural changes that affect the mechanical properties. Thermal models can be applied for a fast assessment of the dimensions of melted zones and HAZ (Figure 14.12).

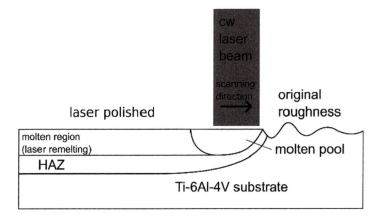

FIGURE 14.11 Schematic of the polishing process on the surface of the additively manufactured Ti-6Al-4V part using the continuous wave (cw) laser beam.

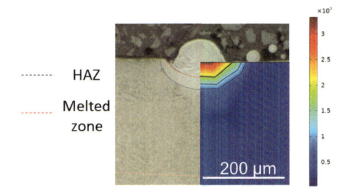

FIGURE 14.12 Comparison of the molten pool and HAZ morphology: cross section of a laser generated melt pool in AM Ti-6Al-4V and numerical simulation of the laser generated temperature field. Reprinted with permission from Solheid, J.S., Mohanty, S., Bayat, M., Wunsch, T., Weidler, P.G., Seifert, H.J., and Pfleging, W., *Journal of Laser Applications*, 32(2), 022019, 2020. Copyright 2020, Laser Institute of America.

The work on modeling the laser treatment process also includes simulations of the mentioned specific features of the laser parameters to predict the melt pool geometry and free surface characteristics to make a comparison with the experimental optimization.

In order to understand the microstructure evolution during laser remelting or heat treatment of titanium and its alloys to be produced in the frame of SLM or LMD processes, the thermal models can also be coupled with metallurgical models to predict the grain size and phase fractions on the assessed HAZ. Finally, experimental studies need to be correlated with the evaluation of material hardness and residual stresses after the laser treatment.

The laser functionalization process consists of modifying the surface of a workpiece to obtain characteristics that will serve different purposes in terms of applications. Ultrafast lasers have been widely used for the functionalization of metallic parts for their versatility in terms of process parameters and highly controllable ablation rates. When compared to cw lasers normally used for laser polishing, the mean laser spot has a reduced diameter with values of about 60 μm, which can also be increased by altering the laser focusing offset but in considerably smaller ranges due to the Rayleigh length. The remaining process parameters that highly influence the processing outcome are the same as in the laser polishing, namely laser scanning speed, hatch distance, and laser power, with the addition of the pulse duration parameter. With this kind of technique, distinct structures can be applied to the surface of the parts, which result in varied behaviors. Two types of structures were investigated in SLM-built Ti-6Al-4V at various stages of the process chain, including after laser polishing, and different functionalities were assessed. The processing parameters adopted were the average laser power of about 4 W, scanning speed of 400 mm/s, pulse duration of around 450 fs, and repetition rate of 1,000 kHz. The resulting structures presented nano-sized ripples and porous topographies and were obtained by repeating the process with the described parameters 1 and 5 times, respectively. For both surfaces, a highly hydrophobic functionality was achieved with contact angles above 100°, while surfaces previously submitted to laser polishing presented a contact angle of around 60° [9].

Due to the current research work, already expertise in the field of laser modification of titanium and its alloys regarding control of biomedical aspects could be achieved [9,36,37]. The proposed laser postprocesses for smoothening and texturing can be applied to ventricular assist devices (VADs), which have the potential to be 3D manufactured by SLM or LMD with improved material properties. The design of one type of centrifugal VAD is presented in Figure 14.13. Based on the results obtained in the laser postprocessing investigations, laser polishing is a suitable technique for the fast smoothening of upper and down shells, while maintaining the desired biocompatibility of titanium and its alloys [9]. Still preserving the biocompatibility feature, laser texturing is a suitable option for processing the surfaces of the rotor, in which hydrophobic characteristics are desired.

For a thorough investigation of the suitability of AM techniques for the manufacturing of VADs, CARoL (cardiac assistant recovery of life) centrifugal blood pumps [38] were printed using a titanium alloy "LaserForm Ti Gr23 (A)" (3D Systems, Leuven) with high strength and biocompatibility. The SLM machine used was a

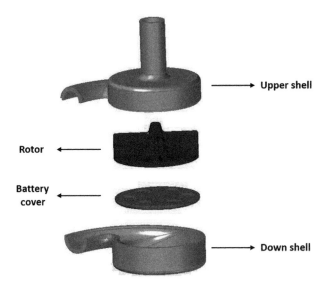

FIGURE 14.13   Exploded view with the main components of CARoL centrifugal VAD.

DMP Flex 350 and the outcome is presented in Figure 14.14. To manufacture the chosen VAD via SLM without altering its design, the abundant use of support structures is necessary due to the occurrence of several overhang areas with critical angles. Even when the limit angle of 45° is obeyed, the use of support structures

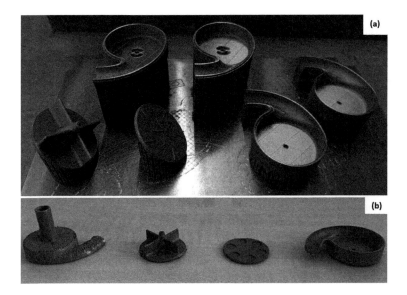

FIGURE 14.14   (a) CARoL VAD on the building platform displaying the supports structures necessary for their production via SLM. (b) CARoL VAD main components after heat treatment and operations for building platform and support structures removal. The rotor and the shell have a diameter of 43.6 mm and 48 mm, respectively.

is justified by the need of dissipating the heat and avoiding the warping that can occur due to the dimension of the part. These support structures must be removed from the parts manually and sometimes with great effort, which affects considerably the resulting surface quality and dimensional accuracy, as shown in Figure 14.14b. Commonly, mechanical operations such as sandblasting, grinding, and machining are adopted as postprocesses, although the use of nonconventional processes has increased significantly over the years.

Hemodynamic tests of the centrifugal blood pumps are going to be performed for the evaluation of the suitability of AM parts and advanced titanium alloys with adjusted material properties and surface functionalities.

14.5 MATERIAL SCREENING

Recently, however, LMD (Figure 14.15a and b) has been developed very successfully as a highly suitable method for high-throughput screening of alloys and at the same time for additive 3D manufacturing of larger components [23–25]. With the LMD process, numerous material variants with a wide variety of chemical compositions and microstructural designs can be combined within a single sample or component.

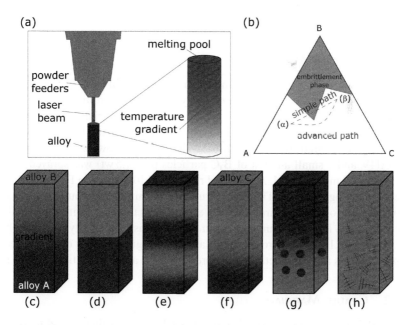

FIGURE 14.15 LMD process for producing of new types of alloys: (a) Schematic view of the LMD process. (b) Schematic view of a ternary phase diagram showing possible metallurgical pathways from one alloy (α) to another alloy (β). Advanced routes avoiding brittle phases are preferred. (c -h) Schematics of some of the different compositionally graded alloys which are possible by applying LMD processes [Ref. 42].

As previously described, the samples/components are built up individually by successive individual layers. Each layer can be individually adjusted in terms of its chemical composition and microstructural characteristics. Only small layer thicknesses of 0.3–0.6 mm are required for the high-resolution analyzes. The LMD process can be automated and carried out quickly in the sense of a high-throughput process. Another very big advantage of the LMD method is that, thanks to the high material deposition rates of up to 1.5 kg/h, large volumes of materials can also be produced in a short time, and therefore larger components can be realized. The methodical advances in LMD control and regulation thus also make additive 3D manufacturing fully accessible. Alloys and metal–ceramic composites (Figure 14.15c–h), which turn out to be particularly suitable for certain applications with the high-throughput method, can be processed into larger components with the same LMD system. This means that the material screening approach can be directly coupled with laser AM for the production of larger components. In order to avoid brittle phases during the LMD process, phase diagrams should be used as guiding maps for the LMD process (Figure 14.15i). The red line in Figure 14.15i indicates the simple approach for moving from one alloy to another by linearly changing the powder composition during LMD. In the presented case, the brittle phase will be crossed, leading to crack formation in the deposited component. To avoid the brittle phase and to achieve a well-designed object with the properties of alloy-end members, the powder composition has to be adjusted during LMD as described by the green line (Figure 14.15i). The following three are the examples of material screening presented, namely the development of composite materials, graded alloys, and HEAs.

14.5.1 COMPOSITE MATERIALS

Ti6Al4V is one of the most established titanium alloys in AM. For achieving an increase in the mechanical strength, especially for use in environments with elevated temperatures up to 500°C, the development of composite materials based on Ti6Al4V matrix with embedded TiB_2 and TiC was investigated by using LMD [40]. For this purpose, a powder mixture (Figure 14.16a)—the so-called powder blend—consisting of Ti6Al4V and a small amount of B_4C particles (0.5–1.5 wt) was sprayed into the laser-generated melting pool. A chemical reaction as illustrated in Figure 14.1b took place by forming TiB and TiC microstructures within the titanium alloy matrix. In comparison to the standard Ti6Al4V alloy, a severe grain refinement could be achieved finally, leading to an increase in the modulus of elasticity and microhardness (Figure 14.16b). The cross-section analysis (Figure 14.16c) of the generated composite shows no imperfections like pores or cracks along the entire building path.

14.5.2 GRADED MATERIALS

In the LMD process, powders of different particle size distribution and topography are used, each of which also requires different nozzle concepts (e.g., annular gaps and bores). The use of small powder sizes in the range below 100 μm, e.g., 40–90 μm, is recommended for creating gradient layers or material alloys of varying compositions. The powder flow is in general guided coaxially to the laser beam.

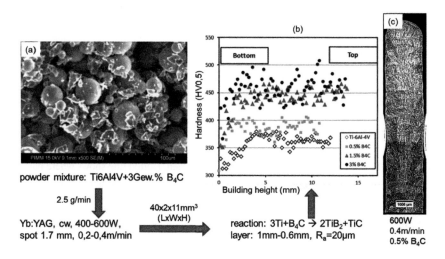

FIGURE 14.16 Process sequence for LMD fabrication of Ti6Al4V-B4C composite with outer dimension of 40x2x11 mm³ (length x width x height). Typical Yb:YAG laser and process parameters are illustrated (laser power, spot size, scan speed). Single layer thicknesses are in the range of 0.6-1 mm. (a) SEM picture of Ti-6Al-4V / B_4C (3wt.%) powder blend. (b) Microhardness values of LMD composite material as function of building height and B_4C content in powder blend (c) Cross-sections of manufactured walls for 0.5wt.% B_4C in powder blend. Reprinted with permission from Tang, Y., Zhang, Y., and Liu, Y., *Journal of Alloys and Compounds*, 727, 196–204, 2017. Copyright 2016, Elsevier.

In the current state of research in the field of laser AM of titanium alloys, the main topic is the evolution and determination of grain texture with its impact on mechanical properties, such as hardness, ductility, yield strength, and elongation at fracture [41]. Numerical simulation can be used to describe the grain growth during the laser AM process. The grains are found to be elongated and columnar after solidification which gives rise to anisotropic properties [42]. For as deposited titanium alloys, defined phase composition transformations could be observed along the deposition direction as well as a change in microhardness as the function of structure height [43]. During laser processing, low or high cooling rates up to 10^7 K/s can be used to design the surface but also the entire material properties along three dimensions. This type of functional grading based on the microstructure control for every single layer can be coupled with a change in composition and phase along the BD.

A prominent LMD example for the connection of steel alloys with different properties is a combination of 304L stainless steel (Fe68Cr20Ni10Mn1Si0.3) with Inconel 625 (IN625) [3]. While 304L is of lower cost and mass, IN625 shows enhanced mechanical strength and corrosion resistance at elevated temperatures. Both of these materials seem to be ideal for establishing tools with graded composition due to the fact that both alloys have a face-centered cubic crystal structure from melt to room temperature without allotropic phase transformations. Furthermore, the main components of the alloys such as Fe, Cr, and Ni show good solubility. During the LMD production of the graded component (Figure 14.17a and b), the powder blend composition containing 304L and IN625 particles was gradually changed along 24 layers (Figure 14.17a).

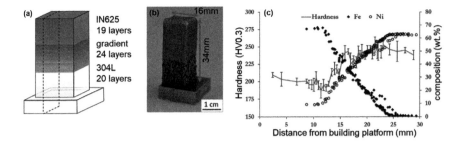

FIGURE 14.17 (a) Schematic of gradient alloy specimen. Dotted line shows where part was cut for subsequent elemental and hardness measurements. (b) Photograph of specimen after LMD fabrication. (c) Microhardness of the gradient alloy overlaid on Fe and Ni composition. Reprinted with permission from Carroll, B. E., Otis, R. A., Borgonia, J. P., Suh, J.-O., Dillon, R. P., Shapiro, A. A., Hofmann, D. C., Liu, Z.-K., and Beese, A. M., *Acta Materialia*, 108, 46–54, 2016. Copyright 2016, Elsevier.

Twenty layers of pure 304L were deposited onto the building platform and after the graded section of 24 layers, pure IN625 was deposited for 19 layers, each layer with a thickness of about 500 μm and a total component height of 34 mm (Figure 14.17b). The Fe and Ni composition gradually changed as expected (Figure 14.17c) and an increase in hardness of about 50 HV above the manufacturer's specifications of the starting material could be achieved. However, a slight drop in hardness at the beginning of the graded zone could be detected which is due to crack formation related to the formation of monocarbides (containing Mo and Nb) at the transition zone from the 304L to the gradient. It is obvious as described earlier that a simple linear change in powder blend composition is in general not an appropriate procedure for establishing graded materials and a controlled bypassing of possible brittle compositions becomes necessary (see Figure 14.15i). As shown in Figure 14.17c, a slight decrease in hardness is also observed in the upper range of the component which is caused by enforced grain growth by heat accumulation along the tip. The maximum hardness was achieved in the center of the gradient zone (Figure 14.17c).

14.5.3 HIGH ENTROPY ALLOYS

Compared to the classic concept of single-base alloys, such as steels or Ni super-alloys, there has been an intensive search for new alloys based on the concept of HEAs for around 15 years. According to this concept, several elements are mixed together in almost equal proportions. The term entropy alloy is derived from the high-configuration entropy resulting from the random mixing of the elements in the alloys. When developing alloys, researchers focused on the corners of a phase diagram to develop a conventional alloy. These alloys only take up a small part of the design space in the phase diagram. The focus at HEAs has now been shifted to the central region. There is still no uniformly recognized definition of HEAs [44]. Originally, alloys with high entropy were defined as alloys that consist of at least five elements with an atomic fraction of 5–35 atomic percent. However, another definition states that for being denoted as HEAs it is necessary that those alloys only

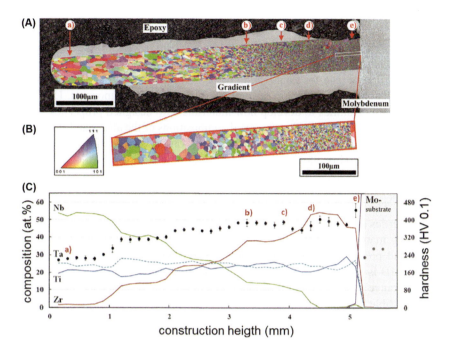

FIGURE 14.18 Top: SEM image with an overlaid color-coded grain orientation map of a cross-section of a LMD produced structure (building platform on the right side is made of Mo). The colours in the grain orientation map indicate the crystal orientations (bcc unit cell) parallel to the building direction (BD) displayed in the stereographic triangle (middle left). Bottom: Composition gradient and respective micro-hardness along building direction. Reprinted with permission from Dobbelstein, H., Gurevich, E. L., George, E. P., Ostendorf, A., and Laplanche, G., *Additive Manufacturing*, 25, 252–262, 2019. Copyright 2019, Elsevier.

form mixed crystals without intermetallic phases which reflects the general meaning of providing high entropy. Therefore, HEAs with less than five elements can be created. But why dealing with HEAs? The main reason is the superior mechanical performance at elevated temperatures in comparison to the well-known steels and superalloys [44].

In situ alloying by LMD provides unique prospects regarding the development of new and advanced HEAs as shown by recent research activities [4,45,46]. Besides the formation of new HEAs by establishing a defined composition [46], it is also possible to realize HEAs with graded composition as shown for the very first time in 2019 by Dobbelstein et al. [45]. In that work, they synthesized TiZrNbTa HEA by varying the concentration of Nb and Zr along the BD as shown in Figure 14.18. The compositionally graded material was built by LMD using five powder blends and by changing the chemical composition from $Ti_{25}Zr_{50}Nb_0Ta_{25}$ at building platform to $Ti_{25}Zr_0Nb_{50}Ta_{25}$. Due to the formation of secondary phases, a solid solution strengthening could be induced, resulting in a microhardness increase with the proportion of Zr (Figure 14.18C). The increase in grain size at the end of construction is again related to heat accumulation which is increased with increasing structure height.

14.6 CONCLUSION

With laser AM, i.e., SLM and LMD, extensive research work on the development of 3D components for different types of applications was performed. While SLM is the most appropriate for establishing devices with high accuracy as required for the development and production of implants such as VAD components, LMD provides new opportunities to develop new materials with designed properties such as graded materials or HEAs. The chemical compositions of the alloys and the process of engineering manufacturing conditions can be varied very flexibly within a wide parameter range. This allows phase and microstructures as well as local chemical compositions and the resulting physical and mechanical properties to be researched efficiently. In addition, ceramic powders can be introduced to produce composite materials. The chemical compositions, the microstructures, and the resulting material properties can be changed in a controlled manner from layer to layer. The most promising materials for the respective applications can thus be efficiently determined and processed with the LMD system into larger, complex-shaped components. LMD is a powerful tool to produce 3D components if the required accuracy is in the range of 500 µm and if surface finishing through subsequent postprocessing is possible. Laser postprocessing via laser polishing and laser functionalization were presented to be a versatile tool for the development of biocompatible surfaces. Similarly, the combination of SLM and subsequent laser surface postprocessing is a powerful approach for the development of advanced and long operational lifetime VAD devices.

ACKNOWLEDGMENTS

This work has received funding from the European Union's Programme PAM2 within Horizon 2020 under grant agreement No. 721383.

REFERENCES

1. Kok, Y., X.P. Tan, P. Wang, M. Nai, N.H. Loh, E. Liu, and S.B. Tor, Anisotropy and heterogeneity of microstructure and mechanical properties in metal additive manufacturing: A critical review. *Materials & Design*, 2018. 139: pp. 565–586.
2. Weng, F., C. Chen, and H. Yu, Research status of laser cladding on titanium and its alloys: A review. *Materials & Design*, 2014. 58: pp. 412–425.
3. Carroll, B.E., R.A. Otis, J.P. Borgonia, J.-O. Suh, R.P. Dillon, A.A. Shapiro, D.C. Hofmann, Z.-K. Liu, and A.M. Beese, Functionally graded material of 304L stainless steel and inconel 625 fabricated by directed energy deposition: Characterization and thermodynamic modeling. *Acta Materialia*, 2016. 108: pp. 46–54.
4. Melia, M.A., S.R. Whetten, R. Puckett, M. Jones, M.J. Heiden, N. Argibay, and A.B. Kustas, High-throughput additive manufacturing and characterization of refractory high entropy alloys. *Applied Materials Today*, 2020. 19: p. 100560.
5. Brenne, F. and T. Niendorf, Load distribution and damage evolution in bending and stretch dominated Ti-6Al-4V cellular structures processed by selective laser melting. *International Journal of Fatigue*, 2019. 121: pp. 219–228.
6. Solheid, J., H.J. Seifert, and W. Pfleging, Laser surface modification and polishing of additive manufactured metallic parts. *Procedia Cirp*, 2018. 74: pp. 280–284.

7. Solheid, J., A. Elkaseer, T. Wunsch, A. Charles, H.J. Seifert, and W. Pfleging. Effect of process parameters on surface texture generated by laser polishing of additively manufactured Ti-6Al-4V. in U. Klotzbach, A. Watanabe, and R. Kling (Eds), *Laser-Based Micro-and Nanoprocessing XIV*, 11268. 2020. International Society for Optics and Photonics: Bellingham, WA.

8. Solheid, J.S., S. Mohanty, M. Bayat, T. Wunsch, P.G. Weidler, H.J. Seifert, and W. Pfleging, Laser polishing of additively manufactured Ti-6Al-4V: Microstructure evolution and material properties. *Journal of Laser Applications*, 2020. 32(2): p. 022019.

9. Solheid, J.S., T. Wunsch, V. Trouillet, S. Weigel, T. Scharnweber, H.J. Seifert, and W. Pfleging, Two-step laser post-processing for the surface functionalization of additively manufactured Ti-6Al-4V Parts. *Materials*, 2020. 13(21): p. 4872.

10. Whitaker, M., The history of 3D printing in healthcare. *The Bulletin of the Royal College of Surgeons of England*, 2014. 96(7): pp. 228–229.

11. Kawata, S., H.-B. Sun, T. Tanaka, and K. Takada, Finer features for functional microdevices. *Nature*, 2001. 412(6848): pp. 697–698.

12. Jackson, R., S. Curran, P. Chambon, B. Post, L. Love, R. Wagner, B. Ozpineci, M. Chinthavali, M. Starke, and J. Green. Overview of the oak ridge national laboratory advanced manufacturing integrated energy demonstration project: Case study of additive manufacturing as a tool to enable rapid innovation in integrated energy systems. in *ASME 2016 International Mechanical Engineering Congress and Exposition,* Phoenix, Ariz. 2016. American Society of Mechanical Engineers Digital Collection.

13. Dai, Q., China and the next production revolution. in *The Next Production Revolution*. 2017. OECD: Paris, pp. 397–432.

14. Sun, C. and G. Shang, On application of metal additive manufacturing. *World Journal of Engineering and Technology*, 2020. 9(1): pp. 194–202.

15. Kumar, L.J. and C.K. Nair, Current trends of additive manufacturing in the aerospace industry, in L.J. Kumar, P.M. Pandey, and D.I. Wimpenny (Eds), *Advances in 3D Printing & Additive Manufacturing Technologies*. 2017, Springer: Berlin, Germany, pp. 39–54.

16. Hipolite, W. Beijing University unveils enormous 3D printed aircraft frames & more, created with SLS technology. *The Voice of 3D Printing/Additive Manufacturing 2017*. Available from: https://3dprint.com/82169/3d-printed-aircraft-parts/.

17. Liu, R., Z. Wang, T. Sparks, F. Liou, and J. Newkirk, Aerospace applications of laser additive manufacturing, in *Laser Additive Manufacturing*. Milan Brandt (ed.). 2017, Elsevier: Amsterdam, pp. 351–371.

18. Seabra, M., J. Azevedo, A. Araújo, L. Reis, E. Pinto, N. Alves, R. Santos, and J.P. Mortágua, Selective laser melting (SLM) and topology optimization for lighter aerospace componentes. *Procedia Structural Integrity*, 2016. 1: pp. 289–296.

19. Gibson, I., D.W. Rosen, and B. Stucker, Sheet lamination processes, in *Additive Manufacturing Technologies*. 2010, Springer: Boston, MA, pp. 223–252.

20. Yang, L., K. Hsu, B. Baughman, D. Godfrey, F. Medina, M. Menon, and S. Wiener, Introduction to additive manufacturing, in *Additive Manufacturing of Metals: The Technology, Materials, Design and Production*. 2017. Springer International Publishing: Cham, pp. 1–31.

21. Zäh, M.F. and S. Lutzmann, Modelling and simulation of electron beam melting. *Production Engineering*, 2010. 4(1): pp. 15–23.

22. SLM 280. Robust selective laser melting: Multiple lasers and process stability for demanding applications, 2021. Available from: www.slm-solutions.com/fileadmin/Content/Machines/SLM_R_280_Web.pdf.

23. Hofmann, D.C., S. Roberts, R. Otis, J. Kolodziejska, R.P. Dillon, J.-O. Suh, A.A. Shapiro, Z.-K. Liu, and J.-P. Borgonia, Developing gradient metal alloys through radial deposition additive manufacturing. *Scientific Reports*, 2014. 4(1): pp. 1–8.

24. Haase, C., F. Tang, M.B. Wilms, A. Weisheit, and B. Hallstedt, Combining thermodynamic modeling and 3D printing of elemental powder blends for high-throughput investigation of high-entropy alloys: Towards rapid alloy screening and design. *Materials Science and Engineering: A*, 2017. 688: pp. 180–189.

25. Knoll, H., S. Ocylok, A. Weisheit, H. Springer, E. Jägle, and D. Raabe, Combinatorial alloy design by laser additive manufacturing. *Steel Research International*, 2017. 88(8): p. 1600416.

26. Hoffmann, P. and R. Dierken, Laser technology for tool production: development of laser surface treatment–system technology and examples of application. *Laser Technik Journal*, 2018. 15(3): pp. 32–35.

27. Mahamood, R.M., E.T. Akinlabi, M. Shukla, and S. Pityana, Scanning velocity influence on microstructure, microhardness and wear resistance performance of laser deposited Ti6Al4V/TiC composite. *Materials & Design*, 2013. 50: pp. 656–666.

28. Lu, L., Y. Shi, C. Xu, G. Xu, J. Wang, and B. Xu, The influence of pulse width and energy on temperature field in metal irradiated by ultrashort-pulsed laser. *Physics Procedia*, 2012. 32: pp. 39–47.

29. Gattass, R.R. and E. Mazur, Femtosecond laser micromachining in transparent materials. *Nature Photonics*, 2008. 2(4): pp. 219–225.

30. Sugioka, K., Ultrafast laser processing of glass down to the nano-scale. Springer *Series in Materials Science*, 2010. 130: pp. 279–293.

31. Sugioka, K., Y. Hanada, and K. Midorikawa, Three-dimensional femtosecond laser micromachining of photosensitive glass for biomicrochips. *Laser & Photonics Reviews*, 2010. 4(3): pp. 386–400.

32. Li, R., J. Liu, Y. Shi, L. Wang, and W. Jiang, Balling behavior of stainless steel and nickel powder during selective laser melting process. *The International Journal of Advanced Manufacturing Technology*, 2012. 59(9): pp. 1025–1035.

33. Niendorf, T., S. Leuders, A. Riemer, F. Brenne, T. Tröster, H.A. Richard, and D. Schwarze, Functionally graded alloys obtained by additive manufacturing. *Advanced Engineering Materials*, 2014. 16(7): pp. 857–861.

34. Nüsser, C., I. Wehrmann, and E. Willenborg, Influence of intensity distribution and pulse duration on laser micro polishing. *Physics Procedia*, 2011. 12: pp. 462–471.

35. Temmler, A., E. Willenborg, and K. Wissenbach. Laser polishing. in G. Hennig, X. Xu, B. Gu, Y. Nakata (Eds), *Laser Applications in Microelectronic and Optoelectronic Manufacturing (LAMOM) XVII*, 23–26. 2012. International Society for Optics and Photonics: Bellingham, WA.

36. Kumari, R., T. Scharnweber, W. Pfleging, H. Besser, and J.D. Majumdar, Laser surface textured titanium alloy (Ti–6Al–4V)–Part II–Studies on bio-compatibility. *Applied Surface Science*, 2015. 357: p. 750–758.

37. Kumari, R., W. Pfleging, H. Besser, and J.D. Majumdar, Microstructure and corrosion behavior of laser induced periodic patterned titanium based alloy. *Optics & Laser Technology*, 2019. 116: pp. 196–213.

38. Marquiori, D.S., P.C. Florentino, S.Y. Araki, I.K. Fujita, R.L.D.O. Basso, A. Babetto, B.C. Bonse, J.R. Moro, T. Leao, A.J. Andrade, and E.G.P. Bock, Tribology and crystallinity in pivot bearings of ventricular assist devices. *The Academic Society Journal*, 2020. 4(1): pp. 52–62.

39. Hofmann, D.C., J. Kolodziejska, S. Roberts, R. Otis, R.P. Dillon, J.-O. Suh, Z.-K. Liu, and J.-P. Borgonia, Compositionally graded metals: A new frontier of additive manufacturing. *Journal of Materials Research*, 2014. 29(17): pp. 1899–1910.

40. Pouzet, S., P. Peyre, C. Gorny, O. Castelnau, T. Baudin, F. Brisset, C. Colin, and P. Gadaud, Additive layer manufacturing of titanium matrix composites using the direct metal deposition laser process. *Materials Science and Engineering: A*, 2016. 677: pp. 171–181.

41. Li, G.-C., J. Li, X.-J. Tian, X. Cheng, B. He, and H.-M. Wang, Microstructure and properties of a novel titanium alloy Ti-6Al-2V-1.5 Mo-0.5 Zr-0.3 Si manufactured by laser additive manufacturing. *Materials Science and Engineering: A*, 2017. 684: pp. 233–238.

42. Dezfoli, A.R.A., W.-S. Hwang, W.-C. Huang, and T.-W. Tsai, Determination and controlling of grain structure of metals after laser incidence: Theoretical approach. *Scientific Reports*, 2017. 7(1): pp. 1–11.

43. Tang, Y., Y. Zhang, and Y. Liu, Numerical and experimental investigation of laser additive manufactured Ti2AlNb-based alloy. *Journal of Alloys and Compounds*, 2017. 727: pp. 196–204.

44. Ye, Y., Q. Wang, J. Lu, C. Liu, and Y. Yang, High-entropy alloy: Challenges and prospects. *Materials Today*, 2016. 19(6): pp. 349–362.

45. Dobbelstein, H., E.L. Gurevich, E.P. George, A. Ostendorf, and G. Laplanche, Laser metal deposition of compositionally graded TiZrNbTa refractory high-entropy alloys using elemental powder blends. *Additive Manufacturing*, 2019. 25: pp. 252–262.

46. Dobbelstein, H., E.L. Gurevich, E.P. George, A. Ostendorf, and G. Laplanche, Laser metal deposition of a refractory TiZrNbHfTa high-entropy alloy. *Additive Manufacturing*, 2018. 24: pp. 386–390.

15 Biosensors

Bruno Jesus dos Santos and
Henrique Stelzer Nogueira
Instituto Federal de São Paulo

CONTENTS

15.1 INTRODUCTION

With the increase in the duration of left ventricular assist device (LVAD) support, attention is shifting to improve patients' quality of life. An important step is the optimization of the assistance provided with LVAD, which depends on the complex interaction between patients' individual pathophysiology and the characteristics of the pump. On the patient side, ventricular contractility and volume status, together with pulmonary and systemic vascular properties, are important factors. On the other hand, the characteristics of the pump are quantified by pressure–flow relations dependent on speed (Uriel et al., 2016).

According to Uriel et al. (2019), although it is well established that LVADs significantly improve the longevity and quality of life in patients with advanced heart failure (HF), only a small percentage of potentially eligible HF patients receive an LVAD, and it is believed that this is mainly due to the high rate of complications and readmissions that limit the acceptance of this form of therapy between patients and referring physicians.

In the recent study of the most modern ventricular assist devices (VADs) on the market MOMENTUM 3 (multicenter study of MagLev Technology in Patients Undergoing Mechanical Circulatory Support Therapy With HeartMate® 3), there were 2.1 hospitalizations per patient-year, with a 10% incidence of stroke, 27% of

DOI: 10.1201/9781003138358-17

297

gastrointestinal bleeding, 24% of ventricular arrhythmias (VAs), and 24% of drive-line infections (Mehra et al., 2018a–c; Uriel et al., 2019).

The most current guidelines of the International Society for Heart and Lung Transplantation for implanted patients focus on increasing the quality of life of patients by reducing the occurrence of adverse events throughout the entire support. The conventional clinical protocol for adjusting the speed of rotation of the LVAD pump based only on adequate decompression of the left ventricle and intermittent opening of the aortic valve (ramp test) is not sufficient to prevent the occurrence of neurological adverse events according to data provided by INTERMACS; to this end, clinical studies point to the need to also take into account variations in hemodynamic data (Uriel et al., 2019).

15.2 IMPLANTABLE SENSORS DEDICATED FOR USE IN TREATMENT WITH VADs

To improve the flow optimization capacity of LVADs, it is required to implement an active flow adjustment scheme that can automatically adapt and adjust the pump speed based on demand, without requiring manual inputs. For this, it is necessary to identify a measurable control variable that can be used to guarantee the ideal perfusion, avoiding the risk of overcoming the venous return. This strategy can allow the development of a Frank–Starling type controller, which can allow a true physiological adjustment of the flow of LVADs. To this end, several physiological control systems for LVADs were developed, each with different control objectives (Tchantchaleishvili et al., 2017).

The work by Pauls et al. (2016) aimed to rigorously evaluate several physiological control strategies previously presented in the literature under identical conditions during *in vitro* simulations in a circulation simulation circuit. This study investigated the ability of each control system to improve LVAD's preload and afterload sensitivities, avoid ventricular suction, and prevent pulmonary congestion during vascular resistance and simulated postural changes. The eight physiological control strategies reported in the literature that were validated in this study are:

- Constant inlet pressure controller (CIP), whose objective is to keep the left ventricular end-diastolic pressure (LVEDP) constant (Bullister et al., 2002);
- Constant differential pressure controller (ΔP), whose objective is to maintain the mean pressure difference between the left ventricle and the aorta close to a specified reference differential pressure (ΔP_{ref}) (Giridharan and Skliar, 2003);
- Controller of constant aortic pressure and differential pressure (AoP/ΔP), with two control objectives, whose main control objective is to keep the aortic pressure constant at a defined value, while the secondary control objective is to maintain the differential pressure of the pump ΔP constant in a defined value (Wu et al., 2004);
- Constant flow controller (CQ), which aims to maintain the pump flow at a predefined reference flow rate (Casas et al., 2007);
- Constant afterload impedance controller (CAI), which uses a linear relationship between LVEDP (a preload measurement) and the target flow of LVAD to maintain a constant afterload impedance, thus imitating the Starling relationship between flow and preload (Moscato et al., 2010);

- Starling LVEDP controller (S-LVEDP), which adjusts the speed of the LVAD pump to achieve a flow rate defined according to the preload (represented by LVEDP) (Stevens et al., 2014);
- Starling pulsatility controller (SP), which defines a target flow rate as a function of preload using LVAD flow pulsatility (difference between the maximum and minimum flow rate during each cardiac cycle) as a substitute for preload (Gaddum et al., 2014); and
- LVAD's inlet cannula (IC) compliance controller, this being a flexible section of tubing placed at the LVAD inlet to passively restrict the inner diameter as the preload decreases, thereby increasing the resistance of the circuit and decreasing the flow of the LVAD to avoid ventricular suction (Gregory et al., 2012).

The work by Pauls et al. (2016) demonstrated that of the eight control strategies tested, four (IC compliance, CIP, CAI, and S-LVEDP) prevented ventricular suction events during all changes in pulmonary vascular resistance and systemic vascular resistance and during passive postural change, increasing the preload sensitivity and decreasing the afterload sensitivity of the LVAD. While IC compliance responded similarly to the constant speed mode during exercise simulations, active control systems capable of increasing the speed of the LVAD (CIP, CAI, and S-LVEDP) reduced the LV systolic work when compared to other control systems and the pump running in constant speed mode. Of all the physiological control systems evaluated in this study, the three active control systems dependent on LVEDP as a substitute for preload (CIP, CAI, and S-LVEDP) performed better in all experiments. These results were later confirmed in the work by Petrou et al. (2018).

Pauls et al. (2016) point out in their study that despite the promising results found in physiological control, one of the limitations of the active control systems evaluated is the dependence on pressure and flow sensors. In the original works (AoP/ΔP, CQ, and CAI), flow and pressure estimation strategies were used based on the LVAD power variables (current, voltage) due to the good correlation between power and the torque of motors used in this application (Wu et al., 2004; Casas et al., 2007; Moscato et al., 2010). However, estimators, particularly flow estimators used in clinics, have proved to be inaccurate in some cases (Slaughter et al., 2010), so estimators have been deliberately omitted and sensors have been used in the study by Pauls et al. (2016) to compare the merits of the control strategy alone, without the risk of errors introduced by inaccurate estimators.

The need to develop sensors to provide physiological control of VAD was also pointed out in the literature review work by Tchantchaleishvili et al. (2017), where of the ten different strategies for physiological control of VAD described in the literature, five of them require the use of sensors to be clinically applicable, being:

- A long-lasting implantable pressure sensor for the constant flow strategy (volume decompression) based on LVEDP (Guyton, 1955);
- One long-term implantable pressure sensor and one flow sensor for the constant flow strategy based on the pressure of the left atrium (Salamonsen et al., 2011; Stevens et al., 2011);

- A long-term implantable pressure sensor for the constant flow strategy based on LV volume (Ochsner et al., 2014);
- Long-lasting pressure and volume sensor for the constant flow strategy based on the LVED pressure–volume ratio (Laird, 1976; Jacob, 1989; Levin et al., 1995; Heerdt et al., 2000; Klotz et al., 2006);
- An implantable long-term pressure sensor and a flow sensor for the constant pressure head (pulsatility) strategy based on pulsatility ratio (Choi et al., 2007; Salamonsen et al., 2012; Bakouri et al., 2014; Gaddum et al., 2014); and
- Two long-term implantable pressure sensors for the constant pressure head strategy based on the constant mean pressure difference between the aorta and the left atrium (Waters et al., 1999; Giridharan and Skliar, 2003; Giridharan et al., 2002, 2004).

As pointed out by Schima et al. (1992), at the beginning of the research on VAD controllers designed to work in harmony with the physiological system, commercial sensors were not reliable enough for presenting severe failures due to the aggressive interaction environment of the physiological system, instigating closed loop control and being able to take patients to a critical state of health, due to such a problematic scenario, the variables of VAD's pump motor (voltage, current, and rotation) were used to the greatest extent possible to estimate the hemodynamic state variables necessary to control the device, and many researchers have worked on control techniques for various types of VADs based on the use of models for estimating hemodynamic variables (Tchantchaleishvili et al., 2017). However, it has been proven that the estimators lack robustness and precision for clinical use (Petrou et al., 2018).

In general, in physiological control the farther from the LV the "substitute" is measured, the less accurate it is (Tchantchaleishvili et al., 2017):

> central venous pressure <right atrial pressure <pulmonary artery pressure (PAP) < pulmonary capillary wedge pressure (PCWP) <left atrial pressure <LVEDP.

A precise means to remotely and frequently assess cardiopulmonary filling pressures and flows in patients with LVADs using sensors can advance control systems toward more physiological control (Tchantchaleishvili et al., 2017).

15.3 IMPLANTABLE SENSOR APPLICATIONS

In the review work carried out by Tchantchaleishvili et al. (2017), implantable sensors are classified into two types:

- Passive implantable sensors (Fonseca et al., 2006; Friyz et al., 2010; Abraham et al., 2011; Hubbert et al., 2017) and
- Battery-operated implantable sensors (Magalski et al., 2002; Hoppe et al., 2009).

Passive implantable sensors are resonant devices capable of detecting physical properties in inaccessible locations, without the need to embark on a power source. These devices are flexible and can be rolled or folded into compact forms, suitable for delivery to the body via a catheter (Fonseca et al., 2006). Potential problems with these devices include deviation from monitoring, less accuracy over time, and thrombus formation (Friyz et al., 2010).

A clinical study with 12 patients using the CardioMEMS sensor in a scientific research phase (St. Jude Medical Inc., St. Paul, MN) showed a good correlation ($r^2 = 0.88$) of the pressure readings of the diastolic pulmonary artery between the implanted sensor and the Swan-Ganz catheter (Edwards Lifesciences, Irvine, CA), but only 60 days later, the correlation was significantly reduced ($r^2 = 0.48$) (Verdejo et al., 2007).

Implantable monitoring systems that operate on batteries despite the intrinsic problems associated with this technology (toxicity, depletion, and larger dimensions) have the advantage of less deviation in measurement over time. For the ImPressure direct PAP monitoring system (Boston Scientific Inc., Natick, MA), the pressure monitoring after 6 months was almost identical to that obtained simultaneously by the Millar catheter (Millar Instruments, Houston, TX) (Hoppe et al., 2009).

Another example of a battery-operated implantable sensor is the chronic implantable hemodynamic monitor (Medtronic Inc., Minneapolis); it is similar to a modified pacemaker and, in addition to a pressure sensor, it has a piezoelectric activity sensor similar to those used in pacemakers adaptive to frequency. The device allows continuous recording of heart rate, patient activity levels, and right ventricular (RV) systolic, RV diastolic, and estimated PAP (Magalski et al., 2002).

Systems based on extra-arterial pressure sensors are investigated due to the lower (Potkay, 2008): (i) risk of blood clotting; (ii) deviation from the measured outlet pressure; and (iii) blood clotting. In this strategy, pressure is measured indirectly through the arterial wall: a cuff is wrapped around the artery and used to detect the expansion and contraction of the vessel.

In the work of Ziaie and Najafi (2001), an extra-arterial blood pressure sensor was manufactured. The micromachined silicone capacitive pressure sensor was incorporated into a titanium clamp ($10 \times 6.5 \times 3$ mm) together with the integrated electronics. The device had a resolution of 0.5 mmHg. In the work by Cong et al. (2010), a clamp prototype ($5 \times 2 \times 0.1$ mm) of soft biocompatible rubber filled with a low-viscosity biocompatible liquid was developed. The implantable system dissipates around 300 µW, provided by an external adaptive power supply by radiofrequency (RF). The concept was verified *in vitro* with the cuff wrapped around a simulated artery and *in vivo* in laboratory rats, showing promising results (Cong et al., 2010).

A solution for the development of sensors for VAD is to incorporate it in the cannulas of the device. In the work of Bullister et al. (2001) and Fritz et al. (2010), pressure sensors are developed with this strategy, where a pressure-sensitive diaphragm is designed to be an integral part of a titanium tube to be positioned in the VAD cannula. For transduction, strain gauges (voltage meters by reference) then at the edges of the thin diaphragm sensitive to pressure variation to detect variations in blood pressure in the form of a difference in tension. However, in this strategy, losses are associated between the physical connection of the extensometers and the diaphragm, establishing a low sensitivity (1 μV/V/mmHg). The deviation of the sensors over time was investigated *in vitro* in both studies, in the work of Bullister et al. (2001) was considered low (1.4–2 mmHg/year), and in the work by Fritz et al. (2010) suffered a very large deviation (−180 to 140 mmHg), attributed to the aging of the connection between the extensometers and the diaphragm.

In the work by Saito et al. (2008), a micromachined sensor was packaged in a cylindrical capsule filled with silicone oil, which was sealed with a thin segmented polyurethane film (thickness around 50 μm). Only the polyurethane film was in contact with the blood flow. The total package has external dimensions of 11 by 12 mm. The sensor was tested *in vivo* with a deviation of 24 mmHg for a period of 5 months (Wei et al., 2008).

In the work by Tortora et al. (2015), a physiological VAD controller is presented based on the acquisition of continuous parameters of pressure and flow sensors implanted in the VAD cannula and provided by noninvasive wearable devices. The MagIC and Winpack wearables provide data on heart rate (electrocardiogram derivation), blood oxygenation (oximetry), temperature (resistance variation), and patient activity (triaxial accelerometer) (Tortora et al., 2015).

The TitanLAP® monitoring system (ISS Inc., Ypsilanti, MI) is an implantable microelectromechanical pressure sensor (MEMS) that has wireless communication with an external monitor for online monitoring of left atrial pressure (LAP). It can be inserted during the implantation of an LVAD, taking >15 minutes to the surgical procedure. The system comprises two main parts: a passive implantable telemetric sensor and an external reading system (Hubbert et al., 2017).

The implantable device consists of a polyether-ether-ketone (PEEK) anchor and a cylindrical probe with a pressure sensor placed inside the anchor. The probe contains a miniature MEMS, along with custom electronics and a telemetry antenna. There are four different lengths for the implantable device, ranging between 18 and 30 mm. The implant can be fixed in the correct position with sutures through four small holes in the flat upper part of the anchor (Hubbert et al., 2017).

Using RF magnetic telemetry, the external reading system transmits energy to and communicates with the implantable device. The RF interface is obtained with a very low power, many times less than commercial RF scanners. Wireless communications include detailed heart pressure waveforms and implant information (Hubbert et al., 2017). Patient data are stored and transmitted at the same time to a central server, where clinicians are able to quickly access and assess potentially dangerous hemodynamic conditions (Hubbert et al., 2017).

In the clinical use of the TitanLAP® monitoring system, the correlation coefficients were 0.99 for LAP, pump speed, LV volume, and left atrial diameter in two patients for 10 weeks (Hubbert et al., 2015). In addition to instantaneous filling pressure monitoring, other parameters on which the TitanLAP® monitoring system has shown benefits include early buffer detection; rapid and effective adaptation and adjustment of drugs; arrhythmia detection; and decreased duration of hypotension, anuria, and oliguria during ICU stay (Hubbert et al., 2015).

The TitanLAP® monitoring system has been shown to successfully capture normal pressure waves (mean LAP of 14.2 mmHg) as well as abnormal pressure waves (an increase in filling pressure corresponding to 27.6 mmHg demonstrated during home monitoring, suggestive of a thrombus in the LVAD in an asymptomatic patient).

Given an early warning in the monitoring of the pressure sensor, LVAD sound, and laboratory markers consistent with a thrombus pump, the patient was accepted for prophylactic surgery to replace the LVAD, demonstrating a thrombus in the LVAD.

In this real patient example, the TitanLAP® monitoring system was able to provide an early warning signal for a potentially fatal complication (Hubbert et al., 2015). These results indicate that the TitanLAP® monitoring system can be useful in regulating and monitoring the ideal pump speed (Tchantchaleishvili et al., 2017). The company that develops the monitoring system TitanLAP® offers a platform for developing an integration technology between the sensor and the LVAD, which in this way can autonomously adjust the LVAD settings according to patients' real-time status (Hubbert et al., 2017).

In 2011, the CardioMEMS® HF heart failure system (Abbott Medical Inc., Abbott Park, IL) was tested in a study called CHAMPION (wireless pulmonary artery hemodynamic monitoring in chronic heart failure). The CHAMPION multicenter clinical trial was a prospective, randomized, single-blind clinical trial. A total of 550 patients with New York Heart Association (NYHA) functional class III HF, regardless of left ventricular ejection fraction, and with a previous hospital stay for HF in the last 12 months were registered in 64 centers (Abraham et al., 2011).

Based on the safe and promising clinical results obtained in the CHAMPION study in 2014, the USFDA approved the CardioMEMS® HF device for NYHA class III HF patients who were hospitalized for HF in the previous year under the guidelines of the European Society for Heart Failure (HFA - European). Cardiology 2016, CardioMEMS® HF received a class IIb recommendation for targeted management and monitoring of tool therapy in patients with HF (Ponikowski et al., 2016).

The CardioMEMS® HF heart failure system provides hemodynamic information of the pulmonary artery (PA) used for the monitoring and management of HF and includes (Ayyadurai et al., 2019):

- A delivery catheter (used during standard catheterization of the right heart) containing an implantable hermetically sealed wireless sensor, where two nitinol loops at the sensor ends serve as anchors and allow automatic sizing of the device across the width of the vessel;
- Hospital electronic unit, used to calibrate the sensor using simultaneous measurements of a PA catheter during the implantation procedure and also to obtain pulmonary arterial pressure (PAP) data, while patients are still in the hospital or during visits subsequent outpatient clinics;
- An electronic patient unit (PU), which is used to passively measure biological data in patients' home; and
- A database for telemetry and telemedicine for patients.

The CardioMEMS® HF wireless sensor was designed for permanent implantation in the distal PA (a branch >7 mm from the left PA). The PA sensor consists of a three-dimensional coil and a pressure-sensitive capacitor wrapped between two fused silica wafers. The set of fused silica is encased in silicone. The sensor body has dimensions of $15 \times 3.4 \times 2$ mm, is biocompatible, and has a service life of more than 3 years (Ayyadurai et al., 2019).

The CardioMEMS® HF system electromagnetically couples a pressure-sensitive capacitor (wireless sensor coil) to an external coil located in the PU electronic system. The capacitance of the sensor coil causes a change in the resonance frequency (principle based on a passive inductor–capacitor oscillator circuit; LC tank) used as a reference for obtaining biological data: PAP waveforms and pressures (Ayyadurai et al., 2019).

The PU consists of an antenna fitted to a pillow on which patients are in supine position and trigger the monitoring procedure. PU allows standardization of the position of the body to guarantee reproducible conditions. PU automatically subtracts the ambient pressure from that measurement from the implanted sensor. PU encrypts the data sent and transmits the information to the protected site, which allows the remote review of the monitored data (Ayyadurai et al., 2019).

Medical knowledge of hemodynamic information can allow a more dynamic and optimized management of LVAD settings before and after implantation when compared to current methods (Feldman et al., 2018a; Veenis et al., 2019a).

Although several clinical variables are involved in the decision to provide support for LVAD, the implantation of a wireless hemodynamic monitoring system in patients with advanced HF can provide physicians with the necessary physiological information to improve the time of LVAD implantation. In the study by Feldman et al. (2018b), an analysis of the characteristics of patients was performed in the CHAMPION clinical study who developed HF with worsening despite the best medical therapy during the follow-up period and deteriorated to the point of requiring an LVAD implant. In this study, the authors concluded that the findings reported in the retrospective analysis suggest that PAP monitoring can early identify patients in need of an LVAD implant.

In pre-LVAD management, clinical signs, laboratory results, and echocardiography are currently used to guide pre-LVAD optimization. However, data are lacking to describe the accuracy of these techniques. Additional daily hemodynamic information is very important to achieve true pre-LVAD optimization (Veenis et al., 2019b). In the study by Veenis et al. (2019b), he points out that an interesting preimplantation goal of LVAD for the advancement of surgery is a reduction in PAP, ideally aiming for an average PAP (mean PAP) of <25 mmHg, as this, according to the authors, is an indication of ideal RV decongestion, potentially decreasing the associated operative risks.

Currently, postimplantation monitoring of LVAD is limited to parameters defined by the pump controller, which display a fixed number of revolutions, calculated pump flow, and pulsatility index. The addition of hemodynamic changes measured with CardioMEMS® HF can lead to earlier detection of complications, such as major bleeding, tamponade, RV failure, decompensation, or arrhythmia. Early detection facilitates early treatment, potentially improving the outcome (Veenis et al., 2019b).

The work by Veenis et al. (2019b) is the first prospective pilot study (HEMO-VAD) to explore the safety and feasibility of using CardioMEMS® HF to optimize LVAD therapy with additional (remote) hemodynamic information. This study will include ten patients with NYHA class IIIb or IV and INTERMACS classes two to five with surgery scheduled for the implantation of an LVAD HeartMate® 3. The objectives will be to assess whether hemodynamic information: (i) before implantation, was used to improve the hemodynamic status and optimize surgery time; (ii) after LVAD implantation, they had an additive value in detecting possible complications at an early stage (bleeding and tamponade); and (iii) during the outpatient phase, made it possible to optimize the settings of the LVAD, detect possible complications, and adapt the clinical management of these patients (Veenis et al., 2019b).

Patients with LVAD have a high incidence of VA and have demonstrated reduced mortality when treated with an implantable cardioverter defibrillator (ICD) (Vakil et al., 2016). PAP monitoring can be used as a substitute for RV function, therefore hemodynamic stability during VA (Harris et al., 2017). As modern ICDs communicate via RF, it can be speculated that implantable sensors can be incorporated so that there is interaction and together they can be used in LVAD physiological control algorithms (Harris et al., 2017).

In the work of Brancato et al. (2016), implantable sensors were implemented using a commercially available absolute pressure sensor SM5108C (Silicon Microstructures, Inc., Milpitas, CA). The SM5108C micromachined silicon sensor has dimensions of $650\,\mu m^3$ and a scale of $1,550\,mmHg$ and consists of a piezoresistive bridge of 5 KW with four active elements on top of a thin square silicon membrane with a side length of $250\,\mu m$. In the SM5108C sensor, a biocompatible encapsulation strategy was implemented based on a thick ceramic film process (alumina substrate) and a double coating of polydimethylsiloxane and parylene C (trade name of several polymers of the poly family [p-xylylene]), increasing the dimensions of the device to $2.6\times3.6\times1.8\,mm$. The device had low energy consumption ($>14.5\,mW$ in continuous mode) and exhibited a temperature-independent sensitivity ($12\,\mu V/V/mmHg$) and good *in vitro* stability when exposed to a continuous flow of saline solution (deviation >0.05 mmHg/day after 50 h). During *in vivo* validation, the transducer was successfully used to record a sheep's BP waveform (Brancato et al., 2016).

In the work by Staufert & Hierold (2016), the implantable sensors were implemented using a commercially available absolute pressure sensor LPS25HB (STMicroelectronics, Geneva, Switzerland). The LPS25HB sensor is micromachined in silicon with an integrated digital interface (I2C), fully packaged and with dimensions of $2.5\times2.5\times0.76\,mm$ and a measuring range from 26 to $126\,kPa$. Similar to conventional pressure sensors for hazardous environments, this design uses a flexible media separation diaphragm as a detection interface. In order to minimize sensor intrusion, the diaphragm is formed as an integral part of a conformal coating, covering the entire cannula of the VAD. The integration of the soft detection interface aims to eliminate the risk of increased thrombogenicity and hemolysis, introduced by obstructions in blood flow. In addition, this design minimizes the deviation of the sensor, preventing the accumulation and deposition of biological material at the interface. The diaphragm is suspended over a recess in the sidewall of the cannula where the real pressure sensor is located later. The recess is also filled with a pressure transmission liquid (silicone oil) and the changes in blood pressure are therefore transmitted to the pressure sensor by deflection of the diaphragm and through the resulting increase in the pressure of the transmission liquid. The first characterization measurements show that the resulting sensor assembly behaves linearly and has an absolute measurement error below 104.2 Pa (0.21% FullScale) in a measurement range of $80–130\,kPa$ (Staufert & Hierold, 2016).

Traditionally, echocardiography has been used to adjust the speed of an LVAD to obtain adequate LV decompression, but its high computational complexity makes it difficult to integrate its application in real-time monitoring of the physiological control of LVADs. In the work of Dual et al. (2019), it demonstrated the feasibility of developing an LV volume sensor based on a simplified ultrasonic monitoring module to be fitted to the LVAD cannula. In this approach, two ultrasonic transducers were used and the LV volume was estimated using the LV end-diastolic diameter; despite the simplification, an accuracy comparable to 2D echocardiography was achieved (Dual et al., 2019).

15.4 IMPLANTABLE SENSOR DEVELOPMENT

In the area of VADs, the most interesting data to be obtained are initially related to the assistance of the VADs (blood flow and differential pressure) because based on these data and the aid of mathematical techniques implemented in the controller, it is possible to estimate the minimum flow of blood to prevent suction and mean arterial pressure (MAP) (oriented to be ≤ 80 mmHg to avoid complications), these being essential variables for the control of VADs more harmonious with the physiological system (Leao et al., 2020).

For hemodynamic control of a patient with LVAD, pressure values are required (Uriel et al., 2019): "central venous pressure; systolic, diastolic, and mean PAP; and

Pulmonary Capillary Wedge Pressure (PCWP)" and "APs; APd; and MAP." Obtained in clinical practice, respectively, by (Chatterjee, 2009; Bennett et al., 2010):

- PA catheterization techniques by Swan-Ganz, this catheter (made up of polyurethane and flexible) for accurate measurements is introduced through a central vein (of suitable caliber) until it reaches the cardiac and pulmonary structures. It is indicated in therapy for the control of the hemodynamic state of a critical patient and, above all, if he is in shock (maximum indication). It is used to detect HF, monitor applied therapy, and evaluate the effect of the drugs administered and
- Doppler ultrasound, where the measurement is performed using an ultrasound of the brachial artery after deflating an arm cuff and recording the audible restoration of the flow as blood pressure by Doppler effect. This technique has an excellent correlation of blood pressure measurements in implanted patients, unlike traditional methods of noninvasive measurements.

The measurement of cardiac output is essential to know about cardiac performance and a very important data for the treatment of a patient with HF, but there is no precise method for measuring it, with estimation techniques such as dilution method, thermodilution, Fick's method, angiographic method and Doppler ultrasonography. In clinical use, this data is obtained mainly by the thermodilution estimation technique using the Swan-Ganz catheter.

In the literature, a good correlation has already been reported between data readings from an implanted sensor and catheterization technique (Ayyadurai et al., 2019; Hubbert et al., 2017).

Important notes regarding monitoring with implantable sensors are:

- Sensors based on strain gauges (differential voltage meters) are simpler to develop; however, they have associated losses in the electrical connection and require a constant electrical supply for operation;
- Capacitance-based sensors are more complex to design but work wirelessly and with low-energy consumption. They need an electronic resonance circuit (external to a patient's body) for operation;
- Sensors designed to be a module attached to the VAD cannula guarantee a convenient sensor implantation strategy, in contrast limit the data that can be measured in the coupling regions of the VAD's inlet and outlet cannulas;
- Sensors detached from the VADs require a rigorous implant design and functioning in a patient's organism, but they present a great advantage in the reading of interesting data (pulmonary and atrial artery) for the hemodynamic control of an implanted patient; and
- An interesting direction is the combination of several types of sensors for improved detection of physiological parameters through cross-checking of the sensor, but for this, an intelligent data integration system is required.

Regardless of the monitoring strategy, for the proper functioning of the sensor, the wide use of: (i) computational analysis by finite elements is necessary to develop the format of the module and identify the ideal transduction points; (ii) computational analysis of fluid dynamics so as not to restrict or significantly alter patients' hemodynamics during monitoring; and (iii) electromagnetic computational simulation to assess adequate and reliable measurement of data.

15.4.1 STANDARDS

Medical devices that come into contact with patients must meet high standards, and those that have long-term contact (such as implantable devices) must conform to the highest standards of all. The development of implantable biocompatible sensors, therefore, requires extensive knowledge in the design and manufacturing stages, as well as installations and machines with the capacity to produce components that meet rigorous parameters (ANSS, 2020; Proven Process, 2020).

The manufacture of medical devices is covered by ISO 13485: 2016. These standards also apply to implantable devices. However, due to the internal nature of the devices and their long-term life cycle, additional standards also apply. These include:

- ISO 14708-1: 2014—General requirements for safety, marking, and for information to be provided by the manufacturer;
- ISO 14708-2: 2012—Cardiac pacemakers;
- ISO 14708-3: 2017—Implantable neurostimulators;
- ISO 14708-4: 2008—Implantable infusion pumps;
- ISO 14708-5: 2010—Circulatory support devices;

- ISO 14708-6: 2010—Particular requirements for active implantable medical devices intended to treat tachyarrhythmia (including implantable defibrillators);
- ISO 14708-7: 2013—Particular requirements for cochlear implant systems;
- ISO 14117: 2012—Electromagnetic compatibility test protocols for implantable cardiac pacemakers, implantable cardioverter defibrillators, and cardiac resynchronization devices; and
- EC 62304: 2006—Medical device software.

For devices to be used in the United States, additional regulations must be followed. Most of them are administered by the Food and Drug Administration. The FDA ensures that implantable devices conform to the appropriate standards before being released to the market through its Devices and Radiological Health Center. Some products (including implantable devices that communicate wirelessly with external devices) are also within the competence of the Federal Communications Commission. The European Union stipulates its regulations in the MDR 2017/745, adopted in 2017.

In addition to the adequate and reliable transduction of physiological data, the following goals in accordance with the above standards are part of the development project for implantable sectors:

I. That the cooking materials are resistant enough to last the intended period (5 years) and stable enough to provide reliable functionality throughout the life cycle of the device;
II. That the material of the surface of direct contact with the patient (encapsulation) has toxicity below the levels that would affect it, even in the long term;
III. That the external surface of the device (body) is free of sharp edges or corners that may cause irritation or inflammation in patients;
IV. That the package and body of the device is electrically neutral;
V. That the device does not operate more than 2°C above normal body temperature (37°C);
VI. That the communication and power supply system is preferably wireless, and in the case of the use of batteries, that they have a long useful life and with a system to notify patients and doctors about the exhaustion well in advance; and
VII. That the operation has electromagnetic compatibility in order to function even when it encounters interference in the form of electromagnetic energy and that its own emissions do not cause significant interference with other devices.

15.4.2 Bio-Hemocompatibility

The main difficulties in using implantable sensors to collect biological data in a stable manner over time (and also without causing any adverse reactions) are associated with (Ratner et al., 2004; Wang, 2013): (i) the defenses of the immune system, constituted by an intricate network of organs, cells, and molecules, which aims to maintain the homeostasis of the organism, combating aggressions in general and (ii) the strong corrosion reaction caused by the internal organic constitution of the human body.

The physiological response of the human immune system when a foreign material is immersed in the blood flow includes (Werner et al., 2007): protein adsorption, thrombin activation, surface clotting, complement activation, platelet activation, and platelet adhesion. Together, they define the hemocompatibility of the material. On the other hand, the device itself cannot present the occurrence of adverse reactions of toxicity as (Makovey et al., 2015): toxic, irritating, inflammatory, allergic, mutagenic, and carcinogenic background. In order to prevail over hemodynamic adversities and have an adequate response, the design of implantable sensors must have bio-hemocompatibility as a key feature.

In the literature on the clinical applications of implantable medical devices, the use of a protective layer (passivation) against corrosion is reported, based on the chemically inert coating of (Werner et al., 2007): metal oxides (TiO); nitrides (TiN); silicon carbide; and inorganic carbon-based materials (hydrogenated amorphous carbon, DLC). The biocompatibility of a specific coating can be improved in three ways (Krishnan et al., 2008): (i) passivation of the surface by long-chain hydrophilic polymers (poly [ethylene glycol], poly [ethylene oxide]) or biopolymers inert (albumin); (ii) immobilization of active molecules to interact with proteins and blood cells (inhibitors to prevent thrombus formation, e.g., AT III, thrombomodulin); and (iii) promoting the growth of endothelial cells. Polymers are easily adapted to specific chemical properties in order to improve hemocompatibility; however, organic molecules are more susceptible to hydrolytic modification and degradation compared to inorganic substrates, which have better long-term stability (Brancato et al., 2016).

In the work of Weisenberg and Mooradian (2002), the *in vitro* hemocompatibility of materials used in MEMS systems (Si, SiO_2, Si_3N_4, and SU-8) was studied based on platelet adhesion and morphology. Platelet adhesion in Si, Si_3N_4, and SU-8 was significantly higher than platelet adhesion in polyurethane (reference material), while in parylene and SiO_2 it was not significantly different. The use of parylene as a dielectric and moisture barrier has been reported through the deposition of chemical vapor from a thin film (Brancato et al., 2016).

The works of Brancato et al. (2016) and Staufert & Hierold (2016) presented a feasibility study for the development of MEMS sensors encapsulated in parylene. In this study, the authors point out that although the literature serves as an indication of the factors that influence the bio-hemocompatibility of materials and the covering of MEMS systems, the conclusions drawn depend on many experimental parameters (sterilization technique, process flow, parameters, and test procedure) and the fluidic conditions used during the preliminary tests do not compare to the hemodynamic flow inside the blood circulatory system (Brancato et al., 2016).

15.5 PHYSIOLOGICAL PARAMETER ANALYSES THAT ARE CHANGED IN PATIENTS WITH VADs

Bronzino (2000) approaches biomedical engineering as an area that has a clear interdisciplinarity because, by applications of principles of electricity, mechanics, chemistry, and others, it is an area of development of materials, devices, and techniques to be used in the clinical/hospital environment (clinical engineering).

One of the applications of biomedical engineering is the development of biosensors for measuring physiological variations and for biological analysis in general, in which this application occurs in obtaining an electrical signal through a biological reaction in cells and consequently in tissues (bioelectric signal) (Barr, 2000).

Commonly, bioelectric sensors act similarly to basic electrical sensors (physical sensors), like the variable resistors that are used in circuits that measure resistance or electrical voltage, as there is a displacement of the sliding knob of these types of sensors (Neuman, 2000).

In communion with this context, we note another type of sensors used in biomedical engineering, which are electrochemical sensors, which are also categorized as to the electrical properties of conductivity and capacitance. These electrochemical sensors are constituted by electrodes inserted in surfaces containing components that interact with specific elements of a sample (Liu, 2000).

Thus, bioelectric sensors can be considered as the result of associations between other sensors, more specifically the physical and electrochemical sensors, in order to obtain signals corresponding to biological processes (Buck, 2000).

When considering what signal is defined as "…a variable phenomenon that can be measured." (Costa, 2017, p. 14), and which is mathematically represented as a function, which can contain one or more independent variables (Costa, 2017), in the case of biosensors this signal is obtained by means of biomaterials and which basically contains three components: (i) receptors (chemoreceptors) to which the sample element to be analyzed connects; (ii) transducers that convert the result of the interaction between the element to be analyzed and the receiver into a measurable signal and; (iii) signal processing.

This combination of components changes the name of this biosensor to a bioanalytical sensor (Buck In: Bronzino, 2000).

15.5.1 BLOOD CLOTTING MEASUREMENT

An important hematological parameter to be measured in clinical cases is blood clotting, especially in patients undergoing treatment for serious cardiovascular diseases, such as atrial fibrillation, pulmonary embolism, heart valve replacement, and HF (Boos & Brown, 2016; Kim et al., 2016; Pozzi et al., 2016).

Blood coagulation is an important monitoring parameter in patients with systolic HF who have a VAD, due to the possibility of hemorrhage and thrombosis, which can negatively affect the functioning of this implanted device and can also impair the health of these patients (Shah et al., 2017).

Bone marrow is responsible for the production of several hematological components, and that includes platelets. When the bone marrow is stimulated, activation of pluripotent hematopoietic stem cells occurs, which then differentiate into a common lymphoid parent and a common myeloid parent. Then, the common myeloid progenitor, still in the bone marrow, differentiates into a progenitor of erythrocytes and a progenitor of megakaryocytes. Megakaryocytes are very large cells, so they cannot pass through the capillary pores and thus reach the bloodstream; therefore, fragmentation of megakaryocytes occurs, which gives rise to platelets (Bain, 2016;; Abbas, Lichtman, & Pillai, 2012; Hall, 2011).

In the platelet membranes are found layers of glycoproteins that allow the platelets to adhere to the injured parts of the endothelium, especially through binding with collagen found in these sites (and other vascular structures), whereas this does not occur in the normal endothelium (Hall, 2011).

When a vascular injury occurs, platelets adhere to the injured site, in the context of early blood clotting, which then results in a complex of active substances that act on the activation of prothrombin, a protein produced by the liver and present in blood plasma, and which is a precursor to thrombin, in which it is an enzyme that converts fibrinogen (also produced by the liver) into fibrin fibers, responsible for forming a tangle of platelets, hematological cells, and plasma, to form the clot. Vitamin K acts as a prothrombin activation cofactor in the liver. Furthermore, calcium ions (Ca^{2+}) participate in the formation of clots, as these ions contribute to the conversion of prothrombin to thrombin (Hall, 2011).

Thrombopoietin (TPO) is a glycoprotein hormone produced by the liver and kidneys, is present in the blood, and binds to its receptors (thrombopoietin cell receptors—MPL) present in platelets, megakaryocytes, and CD34 + cells. The plasma level of TPO is inversely proportional to the mass of megakaryocytes and platelets and the TPO is regulated by the MPL. Therefore, it can be seen that there is a clear communication between the vascular and bone marrow for the production of platelets, thus regulating blood coagulation.

After their actions and half-life, platelets are eliminated by macrophages, mostly located in the spleen (Hall, 2011).

Patients using a VAD are susceptible to coagulation dysregulation, as the vascular friction stress can induce the mechanisms described above for the formation of clots that can result in thrombosis. Thrombosis can also be induced by hemolysis caused by the VAD. Smooth muscle relaxation can also occur with arteriovenous dilation, intestinal hypoperfusion, or even coagulation factor syndrome, which can result in gastrointestinal hemorrhage (Shah et al., 2017).

One of the standardized treatments to prevent excess blood clotting is the use of vitamin K antagonist, warfarin or phenprocoumon, with its anticoagulant action. It is added that long-term continuous use of anticoagulant drugs can increase the risk of serious complications, such as hemorrhage and thromboembolism (Boos & Brown, 2016; Kim et al., 2016; Pozzi et al., 2016).

Therefore, the use of these drugs should be controlled according to the results of monitoring the prothrombin activity time, considered the gold standard, and expressed as the international normalized ratio (INR) for the variation limit of the thromboplastin reagent measurement.

Therefore, this monitoring must be constant, and this voluminous practice regarding the frequency of tests in clinical/hospital environments is not viable; thus, self-monitoring through the use of portable coagulation measurement equipment (INR) using reagent strips is a practical solution for this purpose (McCahon, Roalfe, & Fitzmaurice, 2017; Dillinger et al., 2016; Phibbs et al., 2016).

That said, studies have evaluated the accuracy and correlation of portable coagulation measuring equipment using reagent strips with measurements using conventional blood samples in clinical analysis laboratories, in which the results showed strong correlations ($r > 0$, 8- majority >0.9), agreement, and low variability index of the values obtained between the equipment and methods, which attests to this equipment as reliable for blood coagulation measurements (Zenlander et al., 2017; Kalçik et al., 2017; Riva et al., 2017; McCahon et al., 2017; Wee et al., 2016; Dillinger et al., 2016; Saraiva et al., 2016; Leiria et al., 2007), including complying with ISO standards 17593: 2007 (Plesch et al., 2008).

15.5.2   BLOOD GLUCOSE MEASUREMENT

Glycemic control in diabetic patients is an important measure to reduce the risk of complications, in which capillary glycemia self-monitoring is a practical and interesting way to have this control, which allows patients to correct peaks themselves of hyperglycemia or episodes of hypoglycemia in an agile way, positively impacting the health of this audience (Lee et al., 2017).

Diabetes is a risk factor for the development of HF (Bauters et al., 2003; Levy et al., 1996), so a diabetic individual may need a VAD in the future to compensate for HF.

Dysregulation of glycemia resulting from diabetes mellitus alters the functioning of the sarcoplasmic reticulum Ca^{2+} - ATPase (SERCA2) and the sodium–calcium exchanger, proteins involved in the calcium flow between the sarcoplasmic reticulum and myocardial troponin C, therefore influencing the capacity contraction of the cardiac muscle, in addition to other problems related to energy metabolism, oxidative stress, and inflammation in the cardiovascular context (Shah & Brownlee, 2016; Schillinger et al., 2003).

Therefore, patients using VADs who have diabetes need glycemic control to prevent injuries.

For capillary glycemia self-monitoring, equipment (glycometers or glucometers) are used that work by means of reagent strips to carry out blood glucose tests from obtaining a drop of approximately one microliter of capillary blood. These reagent strips contain amperometric electrodes and an enzyme (glucose dehydrogenase [GDH], glucose oxidase [GO], or glucose oxidase/peroxidases[GOP]). As soon as the capillary glucose comes into contact with the enzyme contained in the strip, an electrochemical reaction occurs that will be measured by the equipment (Baynes & Dominiczak, 2011).

15.5.3   BLOOD LACTATE MEASUREMENT

Patients using a VAD may have complications such as formation of thrombosis, in which changes in the isoforms of the enzyme lactate dehydrogenase (LDH) also occur, so these changes in LDH serve as a biomarker to indicate a possible thrombogenic process (Hurst et al., 2019; Gordon et al., 2019; Shah et al., 2014; Weitzel et al., 2013).

Lactate is a by-product of anaerobic glycolytic metabolism (Berg, Tymocsko, & Stryer, 2008) and serves as a marker of metabolic stress in relevant clinical conditions explained below.

Since lactate's action in inflammation and severe inflammation promotes increased use of lactic anaerobic pathway, this relationship between energy metabolism and immunological problems, including those associated with pathologies, is of clinical relevance, even in more serious issues, as in sepsis (systemic inflammation related to infection); therefore, measurement of capillary lactate in patients with suspected severe infection is a practice in hospital emergency departments, as lactate is a marker of mortality risk in these patients, since the increased lactate can represent cardiovascular and respiratory dysfunctions, which can lead to hypoxia and organ failure, which increases the risk of death, thus making the period between screening and decision making as "golden hours" (Mikkelsen et al., 2009; Shapiro et al., 2005; Rivers et al., 2001).

Tanner, Fuller, and Ross (2010) evaluated, from three different manufacturers, portable lactate analysis equipment using reagent strips, which contain the enzyme lactate oxidase, and in one of them, potassium ferrocyanide is added. In this evaluation, a correlation test was performed with conventional measurement performed in a clinical analysis laboratory (Radiometer ABL700), in swimming, cycling, and running athletes in incremental tests. The equipment showed a strong correlation when compared with blood analysis in a clinical analysis laboratory ($r = 0.913, 0.837$ and 0.936).

Exercise physiology is seen as the relevant content for biomedical and biomaterial engineers (Johnson & Dooly, 2000), in which physical exercise in its various manifestations, including sports and health promotion, is a field application of technologies aimed at analyzing physiological variations, both for purposes alone, i.e., for measuring physical/sports performance, monitoring the physical conditions of athletes and physical exercise practitioners, but also because the physical effort is a tool to verify important physiological variables and their thresholds, which support medicine for the diagnosis and prognosis of clinical conditions, in addition to the physical effort being an interesting way to simulate physiological stress conditions for the purposes of studies.

The study by Bonaventura et al. (2015) used five different equipment with these characteristics and a portable standard hospital equipment (i-STAT) to compare the measurements with the clinical analysis laboratory equipment (Radiometer ABL90). In high concentrations of lactate (above the ventilatory threshold 2), some equipment presented incompatible data; despite values in smaller zones, all equipment presented values compatible with the adopted clinical standard. It is noteworthy that the sample was composed of only five subjects, which is an important limitation; therefore, studies with a larger sample, among other methodological issues, are necessary to compare lactate measurements using portable equipment using reagent strips with collections conventional in clinical analysis laboratories for applications in physical exercise.

In the hospital environment, the study by Gaieski et al. (2013) compared the use of portable lactate meter equipment using reagent strips and whole-blood point of care, with conventional collections in a clinical analysis laboratory, in the emergency department to direct sepsis patients to the intensive care unit, and also with conventional blood collection for clinical analysis. The results showed an excellent interclass correlation (ICC = 0.90 and 0.92), with the benefit of using portable equipment to allow analysis and decision-making more quickly (8–13 vs. 65 minutes).

In the review by Lewis et al. (2016), which evaluated seven studies that combined using 2085 patients, there is this reliability of data obtained by portable lactate measurement equipment using reagent strips in the hospital environment for screening patients with sepsis or septic shock, for referral to the intensive care unit, which allows the widespread use of this type of equipment for this purpose.

Since a patient using a VAD may have metabolic and inflammatory problems that result in an increase in lactate, the use of equipment that uses reagent strips to quantify this metabolite may be interesting for indicating the risk of thrombosis, among other complications.

15.5.4 MEASUREMENT OF C-REACTIVE PROTEIN—A FUTURE PERSPECTIVE OF POINT-OF-CARE TECHNOLOGY

C-reactive protein (CRP) is an inflammatory protein, which is present in squares of acute and chronic inflammations. Its action occurs essentially when it binds to its anchoring protein present in the cell membranes, called phosphorylcholine (or phosphocholine), obtaining from this connection the phosphorylcholine–PCR complex, which in turn stimulates the attachment of a complement system protein, which will then result in actions to combat the offending agent, which will stimulate the production and action of pro-inflammatory cytokines. However, PCR suffers degradation by lysosomal enzymes, so it is also an inhibitor of neutrophil activities, superoxide production and chemotactics, which gives the PCR pro-inflammatory and regulatory characteristics (Collares & Paulino, 2006).

CRP concentrations rise 4–6 hours after a stimulus, doubling the value every 8 hours and peaking between 36 and 50 hours, and with a plasma half-life of 19 hours, serial monitoring of CRP values is recommended after an event (Aguiar et al., 2013; Collares & Paulino, 2006).

In healthy subjects, the mean CRP value is up to 0.8 mg/L for a clinical condition that denotes the absence of inflammation; however, almost the entire population has values that indicate mild inflammation, with concentrations below 10 mg/L, and that most cases do not reach 2 mg/L. Already values above 10 mg/L indicate activity of the inflammatory process (Collares & Paulino, 2006). Values between 10 and 40 mg/L indicate mild inflammation or viral infection and between 40 and 200 mg/L indicate severe inflammation or bacterial infection, where the value of 100 mg/L, despite being in the window for a bacterial infection, in some cases may indicate a viral infection (Aguiar et al., 2013).

Chronic inflammation with persistently high CRP levels serves as a marker of increased risk of coronary heart disease and future cardiovascular disorders (Zhuang et al., 2019; Shrivastava et al., 2015; Strang & Schunkert, 2014; Silva & Lacerda, 2012; Buckley et al., 2009; Koenig et al., 1999). The amount of CRP above 1 mg/L denotes an increase in this risk, especially in men (Zhuang et al., 2019; Yousuf et al., 2013).

It is also noteworthy that the methods for measuring CRP have evolved over time. The pioneer method was qualitative by the reaction of precipitation in a capillary tube. Subsequently, the semiquantitative method for agglutination of latex appeared. Both methods are of limited clinical value. More recently, quantitative immunological methods have emerged, such as turbidimetry (immunoturbidimetria) (Collares & Paulino, 2006).

Patients using a VAD due to HF have inflammatory problems that must be monitored, but the precise measurement of PCR requires sending of blood samples for clinical analysis in specialized laboratories, which requires complex logistics and results in cost and high time, which makes quick decisions for interventions or care for the diverse populations in demand unfeasible (Baynes & Dominiczak, 2011).

This process can be optimized by using an electronic system that, by means of reagent strips, allows immediate analysis and more agile decision-making, such as what happens with similar equipment to measure blood glucose, lactate, and coagulation, with a good degree of reliability in its uses, as previously mentioned.

Thus, the study by Nogueira et al. (2020), derived from the master's program by the Federal Institute of São Paulo (IFSP), verified the possibility of developing a prototype of electronic equipment using reagent strips for future application in the measurement of CRP. At that time, the strips were handcrafted with the insertion of 2-methacryloyloxyethyl phosphorylcholine (MPC), in which acquisition of bioelectric signals occurred through a system containing an Arduino© plate (Arduino Uno—microcontroller), environment program development (Arduino IDE®), and Parallax Data Acquisition (PLX-DAQ)® software from Parallax Inc.,© for transferring data obtained by Arduino© to Excel® spreadsheet, thus performing mathematical modeling of the obtained signals.

The results were promising, in which it was possible to acquire the bioelectric signals of the reaction between the PCR with the MPC contained in the reagent strips, and other studies are presented below that also followed the PCR detection line with the use of MPC.

Park et al. (2004) developed a biomaterial that consisted of conjugation of MPC with n-butyl methacrylate and with p-nitrophenyl-oxycarbonyl poly (ethylene glycol) methacrylate (MEONP), thus forming PMBN, to emulsify the surface under polar groups of phospholipids, thus creating a material with polymeric nanoparticles of MPC (MPC-PNP). This experiment resulted in being able to detect PCR by immobilizing anti-PCR in MPC-PNP, which allowed visualization through a scanning electron microscope.

The study by Kurosawa et al. (2004) used cysteamine hydrochloride, glutaraldehyde, and glycine to fix the PCR-specific antibody in three different preparations (anti-PCR-IgG, anti-PCR F (ab') 2-IgG, and anti-PCR Fab-IgG), whether or not containing MPC on a quartz crystal microbalance surface, an instrument that uses a quartz crystal wave oscillator, and with the variation of the signal frequency influenced by the deposit of something that intends to measure, it is possible to measure the mass of this deposited something. The results showed a high detection of PCR in the preparation with anti-PCR F (ab') 2-IgG containing MPC.

The study by Kitayama and Takeuchi (2014) used the method by visible ultraviolet spectrophotometry to identify changes in light absorption (color changes) caused by the presence of PCR in a container containing gold-conjugated MPC nanoparticles. This variation was calculated using the equation Δ $(A/D)/(A/D)$ 0, where A corresponds to the integral of the MPC spectrum conjugated with gold in the range between 550 and 700 nm and D corresponds to the spectrum in the range between 490 and 540 nm. The data showed that the method provided a good detection of CRP.

In a study by Matsuura et al. (2016), a polymer containing phosphorylcholine (poly [2-MPC]—PMPC) was used to bind and react with PCR. This polymer was embedded in a hybrid plasmonic chip (biological/chemical) with a layer ~4.4 nm thick and 0.7 g/cm^3, prepared by thin metal film coating, resulting in a sensing structure of fluorescence (nanotechnology). This form of detection differs from conventional immunosensing chips that use immobilized antibodies to capture target analytes.

After the PCR was captured by the PMPC on the chip, (i) biotinylated anti-PCR antibody (biotinylation—addition of biotin molecules (vitamin B7) for protein labeling) and (ii) streptavidin (protein, purified in the Streptomyces bacteria) were added, with high affinity to biotin) marked with fluorescence. There was also synthesis of Cy5-anti-PCR by means of a coupling reaction between the amine groups of the side chain of lysine residues in the anti-PCR and in the Cy5-NHS (fluorescent bioconjugate ester).

These preparations were performed so that the captured PCR was detected by the intensity of the fluorescence emitted by the reaction between the PCR and the phosphorylcholine contained in the PMPC. In this way, it was possible to analyze 2 forms of PCR detection using the PMPC with an embedded plasmonic chip—one containing biotin-anti-PCR/Cy5-streptavidin and the other containing Cy5-anti-PCR.

The results showed fluorescent activity in the presence of 1 nM of PCR in both methods of PCR detection using PMPC, however, with greater fluorescence in the method with Cy5-anti-PCR. However, the authors considered that the condition they used or prepared with biotin-anti-PCR/Cy5-streptavidin was more interesting, as it showed less nonspecific binding when compared with Cy5-anti-PCR, since it presented a statistical error very large. It is worth mentioning that the biotin-anti-PCR/Cy5-streptavidin method showed a determination coefficient proportional to the PCR concentration ($r^2 = 0.957$).

The study by Díaz-Betancor et al. (2019) used a more sophisticated way to detect PCR in an MPC hydrogel matrix by fluorescence using a surface reader, resulting in good PCR detection.

It is noted that these studies had positive results for the detection of CRP, however, with methods that were not through bioelectric signal, which is the proposal of this work.

The ability of MPC to be used in biosensors is reinforced by the study by Lee et al. (2018), which evaluated the electrical conductivity of three biomaterials classified as zwitterionic hydrogels, with MPC being among them. At that time, in addition to the comparison between biomaterials, a solution with electrolytes was also used as a reference for these analyzes, even with different concentrations. The findings of this study showed good ionic conductivity of the zwitterionic hydrogel made with MPC.

The study by Pinyorospathum et al. (2019) developed a device using a number 1 filter paper of Whatman type containing MPC with thiol termination (MPC-SH) and gold nanoparticle electrodes to detect PCR, whose detection was measured by electric current using differential pulse voltammetry.

It is noteworthy that the gold electrodes were printed on a wax printer on the paper base, even facilitating the deposition and fixation of the MPC-SH in this apparatus. Another aspect is the existence of two side flaps on the device; one of which was used to deposit calcium and later deposit the sample with 100 μL of PCR and the other was used to deposit potassium ferrocyanide ($K_3Fe(CN)_6$) and subsequently deposit potassium nitrate (KNO_3).

The results showed variation in the electrical signal in the presence of PCR. It happens that this whole analysis process took an hour and a half, which indicates that the method presents an important advance, but needs to be improved so that it can be applied in the technological market, as in the manufacture of electronic devices using reagent strips to quantify PCR in real time.

The conclusion is that it is possible to detect PCR by bioelectric signal and these findings suggest that the development of electronic equipment that uses reagent strips containing MPC for quantification of PCR seems to be feasible, in addition to being able to contribute in the future to infection control and inflammation in patients with various health problems, including those using a VAD.

REFERENCES

Abbas, A. K.; Lichtman, A. H.; Pillai, S. *Imunologia celular e molecular*, 7th ed. Rio de Janeiro: Elsevier, 2012.

Abraham, W. T., et al. Champion trial study group: Wireless pulmonary artery haemodynamic monitoring in chronic heart failure: A randomised controlled trial. *Lancet* 377: 658–666, 2011.

Agência Nacional De Saúde Suplementar. Dispositivos Médicos Implantáveis (DMI). ANSS, 2020. Disponível em: http://www.ans.gov.br/temas-de-interesse/dispositivos-medicos-implantaveis-dmi. Acesso em: 29 de jun. de 2020.

Aguiar, F. J. B. et al. Proteína c reativa: aplicações clínicas e propostas para utilização racional. *Revista da Associação Médica Brasileira*, 59(1): 85–92, 2013.

Ayyadurai, P. et al. An update on the cardiomems pulmonary artery pressure sensor. *Therapeutic Advances in Cardiovascular Disease*, 13: 1753944719826826, 2019.

Bain, B. J. *Células sanguíneas: um guia prático*, 5th ed. Porto Alegre: Artmed, 2016.

Bakouri, M. A.; Salamonsen, R. F.; Savkin, A. V.; Al Omari, A. H.; Lim, E.; Lovell, N. H. A sliding mode-based starling-like controller for implantable rotary blood pumps. *Artificial Organs* 38: 587–593, 2014.

Barr, R. C. Basic electrophysiology, cap. 8. In: Bronzino, J. D. (editor chefe), *The Biomedical Engineering Handbook*, 2nd ed. Boca Raton, FL: CRC Press, 2000.

Bauters, C. et al. Influence of diabetes mellitus on heart failure risk and outcome. *Cardiovascular Diabetology*, 2: 1, 2003.

Baynes, J. W.; Dominiczak, M. H. *Bioquímica médica*, 3rd ed. Rio de Janeiro: Elsevier, 2011.

Bennett, M. K.; Roberts, C. A.; Dordunoo, D.; Shah, A.; Russell, S. D. Ideal methodology to assess systemic blood pressure in patients with continuous-flow left ventricular assist devices. *The Journal of Heart and Lung Transplantation* 29: 593–594, 2010.

Berg, J. M.; Tymoczko, J. L.; Stryer, L. *Bioquímica*, 6th ed. Rio de Janeiro: Guanabara Koogan, 2008.

Bonaventura, J. M. et al. Reliability and accuracy for six hand-held blood lactate analysis. *Journal of Sports Science and Medicine* 14: 203–214, 2015.

Boos, C. J.; Brown, L. Anticoagulation in atrial fibrillation and chronic heart failure: The risk and drug of choice. *Current Opinion in Cardiology* 31(2): 229–234, 2016.

Brancato, L. et al. An implantable intravascular pressure sensor for a ventricular assist device. *Micromachines* 7(8): 135, 2016.

Bronzino, J. D. (editor chefe). *The Biomedical Engineering Handbook*, 2nd ed. Boca Raton, FL: CRC Press, 2000.

Buck, R. P. Bioanalytic sensors, cap. 51. In: Bronzino, J. D. (editor chefe), *The Biomedical Engineering Handbook*, 2nd ed. Boca Raton, FL: CRC Press, 2000.

Buckley, D. I. et al. C-reactive protein as a risk factor for coronary heart disease: A systematic review and meta-analyses for the U.S. preventive services task force. *Annals of Internal Medicine*, 151(7): 483–495, 2009.

Bullister, E.; Reich, S.; D'entremont, P.; Silverman, N.; Sluetz, J. A blood pressure sensor for long-term implantation. *Artificial Organs*, 25: 376–379, 2001.

Bullister, E., S. Reich, and J. Sluetz. Physiologic control algorithms for rotary blood pumps using pressure sensor input. *Artificial Organs* 26: 931–938, 2002.

Casas, F.; Ahmed, N.; Reeves, A. Minimal sensor count approach to fuzzy logic rotary blood pump flow control. *ASAIO Journal* 53: 140–146, 2007.

Chatterjee, K.; Swan-Ganz catheters: Past, present, and future: A viewpoint. *Circulation JAHA* 119: 147–152, 2009.

Choi, S.; Boston, J. R.; Antaki, J. F. Hemodynamic controller for left ventricular assist device based on pulsatility ratio. *Artificial Organs* 31: 114–125, 2007.

Collares, G. B.; Paulino, U. H. M. Aplicações clínicas atuais da proteína c reativa. *Revista Médica de Minas Gerais* 16(4): 227–333, 2006.

Cong, P.; Ko, W. H.; Young, D. J. Wireless batteryless implantable blood pressure monitoring microsystem for small laboratory animals. *Sensors* 10: 243–254, 2010.

Costa, C. *Processamento de sinais para engenheiros: teoria e prática*, 1st ed. Rio de Janeiro: Bonecker, 2017.

Díaz-Betancor, Z. et al. Phosphorylcholine-based hydrogel for immobilization of bio-molecules: Application of fluorometric microarrays for use in hybridization assays and immunoassays, and nanophotonic biosensing. *Microchimica Acta* 186(8): 1–11, 2019.

Dillinger, J.-G. et al. Accuracy of point of care caogulometers compared to reference laboratory measurements in patients on oral anticoagulant therapy. *Thrombosis Research* 140: 66–72, 2016.

Dual, S. A. et al. Ultrasonic sensor concept to fit a ventricular assist device cannula evaluated using geometrically accurate heart phantoms. *Artificial Organs* 43: 467–477, 2019.

Feldman, D. S. et al. The utility of a wireless implantable hemodynamic monitoring system in patients requiring mechanical circulatory support. *ASAIO Journal* 64(3): 301–308, 2018a.

Feldman, C. et al. Left ventricular assist devices–a state of the art review. In: Islam, M. (editor), *Heart Failure: From Research to Clinical Practice*. Cham: Springer, 2018b, pp. 287–294.

Fonseca, M. A. et al. Flexible wireless passive pressure sensors for biomedical applications. In: *Technical Digest Solid-State Sensor, Actuator, and Microsystems Workshop (Hilton Head 2006)*, pp. 37–42, 2006.

Fritz, B. et al. Development of an inlet pressure sensor for control in a left ventricular assist device. *ASAIO Journal* 56: 180, 2010.

Gaddum, N. R., et al. Starling-like flow control of a left ventricular assist device: in vitro validation. *Artificial Organs* 38: E46–E56, 2014.

Gaieski, D. F. et al. Accuracy of handheld point-of-care fingertip lactate measurement en the emergency department. *West Journal of Emergency Medicine* 14(1): 58–62, 2013.

Giridharan, G. A.; Skliar, M. Control strategy for maintaining physiological perfusion with rotary blood pumps. *Artificial Organs* 27: 639–648, 2003.

Giridharan, G. A. et al. Nonlinear controller for ventricular assist devices. *Artificial Organs* 26: 980–984, 2002.

Giridharan, G. A.; Pantalos, G. M.; Gillars, K. J.; Koenig, S. C.; Skliar, M. Physiologic control of rotary blood pumps: An in vitro study. *ASAIO Journal* 50: 403–409, 2004.

Gordon, J. S. et al. Clinical implications of LDH isoenzymes in hemolysis and continuous-flow left ventricular assist device-induced thrombosis. *Artificial Organs* 44(3): 231–238, 2019.

Gregory, S. D.; Pearcy, M. J.; Timms, D. Passive control of a biventricular assist device with compliant inflow cannulae. *Artificial Organs*, 36: 683–690, 2012.

Guyton, A. C. Determination of cardiac output by equating venous return curves with cardiac response curves. *Physiological Review* 35: 123–129, 1955.

Hall, J. E. *Guyton e Hall: Tratado de Fisiologia Médica*, 12th ed. Rio de Janeiro: Elsevier, 2011.

Harris, J. R. et al. Pulmonary arterial pressure sensing in a patient with left ventricular assist device during ventricular arrhythmia. *HeartRhythm Case Reports* 3(7): 348–351, 2017.

Heerdt, P. M. et al. Chronic unloading by left ventricular assist device reverses contractile dysfunction and alters gene expression in end-stage heart failure. *Circulation* 102: 2713, 2000.

Hoppe, U. C. et al. Chronic monitoring of pulmonary artery pressure in patients with severe heart failure: Multicentre experience of the monitoring Pulmonary Artery Pressure by Implantable device Responding to Ultrasonic Signal (Papirus) II study. *Heart* 95(13): 1091–1097, 2009.

Hubbert, L. et al. Left atrial pressure monitoring with an implantable wireless pressure sensor after implantation of a left ventricular assist device. *ASAIO Journal* 63(5): e60, 2017.

Hubbert, L.; Baranowski, J.; Delshad, B.; Ahn, H. Change of left atrial pressure, lap measured with a wireless implantable pressure sensor (titan sensor) during echocardiographic Ramp-test in HeartMate II patients. *The Journal of Heart and Lung Transplantation* 34: S218–S219, 2015.

Hurst, T. E. et al. Dynamic prediction of left ventricular assist device pump thrombosis based on lactate dehydrogenase trends. *ESC Heart Failure* 6(5): 1005–1014, 2019.

Jacob, R.; Kissling, G. Ventricular pressure-volume relations as the primary basis for evaluation of cardiac mechanics: Return to Frank's diagram. *Basic Research in Cardiology* 84: 227–246, 1989.

Johnson, A. T.; Dooly, C. R. Exercise physiology, cap. 23. In: Bronzino, J. D. (editor), *The Biomedical Engineering Handbook*, 2nd ed. Boca Raton, FL: CRC Press, 2000, pp. 141–147.

Kalçik, M. et al. Comparison of the INR values measured by CoaguChek XS coagulometer and conventional laboratory methods in patients on VKA therapy. *Clinical Applied Trombosis/Hemostasis* 23(2): 187–94, 2017.

Kim, J. H. et al. Coagulation abnormalities in heart failure: Pathophysiology and therapeutic implications. *Current Heart Failure Reports* 13(6): 319–328, 2016.

Kitayama, Y.; Takeuchi, T. Localized surface plasmon resonance nanosensing of c-reactive protein with poly(2-methacryloyloxyethyl phosphorylcholine)-grafted gold nanoparticles prepared by surface-initiated atom transfer radical polymerization. *Analytical Chemistry* 86(11): 5587–5594, 2014.

Klotz, S. et al. Single-beat estimation of enddiastolic pressure-volume relationship: A novel method with potential for noninvasive application. *The American Journal of Physiology-Heart and Circulatory Physiology* 291: H403–12, 2006.

Koenig, W. et al. C-Reactive protein, a sensitive marker of inflammation, predicts future risk of coronary heart disease in initially healthy middle-aged men: results from the MONICA (Monitoring Trends and Determinants in Cardiovascular Disease) Augsburg Cohort Study, 1984 to 1992. *Circulation* 99(2): 237–242, 1999.

Krishnan, S.; Weinman, C. J.; Ober, C. K. Advances in polymers for anti-biofouling surfaces. *Journal of Materials Chemistry* 18: 3405–3413, 2008.

Kurosawa, S. et al. Evaluation of a high-affinity QCM immunosensor using antibody fragmentation and 2-methacryloyloxyethyl phosphorylcholine (MPC) polymer. *Biosensors and Bioeletronics* 20(6): 1134–1139, 2004.

Laird, J. D. Asymptotic slope of log pressure vs log volume as an approximate index of the diastolic elastic properties of the myocardium in man. *Circulation* 53: 443–449, 1976.

Leao, T. et al. In vitro evaluation of multi-objective physiological control of the centrifugal blood pump. *Artificial Organs* 2020, 44(8), 785–796.

Lee, J. M. et al. Real-world use and self-reported health outcomes of a patient-designed do-it-yourself mobile technology system for diabetes: Lessons for mobile health. *Diabetes Technology and Therapeutics* 19(4): 1–11, 2017.

Lee, C.-J. et al. Ionic conductivity of polyelectrolyte hydrogels. *ACS Applied Material and Interfaces* 10(6): 5845–5852, 2018.

Leiria, T. L. L. et al. Controle de tempo de protrombina em sangue capilar e venoso em pacientes com anticoagulação oral: correlação e concordância. *Arquivos Brasileiros de Cardiologia*, 89(1): 1–5, 2007.

Levin, H. R.; Oz, M. C.; Chen, J. M., Packer, M.; Rose, E. A.; Burkhoff, D. Reversal of chronic ventricular dilation in patients with endstage cardiomyopathy by prolonged mechanical unloading. *Circulation* 91: 2717–2720, 1995.

Levy, D. et al. The progression from hypertension to congestive heart failure. *The Journal of American Medical Association* 275(20): 1557–1562, 1996.

Lewis, C. T. et al. Prehospital point-of-care lactate following trauma: A systematic review. *Journal of Trauma and Acute Care Surgery* 81(4): 748–755, 2016.

Liu, C-C. Electrochemical sensors, cap. 49. In: Bronzino, J. D. (editor), *The Biomedical Engineering Handbook*, 2nd ed. Boca Raton, FL: CRC Press, 2000, pp. 1–6.

Magalski, A. et al. Continuous ambulatory right heart pressure measurements with an implantable hemodynamic monitor: A multicenter, 12-month follow-up study of patients with chronic heart failure. *Journal of Cardiac Failure* 8(2): 63–70, 2002.

Makovey, I. et al. Clinical and regulatory considerations of implantable medical devices. In: Bhunia, S.; Majerus, S.; Sawan, M (editors), *Implantable Biomedical Microsystems*. Norwich, NY: William Andrew Publishing, pp. 137–166, 2015.

Matsuura, R. et al. A plasmonic chip-based bio/chemical hybrid sensing system for the highly sensitive detection of C-reactive protein. *Chemical Communications* 52(20): 3883–3886, 2016.

Mehra, M. R., Goldstein, D. J. Magnetically levitated cardiac pump at 2 years. New England Journal *of* Medicine 379:897, 2018a.

Mehra, M. R. et al. Two year outcomes with a magnetically levitated cardiac pump in heart failure. *New England Journal of Medicine* 378:1386–1395, 2018b.

Mehra, M. R. et al. Healthcare resource use and cost implications in the MOMENTUM 3 long-term outcome study. *Circulation* 138:1923–1934, 2018c.

McCahon, D.; Roalfe, A.; Fitzmaurice, D. A. An evaluation of a coagulation system (Xprecia Stride) for utilization in anticoagulation management. *Journal of Clinical Pathology* 0: 1–7, 2017.

Mikkelsen, M. E. et al. Serum lactate is associated with mortality in severe sepsis independent of organ failure and shock. *Critical Care Medicine* 37(5): 1670–1677, 2009.

Moscato, F., et al. Left ventricle afterload impedance control by an axial flow ventricular assist device: A potential tool for ventricular recovery. *Artificial Organs* 34: 736–744, 2010.

Neuman, M. R. Physical measurements, cap. 47. In: Bronzino, J. D. (editor), *The Biomedical Engineering Handbook*, 2nd ed. Boca Raton, FL: CRC Press, 2000, pp. 1.

Nogueira, H. S. et al. Monitoring the level of infection by COVID 19: An previous experiment to possibility of future application to the C reactive protein detection by bioelectric signals. *TAS Journal* 4(2): 104–22, 2020.

Ochsner, G. et al. A physiological controller for turbodynamic ventricular assist devices based on a measurement of the left ventricular volume. *Artificial Organs* 38: 527–538, 2014.

Park, J. et al. Evaluation of 2-methacryloyloxyethyl phosphorylcholine polymeric nanoparticle for immunoassay of C-reactive protein detection. *Analytical Chemistry* 76(9): 2649–55, 2004.

Pauls, J. P. et al. Evaluation of physiological control systems for rotary left ventricular assist devices: An in-vitro study. *Annals of Biomedical Engineering* 44(8): 2377–2387, 2016.

Petrou, A. et al. Standardized comparison of selected physiological controllers for rotary blood pumps: in vitro study. *Artificial Organs* 42(3): E29–E42, 2018.

Phibbs, C. et al. At-home versus in-clinic INR monitoring: A cost-utility analysis from the home INR study (THINRS). *Journal of General Internal Medicine* 31(9): 1061–1067, 2016.

Pinyorospathum, C. et al. Disposable paper-based electrochemical sensor using thiol-terminated poly(2-methacryloyloxyethyl phosphorylcholine) for the label-free detection of c-reactive protein. *Microchimica Acta* 186(7): 1–10, 2019.

Plesch, W. et al. Results of the performance verification of the CoaguChek XS system. *Trombosis Research* 123(2): 381–389, 2008.

Ponikowski, P. et al. 2016 ESC guidelines for the diagnosis and treatment of acute and chronic heart failure: the task force for the diagnosis and treatment of acute and chronic heart failure of the European Society of Cardiology (ESC). Developed with the special contribution of the Heart Failure Association (HFA) of the ESC. *European Journal of Heart Failure* 18: 891–975, 2016.

Potkay, J. A. Long term, implantable blood pressure monitoring systems. *Biomedical Microdevices* 10: 379–392, 2008.

Pozzi, M. et al. International normalized ratio self-testing and self-management: Improving patient outcomes. *Vascular Health and Risk Management* 12: 387–392, 2016.

Proven Process. Active Implantable Medical Device Expertise, 2020. Disponível em: https://provenprocess.com/active-implantable-devices.

Ratner, D. et al. *Biomaterials Science: An Introduction to Materials in Medicine.* Amsterdam: Elsevier, 2004.

Riva, N. et al. A comparative study using thrombin generation and three different INR methods in patients on vitamin K antagonist treatment. *International Journal of Laboratory Hematology* 39(5): 482–488, 2017.

Rivers, F. et al. Early goal directed therapy in the treatment of severe sepsis and septic shock. *The New England Journal of Medicine* 345(19): 1368–1377, 2001.

Saito, I. et al. Implementation of the natural heartbeat synchronize control for the undulation pump ventricular assist device using the inflow pressure. *In: 7th Asian-Pacific Conference on Medical and Biological Engineering*, Springer, Berlin, Heidelberg, 2008, pp. 62–65.

Salamonsen, R. F.; Mason, D. G.; Ayre, P. J. Response of rotary blood pumps to changes in preload and afterload at a fixed speed setting are unphysiological when compared with the natural heart. *Artificial Organs* 35: E47–E53, 2011.

Salamonsen, R. F. et al. Theoretical foundations of a Starling-like controller for rotary blood pumps. *Artificial Organs* 36: 787–796, 2012.

Saraiva, S. S. et al. Home management of INR in the public health system: Feasibility of self-management of oral anticoagulantion and long-term performance of individual POC devices in determining INR. *Journal of Trombosis and Trombolysis* 42(1): 146–153, 2016.

Schillinger, W. et al. Relevance of Na+-Ca2+ exchange in heart failure. *Cardiovascular Research* 57(4): 921–933, 2003.

Schima, H.; Trubel, W.; Moritz, A.; Wieselthaler, G.; Stohr, H.G.; Thoma, H.; Losert, U.; Wolner, E. Noninvasive monitoring of rotary blood pumps: Necessity, possibilities, and limitations. *Artificial Organs* 6: 195–202, 1992.

Shah, M. S.; Brownlee, M. Molecular and cellular mechanisms of cardiovascular disorders in diabetes. *Circulation Research* 118(11): 1808–1829, 2016.

Shah, P. et al. Diagnosis of hemolysis and device thrombosis with lactate dehydrogenase during left ventricular assist device support. *The Journal of Heart and Lung Transplantation* 33(1): 102–104, 2014.

Shah, P. et al. Bleeding and thrombosis associated with ventricular assist device therapy: A state of the art review. *Journal of Heart and Lung Transplantation* 36(11): 1164–1173, 2017.

Shapiro, N. I. et al. Serum lactate as a predictor of mortality in emergency department patients with infection. *Annals of Emergency Medicine* 45(5): 524–528, 2005.

Shrivastava, A. K. et al. C-reactive protein, inflammation and coronary heart disease. *The Egyptian Heart Journal* 67(2): 89–97, 2015.

Staufert, S., Hierold, C. Novel sensor integration approach for blood pressure sensing in ventricular assist devices. *Procedia Engineering* 168: 71–75, 2016.

Silva, D., Lacerda, A. P. High-sensitivity C-reactive protein as a biomarker of risk in coronary artery disease. *Revista Portuguesa de Cardiologia* 31(11): 733–745, 2021.

Slaughter, M. S. et al. Clinical management of continuous-flow left ventricular assist devices in advanced heart failure. *The Journal of Heart and Lung Transplantation* 29: S1–S39, 2010.

Stevens, M. C. et al. Frank-starling control of a left ventricular assist device. *Conference Proceedings: IEEE Engineering in Medicine and Biology Society* 2011: 1335–1338, 2011.

Stevens, M. C. et al. Physiological control of dual rotary pumps as a biventricular assist device using a master/slave approach. *Artificial Organs* 38: 7–774, 2014.

Strang, F.; Schunkert, H. C-reactive protein and coronary heart disease: All said—is not it? *Mediator in Inflammation* 2014: 1–7, 2014.

Tanner, R. K.; Fuller, K. L.; Ross, M. L. R. Evaluation of three portable blood lactate analysers: Lactate Pro, Lactate Scout and Lactate Plus. *European Journal of Applied Physiology* 109(3): 551–559, 2010.

Tchantchaleishvili, V. et al. Clinical implications of physiologic flow adjustment in continuous-flow left ventricular assist devices. *ASAIO Journal* 63(3): 241–250, 2017.

Tortora, G. et al. A dynamic control algorithm based on physiological parameters and wearable interfaces for adaptive ventricular assist devices. In: *2015 37th Annual International Conference of the IEEE Engineering in Medicine and Biology Society (EMBC)*, Milano, Italy, IEEE, 2015.

Uriel, N. et al. Hemodynamic ramp tests in patients with left ventricular assist devices. *JACC: Heart Failure* 4(3): 208–217, 2016.

Uriel, N. et al. Impact of hemodynamic ramp test-guided HVAD speed and medication adjustments on clinical outcomes: The RAMP-IT-UP multicenter study. *Circulation: Heart Failure* 12(4), e006067, 2019.

Vakil, K. et al. Implantable cardioverter-defibrillator use in patients with left ventricular assist devices: a systematic review and meta-analysis. *JACC: Heart Failure* 4(10): 772–779, 2016.

Veenis, J. F. et al. Design and rationale of haemodynamic guidance with Cardiomems in patients with a left ventricular assist device: The HEMO-VAD pilot study. *ESC Heart Failure* 6(1): 194–201, 2019a.

Veenis, J. F.; Birim, O.; Brugts, J. J. Pulmonary artery pressure telemonitoring by Cardiomems in a patient pre-and post-left ventricular assist device implantation. *European Journal of Cardio-Thoracic Surgery* 56(4): 809–810, 2019b.

Verdejo, H. E. et al. Comparison of a radiofrequency-based wireless pressure sensor to swan-ganz catheter and echocardiography for ambulatory assessment of pulmonary artery pressure in heart failure. *Journal of the American College of Cardiology* 50(25): 2375–2382, 2007.

Wang, X. Overview on biocompatibilities of implantable biomaterials. In: Lazinica, R. (editor), *Advances in Biomaterials Science and Biomedical Applications in Biomedicine.* London: IntechOpen, 2013, pp. 111–155.

Waters, T. et al. Motor feedback physiological control for a continuous flow ventricular assist device. *Artificial Organs* 23: 480–486, 1999.

Wee, H. E. et al. Validation of the use of a point-of-care device in monitoring the international normalized ratio in postoperative cardiac patients. *Annals of the Academic of Medicine* 45(9): 424–426, 2016.

Wei, S. et al. Development of an auto calibration method for the implantable blood pressure sensor in the undulation pump ventricular assist device (UPVAD). In *7th Asian-Pacific Conference on Medical and Biological Engineering (APCMBE)*, Berlin/Heidelberg, Germany: Springer, 2008.

Weisenberg, B. A.; Mooradian, D. L. Hemocompatibility of materials used in microelectro-mechanical systems: Platelet adhesion and morphology in vitro. *Journal of Biomedical Materials Research* 60: 283–291, 2002.

Weitzel, L. B. et al. Left ventricular assist device effects on metabolic substrates in the failing heart. *PLoS One* 8(4): e60292, 2013.

Werner, C.; Maitz, M. F.; Sperling, C. Current strategies towards hemocompatible coatings. *Journal of Materials Chemistry* 17: 3376–3384, 2007.

Wu, Y., et al. A bridge from short-term to long-term left ventricular assist device–experimental verification of a physiological controller. *Artificial Organs* 28: 927–932, 2004.

Yousuf, O. et al. High-sensitivity C-reactive protein and cardiovascular disease. *Journal of the American College of Cardiology* 62(5): 397–408, 2013.

Zenlander, R. et al. Point-of-care versus central laboratory testing of INR in acute stroke. *Acta Neurologica Scandinavica* 14(1): 1–7, 2017.

Zhuang, Q. et al. Association of high sensitive C-reactive protein with coronary heart disease: A Mendelian randomization study. *BMC Medical Genetics* 20(1): 1–7, 2019.

Ziaie, B.; Najafi, K. An implantable microsystem for tonometric blood pressure measurement. *Biomedical Microdevices* 3: 285–292, 2001.

16 Optics and VADs

Isac K. Fujita and Sergio Y. Araki
Instituto Federal de São Paulo

CONTENTS

16.1 INTRODUCTION

Ventricular assist devices (VADs) allow patients to be kept in stable hemodynamic conditions until the heart transplant is performed, which is more efficient in the use of organs and reduces transplantation of patients on the waiting list (Uebelhart et al., 2013; Saito, 2014; Souza, 2019).

VADs are classified into two subtypes: the first being pulsatile, used as a cardiopulmonary bypass, uses a diaphragm that advances by mechanical or pneumatic means to pump blood to the aorta (Slaughter et al., 2009) and the second type, on the other hand, are implantable centrifugal pumps, in which these are characterized by continuous pumping of blood through a rotor. These pumps are smaller than pulsatile and provide a more dynamic flow control system (Bock et al., 2011).

As centrifugal pumps are made up of a shaft rotor and two bearings, these bearings can be of three types of materials: ceramic, magnetic levitation, and polyurethane. One of the analytical studies of these bearings is the relationship of wear to the pump's active time, as this can cause vibrations that are harmful to patients' health, causing blood contamination of the worn-out bearings (Hertz et al., 2005; Bock et al., 2013; Paulo, 2016; Lopes et al., 2017; Souza, 2019).

One for the study of these deformations in the bearings is the use of the moiré projection technique in order to obtain its profile and analyze the bearing profiles to be studied. This technique is characterized by generating deformation or stress maps of the object under study using a multimedia projector, digital camera, and moiré degrees, which can be digital or physical (Porto et al., 2011; Rodrigues et al., 2019).

DOI: 10.1201/9781003138358-18

The moiré method is based on superimposing two lattices, generating an angle of 90° between the direction of the lines. The reticles are made up of light and dark lines of the same dimension. The moiré fringes are generated from the patterns of these lattices as what are the dark lines according to the relative displacement between the lattices (Gazzola, 2011). These experiments test three or four images with small displacements of the fringes to obtain deformation maps and moiré fringes.

The position of the fringes generates maps reproducing the object's topography. This topography obtains the geometric design in a three-dimensional form, providing information on the topographic contours, curvature and shape of the objects, and deformations inside and outside the plane.

Optical methods present data that define greater reality in results (Andonian, 2008) and, in addition, have advantages associated with the low cost of experimental apparatus and simplicity in image processing applied to any type of body, regardless of the shape geometric and color.

16.2   VENTRICULAR ASSIST DEVICES

VADs are devices that help the heart to pump blood from the main pumping chamber of the heart's blood, the left ventricle, to the rest of the body. The devices can be implanted in the body or connected to a pump outside the body and are used by patients who are in a critical stage of cardiac progression, stage D (Braunwald, 2012).

VADs consist of three parts: a pump, an electronic controller, and two batteries. Its pump weighs about a kilogram, being allocated inside the body, if it is permanent, or outside the body, when the patient waits for a permanent pump or for a heart transplant. The electronic controller is a small computer that controls the operation of the pump. The batteries are charged outside the body and are connected to the pump by cables that pass through the patient's body. The devices take from 04 to 06 hours to be implanted. These devices are intended to replace heart pumping functions and are therefore notably important for cases where they become necessary. However, there are two subtypes of VADs: pulsatile and implantable centrifugal pumps (Slaughter et al., 2009). Figure 16.1 shows details on how to use VADs.

VADs have two subtypes: the first is pulsatile, which uses a diaphragm that advances by mechanical or pneumatic means to pump blood to the aorta (Slaughter et al., 2009) and the second type is continuous flow pumps, such as axial and implantable centrifuges. Generally, these pumps are smaller than pulsatile ones and have greater reliability because they are simple and require a more dynamic flow control system (Florentino et al., 2018).

Centrifugal pumps have bearings that can be of three types: ceramic–polymeric (or pivot bearings), magnetic levitation, or hydrodynamic levitation (Bock et al., 2008). Figure 16.2 shows the pivot bearings to be studied.

16.3   OPTICS

Optical methods can provide full-field displacement and deformation fields of structures under static or dynamic conditions. Because of their noncontact nature, optical methods do not alter the response of the objects being studied. Thus, results obtained by optical methods represent reality and can be used to validate computational models.

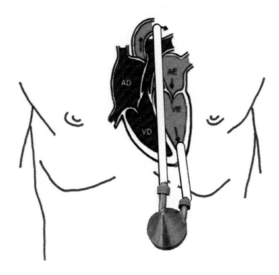

FIGURE 16.1 Details of a ventricular assist device and systems.

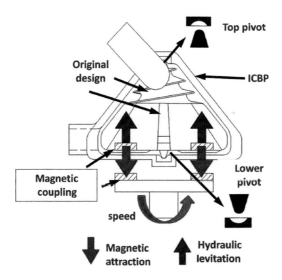

FIGURE 16.2 Ceramic–polymeric pivot bearings studied.

16.3.1 PHOTOELASTICITY

Photoelasticity is one of the oldest optical metrology tools for engineering purposes. It makes use of stress-induced birefringence in transparent materials and provides a relationship between the change in the state of stress or strain at a given point on the structure and the optical data. Photoelasticity can only provide principal stress difference or maximum in-plane shear stress directly. Stress separation techniques need to be used to obtain individual stress and strain components (Figure 16.3) (Andonian, 2008).

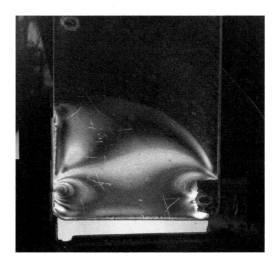

FIGURE 16.3 Image of the specimen under load.

16.3.2 Laser Doppler Vibrometry

Laser Doppler vibrometry is a noncontact measurement technique for measuring velocity and vibrations on moving surfaces. Laser Doppler vibrometers (LDVs) are well suited for measuring vibrations where alternate methods simply cannot be applied. Contacting transducers may fail when attempting to measure high amplitudes. LDVs can measure vibrations up to the 30 MHz range with very linear phase response and high accuracy. Laser Doppler vibrometry can be applied in complex applications, where contact sensors cannot make a measurement, such as making measurements on very hot objects. LDVs use the principle of optical interference, requiring two coherent light beams to overlap (29.31). The resulting interference relates to the path length difference between both beams (Andonian, 2008).

16.3.3 Moiré Methods

Moiré techniques are based on moiré phenomenology and are characterized by an effect resulting from the geometric interference between two or more amplitude grids overlapping near each other, generating patterns of wider and darker lines, which are called moiré pattern fringes (Gazzola et al. 2013). Figure 16.4 illustrates the effect overlapping moiré of two grids.

16.3.3.1 Shadow Moiré

The principle of shadow moiré is shown in Figure 16.5. The grating lying over the curved surface is illuminated under the angle of incidence θ_1 (measured from the grating normal) and viewed under an angle θ_2. From the figure, we see that a point P_0 on the grating is projected to a point P_1 on the surface which by viewing is projected to the point P_2 on the grating.

The experimental apparatus is shown in Figure 16.6.

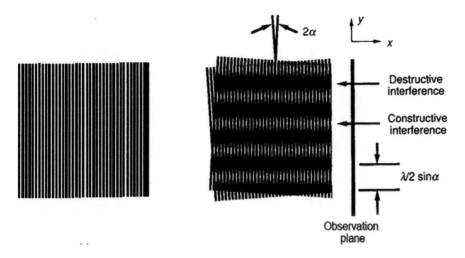

FIGURE 16.4   Overlapping grids and formation of light and dark fringes.

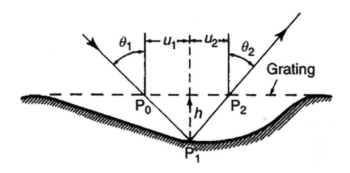

FIGURE 16.5   Shadow moiré (see Gasvik, 2002)

16.3.3.2   Projected Fringes

The moiré method by phase shifting is based on the displacement of grids by 90°, projecting them separately directly onto the object using a multimedia projector. As for the grids, Lino (2002) mentions that this essay requires projection of three or four images, with a small displacement of fringes between them, to obtain the phase and surface map contour of the studied objects. This phase change of the grid can be done with parallel-line reticles or also by sinusoidal grids, both displaced 90° between themselves. Lino (2002) explains that the phase shifting technique is capable of being used in bodies of continuous geometry, such as cubes, fruits, etc. Figures 16.7 and 16.8 show grids used in moiré phase shifting tests by lattice and sinusoidal grids, respectively.

Figure 16.9 illustrates an example of experimental arrangement for the development of moiré technique by phase shifting.

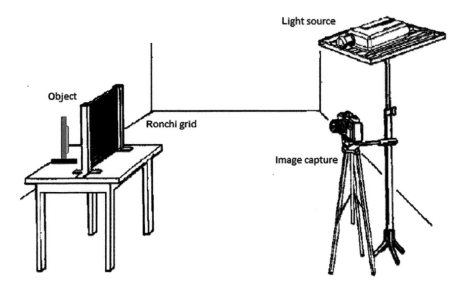

FIGURE 16.6   Apparatus to shadow moiré technique (see Fujita, 2015).

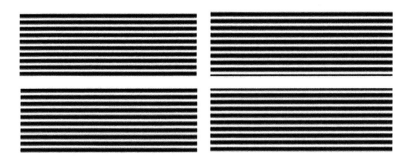

FIGURE 16.7   Grids of phase shifting by reticles, displaced 90° from each other (see Fujita, 2015).

16.3.3.3 Laser Speckle

When a beam of coherent light hits a rough surface, each point of it acts as an emitter of small secondary waves, which start to obtain a different phase in relation to the phase of the incident wave. In any observation plane, the coherent superposition of waves originates at different points on the surface of the origin to an interference pattern whose intensities also vary.

At the points of constructive or destructive interference, there is formation of a spatially distributed granular pattern. These grains found can be considered diffractive elements, which, through image treatment and scale adjustment, reveal irregularities of the piece.

According to the experimental setup, speckles can be divided into two categories: objective and subjective.

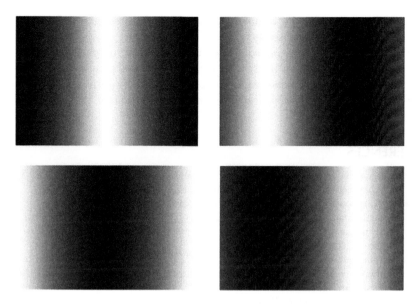

FIGURE 16.8 Phase shifting sinusoidal grid displaced 90° from each other (see Fujita, 2015).

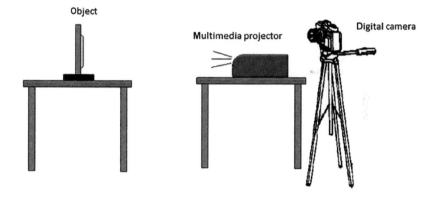

FIGURE 16.9 Experimental moiré arrangement by phase shifting (see Fujita, 2015).

16.4 PROJECTS INVOLVING OPTICS AND VADs

Instituto Federal de São Paulo (IFSP) has the possibility for students and professors to participate in research scholarship programs and to assist with participation in events. Some programs involve research and development. Thus, projects are listed in the sequence:

- Profile analysis on the axis of VADs using the projection moiré technique
- Application of moiré technique in tension testing in a metallic plate with discontinuity
- Application of shadow moiré technique for the survey of metallic surface

- Making educational material to obtain a map of stresses and deformations using classic photoelasticity
- Speckle methodology as an alternative for measuring roughness
- Optical velocimetry using speckle technique in blood pumps
- Surface survey using moiré techniques for orthopedic purposes
- Bibliographic study of a biospeckle and its applications

REFERENCES

Andonian, A. A. T. Optical methods, Chapter 39. In: William N. Sharpe (ed.), *Springer Handbook of Experimental Solid Mechanics*. Baltimore, MD: Springer, 2008, pp. 823–837.

Bock, E., Ribeiro, A., Silva, M., Antunes, P., Fonseca, J., Legendre, D., Andrade, A. New centrifugal blood pump with dual impeller and double pivot bearing system: Wear evaluation in bearing system, performance tests, and preliminary hemolysis tests. *Artificial Organs*, 32(4), 329333, 2008.

Bock, E., Andrade, A., Dinkhuysen, J., Arruda, C., Fonseca, J., Leme, J. Introductory tests to in vivo evaluation: Magnetic coupling influence in motor controller. *ASAIO Journal*, 57(5), 462465, 2011.

Bock, E., Leão, T., Uebelhart, B., Galantini, D., Andrade, A., & Cavalheiro, A. A ceramic pivot bearing implantable centrifugal blood pump. *The International Journal of Artificial Organs*, 36(8), 543, 2013.

Braunwald, E. *Braunwald's Heart Disease: A Textbook of Cardiovascular Medicine*. Boston, MA: Elsevier, 2012.

Florentino, P. C. et al. Dilatometria da Zircônia pelo Processo de Colagem de Barbotina em Moldes de Gesso para Eixos no DAV. *The Academic Society Journal*, 2(3), 113–119, 2018.

Fujita, I. K. Aplicação de técnica de Moiré de sombra na medição de tensões em elementos estruturais submetidos a ensaio de tração. Dissertação de Mestrado em Engenharia Agrícola - Faculdade de Engenharia Agrícola, Universidade Estadual de Campinas, 2015, 64 p.

Gasvik, J. K. *Optical Metrolgy*. England: John Wiley & Sons, Ltd, 2002.

Gazzola, J. Aplicação de Técnica Óptica no Estudo da Distribuição de Tensões em Modelos Reduzidos de Feixe de Toras e Peças Serradas. Dissertação de Mestrado em Engenharia Agrícola – Faculdade de Engenharia Agrícola, Universidade Estadual de Campinas, 2011, 151 p.

Gazzola, J., Affonso, E. A., Fabbro, I. M. Aplicação da técnica óptica de Moiré de sombra na determinação do mapa de deformações de corpos carregados axialmente. *Sinergia, São Paulo*, 14 (3), 211–216, 2013.

Hertz, H. R. G. et al. Desenvolvimento da Técnica de Moiré de Sombra como Alternativa de Baixo Custo para Análise Postural. *Scientia Medica, Porto Alegre*, 15(4), 235–242, 2005.

Lino, A. C. L. "Técnica Óptica de Moiré Visando a Aplicação no Estudo de Superfícies Irregulares." Dissertação de Mestrado em Engenharia Agrícola - UNICAMP. Campinas, São Paulo, 2002.

Lopes, G., Bock, E., Gómez, L. Numerical analyses for low reynolds flow in a ventricular assist device. *Artificial Organs*, 41 (6), E30–E40, 2017.

Paulo, M. F. Ferramenta computacional de supressão do sinal de atividade ventricular em eletrocardiograma. Pós-graduação Stricto Sensu em Automação e Controle de Processos, Instituto Federal de educação ciência e tecnologia de São Paulo, 2016.

Porto, F., Gurgel, J. L. F., de Tarso Veras, P. Topografia de Moiré como método de avaliação postural: Revisão do estado da arte. *Revista Brasileira de Geriatria e Gerontologia* 14 (3), 567–577, 2011.

Rodrigues, M., Cruz, N., Rocha, J., Sá, R., Bock, E. Surface roughness of biomaterials and process parameters of titanium dioxide gritblasting for productivity enhancement. *The Academic Society Journal*, 3 (2), 169–176, 2019.

Saito, Marcia Tiemi. Utilização de técnicas de análise de franjas para a avaliação de dimensões de lesões na pele. Dissertação (Mestrado) - Curso de Física, Instituto de Física, Universidade de São Paulo, São Paulo, 2014, 123, p.

Slaughter, M. S. et al. Advanced heart failure treated with continuous-flow left ventricular assist device. *The New England Journal of Medicine*, 361 (23), 2241–2251, 2009.

Souza, R. L., Chabu, I. E., Drigo, E., Andrade, A. J. P., Leao, T. F., Bock, E. G. P. A strategy for designing of customized electromechanical actuators of blood pumps. *Artificial Organs*, 44 (8): 797–802, 2019.

Uebelhart, B., Silva, B. U., Fonseca, J., Bock, E., Leme, J., da Silva, C., Leão, T. Study of a centrifugal blood pump in a mock loop system. *Artificial Organs*, 37 (11): 946–949, 2013.

Index